THE COMPLETE IDIOT'S GUIDE® TO

Prescription Drugs

by Michael C. Gerald, Ph.D.

ALPHA

A member of Penguin Group (USA) Inc.

ALPHA BOOKS

Published by the Penguin Group

Penguin Group (USA) Inc., 375 Hudson Street, New York, New York 10014, U.S.A.

Penguin Group (Canada), 10 Alcorn Avenue, Toronto, Ontario, Canada M4V 3B2 (a division of Pearson Penguin Canada Inc.)

Penguin Books Ltd, 80 Strand, London WC2R 0RL, England

Penguin Ireland, 25 St Stephen's Green, Dublin 2, Ireland (a division of Penguin Books Ltd)

Penguin Group (Australia), 250 Camberwell Road, Camberwell, Victoria 3124, Australia (a division of Pearson Australia Group Pty Ltd)

Penguin Books India Pvt Ltd, 11 Community Centre, Panchsheel Park, New Delhi—110 017, India

Penguin Group (NZ), cnr Airborne and Rosedale Roads, Albany, Auckland 1310, New Zealand (a division of Pearson New Zealand Ltd)

Penguin Books (South Africa) (Pty) Ltd, 24 Sturdee Avenue, Rosebank, Johannesburg 2196, South Africa

Penguin Books Ltd, Registered Offices: 80 Strand, London WC2R 0RL, England

International Standard Book Number: 1-59257-477-7
Library of Congress Catalog Card Number: 2006922329

08   07   06   8   7   6   5   4   3   2   1

Interpretation of the printing code: The rightmost number of the first series of numbers is the year of the book's printing; the rightmost number of the second series of numbers is the number of the book's printing. For example, a printing code of 06-1 shows that the first printing occurred in 2006.

Printed in the United States of America

Note: This publication contains the opinions and ideas of its author. It is intended to provide helpful and informative material on the subject matter covered. It is sold with the understanding that the author and publisher are not engaged in rendering professional services in the book. If the reader requires personal assistance or advice, a competent professional should be consulted. Moreover, before taking any drug, the consumer should consult the full prescribing information about the drug, along with manufacturer and FDA recommendations.

The author and publisher specifically disclaim any responsibility for any liability, loss, or risk, personal or otherwise, which is incurred as a consequence, directly or indirectly, of the use and application of any of the contents of this book.

Most Alpha books are available at special quantity discounts for bulk purchases for sales promotions, premiums, fundraising, or educational use. Special books, or book excerpts, can also be created to fit specific needs.

For details, write: Special Markets, Alpha Books, 375 Hudson Street, New York, NY 10014.

Publisher: *Marie Butler-Knight*
Editorial Director/Acquiring Editor: *Mike Sanders*
Managing Editor: *Billy Fields*
Senior Acquisitions Editor: *Paul Dinas*
Development Editor: *Jennifer Moore*
Production Editor: *Kayla Dugger*
Copy Editor: *Keith Cline*

Cartoonist: *Shannon Wheeler*
Cover Designer: *Becky Harmon*
Book Designers: *Trina Wurst, Kurt Owens*
Indexer: *Brad Herriman*
Layout: *Becky Harmon, Chad Dressler*
Proofreader: *Mary Hunt*

Contents at a Glance

Contents

Foreword

We've all heard it many times before: If you've got your health, you've got it all. Nothing makes us as happy as feeling well. But what does it take to achieve and maintain good health? How can we minimize illness and maximize wellness? I think it's safe to say that now, more than ever before, information is the key. The more we know, the better able we are to care for ourselves and our loved ones in times of need.

Yet there's so much to learn. Thousands of books have been written about sickness and health, diagnosis and treatment, medicine and surgery. Indeed, the shelves of libraries and bookstores are jammed with every conceivable book and magazine telling us what to do or what not to do to be well. Sadly, many texts read like college theses, while others hold so little useful information that reading them is a waste of time. What's a person to do?

Well, one of the best things you could do for your health and your safety is read *The Complete Idiot's Guide to Prescription Drugs*. It's the perfect place to start your own medical investigation. It's packed with practical information that's really quick to read and easy to understand. It covers the most common and important illnesses you'll face in your life and presents an insider's knowledge of the most powerful weapons you have to combat disease: pharmaceuticals. More than this, it suggests ways of reducing your health-care costs while increasing the safety and effectiveness of the medicines you take. And, it offers a comprehensive list of where to obtain more detailed information once you have gained a rapid base of knowledge about your medical problems and how to manage them.

As a physician, I know how complicated and confusing medicine has become, especially for patients who lack knowledge and experience. Your own questions can drive you crazy. "Did my doctor prescribe the right drug for me? How will I know if it's safe? How will I know if it's working? What if I miss a dose? What happens if I mix drugs? When should I seek immediate help? What are my alternatives?" Worst of all is trying to get answers from your health-care team or private physician. Even if you can reach them, it's easy to feel idiotic when they speak a language you don't understand about a topic that's way over your head. And how will you know if they're right?

The answers to all of these questions and many more can be found in this book. Its author, Michael C. Gerald, Ph.D., is a recognized expert, a professor of pharmacy at the University of Connecticut and formerly at Ohio State University, who has served such prestigious institutions as the World Health Organization and the U.S. Food and Drug Administration. Dr. Gerald has compiled just the right amount of information to start you off on your quest for knowledge about your medical problems and the drugs that can restore your good health. I know you'll find the book helpful and comforting. I highly recommend it.

Albert Marchetti, M.D.
President and Medical Director
Medical Education and Research Alliance of America
Adjunct Professor
University of Medicine and Dentistry of New Jersey

Dr. Marchetti is Founder and President of the Medical Education and Research Alliance of America—Med-ERA, Inc. and Adjunct Professor of Preventive Medicine and Community Health at the University of Medicine and Dentistry of New Jersey. For 15 years, he served as Vice President and Medical Director of Thomson Physicians World, the world's foremost medical communications company, and its education and research divisions. He has authored three contemporary medical books for consumers—*Common Cure For Common Ailments, Dr. Marchetti's Walking Program,* and *Beating the Odds.*

Introduction

We have all taken prescription medicines at one time or another. Most people use medicines to deal with the relief of relatively minor, short-term health conditions, whereas others are obliged to take lifesaving medications for the remainder of their lives.

Because you are reading this book, I assume you have questions about your medicines. Are you interested in knowing how the drugs work and whether you should expect some delay before you begin to improve? Will the medicine cure the condition or just make you feel better? What are some of the common undesirable side effects they produce, and what precautions can you take to reduce the likelihood that they will produce harm?

Or maybe you have questions about how to afford the medicines your doctor has prescribed. Without sacrificing quality, are there any ways to save money on your medications?

There is no shortage of books addressing these kinds of questions. Unfortunately, most are written in medical jargon or assume you have spent the past few years of your life taking science courses intended to prepare you for a career in the health professions. Not to worry. All the scientific information and vocabulary you need will be presented here in plain English.

What's in This Book?

We've divided this book into two major parts.

In **Part 1, "The Basics,"** you'll find six chapters dealing with, well, the basics. This general information applies to all medicines and should help you get off to a running start. We talk about the different kinds of prescription and nonprescription medicines out there and the various ways drugs are given and taken. We also consider factors that account for the different ways we respond to medications, and how we know that the drugs we take are safe and effective.

To prepare you to become more active participants in decisions about the medicines you take, we suggest several questions that you should ask your doctor and pharmacist every time a new drug is prescribed. We talk about selecting reliable sources that you can consult to get more detailed information about your medical conditions and the drugs used to treat them. Finally, we suggest ways to save money on your medicines that won't jeopardize your health.

Part 2, "Directory of Medical Conditions and Their Drug Treatment," consists of several sections devoted to the most common medical conditions and the drugs used to treat them. There are many thousands of prescription medicines out there, and not even experts agree how many. Each of these medicines usually has more than one name.

We could have organized this book according to drugs, starting with those beginning with *A* and concluding with the *Z* drugs. We would soon find, however, that essentially the same information was being repeated many times, since many drugs are very similar. Moreover, using this approach, we wouldn't be able to compare different drugs used for the same condition.

We've taken a different, more reader-friendly approach. We list the most common conditions, and then talk about the different groups of drugs used to treat that condition. In most cases, there are multiple drugs in each group, and drugs within a given group are usually very much alike. Thus, all the essential information about a drug group used for a given condition is located in one place.

How to Use This Book

After reading Part 1, or at least the chapters of greatest interest to you, there are several easy ways you can find the specific information you're looking for.

Using the alphabetized Table of Contents in Part 2 or the very comprehensive index at the back of this book, you can locate the medical condition. After introductory remarks about the medical condition, we talk about the important groups of drugs used to treat it. Each condition is independently considered and can be read in any order.

At the end of each medical condition section, we have compiled a table listing the most important drugs used for its treatment. All these tables contain the generic and trade names of the prescription medicines and, in case you want to save some money, whether an equivalent generic product is available.

A general index is provided for your convenience. In addition, we have prepared a second index that is organized by generic drug name and lists the various conditions each drug is used to treat along with cross-references to the trade name of the drug.

The appendixes at the end of this book contain a glossary and a list of resources you can contact to get additional information about the medical conditions and their treatment.

Throughout the book, you'll find five kinds of sidebars. Here's what to expect from each:

Did You Know That ...?
Interesting information or facts are found here.

def•i•ni•tion
This sidebar contains definitions of terms and jargon.

Warning!
These sidebars highlight particularly significant warnings or precautions associated with the use of the medicine, including drug-drug interactions.

Maximizing Your Medicine
Here we provide money-saving tips or information about the proper use or storage of the medicine.

OTC Alternatives
Although this book focuses upon prescription medicines, sometimes highly effective, and usually less-expensive, over-the-counter (OTC) drugs can be used to treat the medical condition. When there is a good OTC alternative to a prescription drug, we tell you about it here.

Acknowledgments

I extend my warm thanks to my son, Marc, and my wife, Gloria, for their encouragement and support during the course of this project. For her extreme patience and critical assistance in preliminary reviews of this manuscript, I also thank Gloria. Warm thanks are also extended to my editors Paul Dinas and Jennifer Moore for ensuring the project's progress and completion.

Special Thanks to the Technical Reviewer

The Complete Idiot's Guide to Prescription Drugs was reviewed by two experts who double-checked the accuracy of what you'll learn here. Special thanks are extended to Albert Marchetti, M.D., and Monica D. Mehta, PharmD.

Trademarks

All terms mentioned in this book that are known to be or are suspected of being trademarks or service marks have been appropriately capitalized. Alpha Books and Penguin Group (USA) Inc. cannot attest to the accuracy of this information. Use of a term in this book should not be regarded as affecting the validity of any trademark or service mark.

Part 1

The Basics

Before we start talking about specific medical conditions and the prescription medicines used to treat them, some basic information will be helpful. Part 1 will introduce you to some of the terms and concepts that apply to all drugs.

First we'll focus on the different kinds of drugs, how they're used, what happens after they're taken, and how we know that they are safe and really work.

One of the most important messages this book conveys is that you need to take an active role in managing your health care. You can do this by learning more about your medical conditions and the drugs you are taking and also by working as an active partner with your health-care providers. Saving some money on your medical bills wouldn't be such a bad thing either. We'll say a lot more about this.

Now is a great time to get started. If you can't wait, feel free to skip directly to medical conditions of greatest interest to you in Part 2.

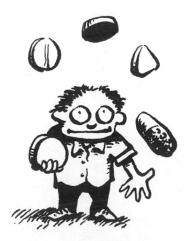

The Medicine Landscape

In This Chapter

- ◆ Using medicines for medical disorders
- ◆ Identifying drugs by trade and generic names
- ◆ Distinguishing between prescription (Rx) and over-the-counter (OTC) drugs
- ◆ Making sense of drug labels
- ◆ Taking a hard look at dietary supplements and homeopathic remedies

Drug companies sell thousands of drugs for treating the many medical disorders that afflict humans. If the malady has a name, chances are there's at least one *drug* for it.

You already knew that. The last time you went into your neighborhood pharmacy you saw a bewildering assortment of thousands of ointments, tablets, and sprays as you walked down the drug aisle or peered at the medicine shelves behind the prescription counter.

def•i•ni•tion

Although subtle differences exist among the terms, I use **medicine, drug,** and **pharmaceutical** interchangeably to refer to any drug that is used for treating medical disorders.

This first chapter starts by taking a look at the general ways all these drugs are used to deal with medical disorders. Drugs can be divided into two major categories: prescription drugs and those that are available without a prescription (over-the-counter, or OTC). Prescription drugs are further distinguished by their trade name and generic name, and knowing the difference between the two may save you some big bucks.

Four General Uses of Drugs

When used by members of a health-care team, drugs have four general uses:

◆ To prevent medical disorders from occurring

◆ To treat medical disorders

◆ To diagnose medical disorders and study their progress

◆ To change the function of the body

With a few exceptions, this book covers drugs that fall into the second category, the treatment of medical disorders. However, in this first chapter, I provide a brief overview of all four categories, beginning with the prevention of medical disorders.

To Prevent Medical Disorders

The primary goal of health care should be to prevent diseases and other medical disorders from occurring in the first place. I think we would all agree that it is far easier—not to mention less expensive—to *prevent* medical problems than to deal with them after they occur.

We use numerous substances to prevent medical disorders, many on a daily basis, often without even realizing it. For instance, a morning dose of multivitamins or enriched foods prevents formerly common vitamin-deficiency diseases such as rickets (caused by vitamin D deficiency) or scurvy (caused by deficiency in ascorbic acid). Iodide, added to table salt, has made goiter, a thyroid gland disorder, a relatively unusual disorder. And thanks to the addition of fluorides to drinking water and toothpaste, tooth decay is a far-less-common affliction than it was in the past.

Far more dramatic has been the use of vaccines to prevent smallpox and such formerly common childhood diseases as measles, mumps, and rubella. And widespread use of the polio vaccine has virtually eradicated polio in developed nations.

To Treat Medical Disorders

Most of the medicines used in health care are intended to treat medical disorders—both life threatening and minor. (Of course, no disorder is really minor when you're the one who has it.) Such treatment can be further broken down into two categories: those used to cure a medical disorder and those used to relieve its symptoms.

When a drug cures a medical disorder, the problem is gone—history … just a bad memory. Antibiotics and other similar drugs can cure many infectious diseases caused by bacteria, fungi, and by the parasites found in many tropical countries. Other medicines check and keep under control viral infections and some cancers, but they cannot cure them.

Most of the medicines we take relieve the symptoms of medical disorders, but do not *directly* produce a cure. Drugs used to treat high blood pressure, diabetes, or osteoarthritis all relieve the symptoms of these chronic disorders. We feel better, and fewer problems arise from these disorders over a long-term period. But the medicines that are now available do not correct their underlying cause and must be taken for a lifetime.

In other cases, although drugs may relieve distressing symptoms or improve an acute disorder, the body must do the heavy lifting and make the necessary repairs or changes for health to be restored to normal. For instance, decongestants relieve nasal stuffiness, letting you breathe easier, but it's up to your body's immune system to bring the common cold under control. Similarly, morphine eases the severe pain caused a broken bone, but the body must heal the fracture on its own.

To Diagnose and Study Medical Disorders

Drugs are sometimes used as tools to diagnose the presence of a medical disorder or to assess whether the disorder is getting better or worse. Drugs are used to detect thyroid gland problems and certain eye disorders.

To Change Body Function

Drugs used to change body function do not necessarily treat a disease or medical disorder. Rather they are used to alter a normal state. For instance, we all know that pregnancy is not a disease, yet thousands of women take oral contraceptives ("the pill") to prevent pregnancy. Other drugs are used to terminate pregnancy.

Did You Know That ...?

Turn on the TV or flip through a magazine and you'll see dozens of ads for drugs intended to treat a variety of lifestyle disorders. These drugs are intended to improve people's quality of life but not necessarily their health. Everyone would agree that lung cancer and stroke are real diseases. Although often causing genuine distress in sufferers, some would question whether baldness, wrinkles, shortness, and sexual performance are also diseases.

Up until now, we've be talking about "drugs" and "medicines" and their uses in disease. Let's start being more specific and talk about real drugs and medicines which have names.

How Drugs Are Named

The naming conventions for drugs can seem downright baffling at times. The confusion is caused, at least in part, by the fact that drugs can be referred to by their chemical name, their generic name, and their trade name. Here's a quick overview of each of these aliases:

Maximizing Your Medicine

The beginnings or endings of the generic name may provide a clue about the nature of the drug. For instance, if a drug ends in "-cycline," it means it's a tetracycline-like antibiotic; "-olol" or "-lol" endings indicate that the drug is a beta-blocker. I point these out as we discuss the use of medicines for various medical disorders in Part 2.

◆ A drug's *chemical* name is usually very lengthy and complex and describes a unique chemistry of the drug in all details. The chemical name is primarily used by laboratory scientists and patent seekers, but is far too cumbersome for us to even think about, much less use.

◆ Fortunately for us, the *generic* (a.k.a. nonproprietary or official) name is much shorter than the chemical name. Generally one or two words long, this serves as the official name used for the drug in the United States. The generic name refers to only a single drug and can be used by anyone and everyone who can legally market that medicine.

To an increasing extent, medicines are being sold to an international patient population. Outside the United States, international nonproprietary names (INN) are used. INNs may be the same, similar to, or very different from the generic name used in the United States. Globe-trotters who may need new supplies of their medicines during the course of their travels should know the INN of any drugs they are taking.

◆ A drug's *trade* (a.k.a. brand or proprietary) name is the unique name chosen by the pharmaceutical manufacturer. The manufacturer has exclusive rights to use this trademarked name and will aggressively safeguard these rights in court. It is in the manufacturer's best commercial interest to make this name short, simple, catchy, and easy for the doctor and consumer to remember. Which is easier to remember: sildenafil citrate, the generic name; or Viagra, the trade name? Same drug, different names. When you travel abroad, keep in mind that the same manufacturer may, and often does, use different trade names in different countries.

As you might have noted, generic names are designated in lower case, whereas trade names have their first letter capitalized.

Maximizing Your Medicine

Patents give the holder (e.g., pharmaceutical manufacturer) exclusive rights to make, use, or sell their invention or product. Free of competition, producers can reap greater profits. Drugs granted patents after 1995 have a 20-year period of market exclusivity; patents granted prior to 1995 have 17 years.

After a patent expires, almost anyone can market the drug using its generic name and compete with the trade-name product. Generic products cost far less than the equivalent brand-name drug, and they are equally effective at treating medical disorders. The Food and Drug Administration (FDA) evaluates generic drugs to ensure that they are equivalent to the trade-name products and can be used interchangeably with them.

Compare the approximate retail cost of trade-name products and their generic equivalents of the same strength and quantity for one 30-day supply:

◆ High blood pressure and heart disorders
   Trade Lopressor: $90
   Generic Metoprolol: $15
◆ Depression
   Trade Prozac: $253
   Generic Fluoxetine: $70

Prescription vs. Nonprescription Medicines

Both prescription-only (Rx) drugs and nonprescription (over-the-counter or OTC) drugs must meet stringent federal requirements for safety and effectiveness. (We return to the notion of safety and effectiveness in Chapter 4, when we consider the drug approval process). So why do you need a prescription for some drugs and not for others?

Did You Know That …?

Prescription drugs are intended to be used under the supervision of a doctor. A prescription is required for a drug if any of the following conditions apply:

♦ Individuals cannot be expected to diagnose the medical disorder themselves or determine whether the disorder is getting better or worse.

♦ The drug causes significant toxic effects or is potentially harmful if not used properly.

♦ The drug is habit-forming.

To make a very long story short(er), a drug can be sold OTC if it can be labeled with directions that permit consumers to safely treat themselves. Sounds pretty simple, but it isn't. It implies that …

♦ Consumers can self-diagnose the medical disorder for which the drug is intended.

♦ The drug is safe for use. Let's quickly qualify this by saying that the OTC drug is only relatively safe—no drug is absolutely safe. The OTC drug causes no toxicity, nor are there any potentially harmful effects when it is used as recommended. Furthermore, its use does not require the supervision of a doctor or other health-care professional.

♦ The drug is not habit-forming.

If a drug does not satisfy these conditions, it can only be sold on a prescription basis.

Prescription Drugs and Their Labels

When doctors write a prescription, they draw upon their training and expertise to select the most appropriate drug and dosage for you and your condition. Doctors are aware of the potential problems that may be caused by the medicine but believe that its benefits outweigh any of its possible risks. In short, the doctor has assumed the responsibility for treating you. With an OTC drug, you make all these decisions.

Ever notice the difference between the labels on a prescription medicine versus those on over-the-counter medications? Sure you have. The prescription label contains …

◆ Your name.

◆ The doctor's name.

◆ The name of the drug and its strength.

◆ Name, address, and phone number of the pharmacy.

◆ The date the prescription was filled.

◆ The number of refills authorized for the prescription, if any.

◆ An expiration date.

◆ Directions for taking the medication. ("Two tablets three times a day after meals," or "Two drops into right eye twice daily.")

In addition, special labels might be attached to the medicine container that might direct you to shake the liquid medication well before using it or to refrigerate the medicine after opening; or they might warn you that the drug might make you drowsy or caution you against taking alcoholic drinks with the medicine.

Many pharmacies provide additional information about the medication, its side effects, and possible hazards. Some of these information sheets are more clearly written (plain English, less jargon) than others. I talk about what you and your pharmacist should be discussing in Chapter 5.

OTC Drugs and Their Labels

OTC drugs are safer than prescription medications. That is, there is a greater margin between safe doses and those that can cause you harm. Nevertheless, keep in mind that OTC drugs can cause health problems if not used as recommended on the label. In addition, their use can interfere with the effects of other medications you may be taking (this is called a drug-drug interaction, and we talk more about it in Chapter 3).

If you look at a bottle of an OTC drug, particularly one intended for internal use, you see a front label and a back label.

The front label has basic identifying information about the product, including the product's trade name, the dosage units, and the dosage form. We return to the topic of dosage forms in Chapter 2.

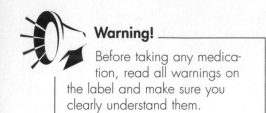

Warning!

Before taking any medication, read all warnings on the label and make sure you clearly understand them.

The back label contains very important information on how the drug should be used safely and effectively. Read the back label before buying the product to make sure that it is right for you or for the intended user. Read it again, prior to its use, to ensure that the correct dose is being taken at the correct interval between doses.

All OTC labels must include the following drug facts, using the same primary sections:

- Active ingredient, its amount, and the purpose each ingredient has in the product.

- Medical disorders or problems for which the product is intended.

- Warnings. This is probably the most important but least frequently read part of the label. Here are some of the warnings you might see on an OTC drug label:

  - Avoid other drugs. Drugs that should not be taken when taking this product, because of the risk of a drug-drug interaction.

  - Allergy alerts. Keep track of your drug allergies, for both prescription and OTC drugs. Make sure your family members, doctors, and pharmacist have noted and recorded this information.

  - Drug warnings. If certain conditions are present (e.g., pregnancy) the drug should never be used. For others (e.g., driving), greater than normal caution should be exercised when taking the drug.

  - Stop drug. "Stop use and ask a doctor if "—may include signs of an allergic reaction to the drug; or, if symptoms get worse or continue for more than _ days, consult your doctor.

  - Side effects. List of common potential side effects, some of which may occur at the usual doses.

  - Dosing and directions. How much, how often can these doses be repeated, when should the product be taken, and the youngest age at which the product can be safely used.

  - Inactive ingredients. List of inactive chemicals that are present in the drug product, which may be of importance for persons with specific allergies.

  - Manufacturer's information and an expiration date. Drugs are typically good for at least 12 months beyond this date.

When a Drug Switches from Rx to OTC

So far I've made the distinction between prescription and nonprescription medicines sound pretty clear. Unfortunately, the situation isn't so simple. Dozens of drugs that were once prescription-only (Rx) have converted to a nonprescription (OTC) status. Here are just a few drugs that have made the Rx-to-OTC switch:

Medical Disorder	Generic Name	Trade Name(s)
Pain	Ibuprofen	Advil, Motrin
	Naproxen	Aleve
Allergy	Chlorpheniramine	Chlor-Trimeton
	Diphenhydramine	Benadryl
	Loratadine	Claritin
Nasal stuffiness	Oxymetazoline	Afrin
	Phenylephrine	Neo-Synephrine
	Pseudoephedrine	Sudafed
	Xylometazoline	Otrivin
Fungal infection (skin)	Clotrimazole	Cruex
	Miconazole	Micatin
	Tolnaftate	Tinactin
Heartburn/indigestion	Cimetidine	Tagamet-HB
	Famotidine	Pepcid-AC
	Ranitidine	Zantac-75
Diarrhea	Loperamide	Imodium A-D
Baldness	Minoxidil	Rogaine

The Rx-to-OTC switch can have a number of consequences, some good, some not so good.

As a consumer, you can assume greater control of your health care because you are now empowered to decide what medications you want to take. You can save money, bother, and time by not having to visit your doctor and getting your prescription filled. OTC products are usually much cheaper than the same product in prescription form.

However, for some 80 to 90 percent of us, a private or public insurance plan pays some portion of our prescription medication bills. OTC drugs are not usually covered. Guess what! If a prescription drug is now available OTC, the insurance carrier is off the hook and doesn't have to pay for it.

Prescription Drug Advertising to Consumers

Before 1997, advertisements for prescription drugs were directed exclusively to doctors and pharmacists. Not only was general information about the drug kept a secret from the patient, so was the drug's name. Now happily, prescription labels routinely bear the name of the medication and its strength.

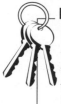

Did You Know That ...?

During the first half of the twentieth century, generations of medical students and doctors learned about drugs by studying Torald Sollmann's classic and highly authoritative textbook *A Manual of Pharmacology*. For many decades, Dr. Sollmann advocated that physicians write their prescriptions in Latin because "it serve[s] to keep the patient in ignorance of the nature of drugs."

Since 1997, the rules changed and manufacturers have been able to advertise their prescription medicines directly to patients. Spending more than $3 billion a year, pharmaceutical manufacturers now advertise directly to consumers, telling us about treatments for everything from allergy and asthma, elevated cholesterol levels, arthritis, heartburn, depression, obesity, anemia caused by anticancer drugs, and erectile dysfunction. These ads are intended to inform us about the prescription medications that are available to improve our health and the quality of our lives.

Manufacturers assert that these ads increase public awareness of chronic medical disorders and encourage us to seek advice from our doctors about their diagnosis and treatment. Opponents counter that direct-to-consumer advertising encourages patients to pressure their doctors to prescribe brand-name medications when other treatment options may be more appropriate and much less expensive.

Back to Nature: Plant-Based Remedies and Homeopathic Cures

The first medicines our ancestors used were natural substances, in particular, plants. Until the early decades of the twentieth century, plants remained the primary source of drugs. Recently, people have taken a renewed interest in alternative therapies based on natural ingredients. If you aren't already aware of the resurgence in interest in natural therapies, all you need to do is visit your neighborhood pharmacy or health-foods store to see how popular they are.

Dietary Supplements

Dietary supplements are natural products that include, but are not limited to, vitamins, minerals, herbs, and other botanical products.

Federal law classifies dietary supplements as food rather than as medicines. This means that, unlike prescription and OTC drugs, dietary supplements don't have to be proved to be safe and effective before they are marketed. We return to this matter in Chapter 3 when we discuss the Food and Drug Administration and the drug approval process.

Because they are not classified as medicines, dietary supplement manufacturers cannot specifically claim that their products are effective for the treatment of a disease. However, they can and do make "structure/function claims." That is, they can describe the role the supplement plays in affecting the normal structure and function of the body. Such a claim might state that this product "reduces joint pain and stiffness due to occasional overuse."

Supporters of dietary supplements—and there are many of them—make a number of claims about why their products are better than traditional medicines. When compared with manufactured drugs, they argue, these products are safer and have fewer side effects. If it's natural, it must be safe, they say. Moreover, natural medicines are more effective, because they permit the body to return to good health by natural means. I talk about such claims in Chapter 3. For now, let me say that such blanket claims are not valid. Proponents of dietary supplements also claim that they are less expensive. Some are, some aren't.

Homeopathic Remedies

The ingredients in homeopathic remedies are also derived from natural sources, namely, extracts of plants and minerals. Homeopathic medicine goes back to the late eighteenth century. Homeopathic remedies are now used for both human and animal patients in the United States and Canada, and even much more extensively in Europe.

Homeopathic medicine is based on the principle that "like cures like." Their doctors believe that if large doses of a substance can cause a medical disorder, then a tiny dose of that substance can also cure the disorder. The more the homeopathic ingredient is diluted, the stronger it gets as a medicine. How can less drug be more effective? What's the bottom line? Most members of the established medical community believe that no reliable evidence supports the concept that these very highly diluted medicines can cure diseases.

The Least You Need to Know

♦ Drugs are used to prevent, treat, and diagnose medical disorders and to change the function of the body in such nonmedical conditions as pregnancy.

♦ Generic equivalents of brand-name prescription drugs are almost always just as good and cost much less.

♦ Unlike nonprescription (over-the-counter, OTC) drugs, prescription (Rx) drugs have a smaller margin of safety and should be used under the supervision of a health-care professional.

♦ The valuable information found on OTC labels should be read carefully to ensure that these medicines are used properly and as intended.

♦ Unlike dietary supplements, the safety and effectiveness of both prescription and OTC drugs must be proven before they can be marketed.

How Medicines Are Given and How They Work

In This Chapter

- Tracking medicine from ingestion to elimination
- Looking at different ways of taking medicine
- Distinguishing between tablets, capsules, caplets, and other drug forms
- Understanding how medicines work in the body
- Demystifying dosage

In this chapter, we follow the steps a drug takes from the time it enters the body until it leaves. Along the way, we consider the different ways medicines can be taken and talk a little about dosages.

We also look at how drugs work to produce their beneficial effects to treat medical conditions and how and why bad effects sometimes happen. We conclude by considering things you might think about when deciding how much medicine to take.

The Fate of Drugs

Let's start off by looking at what happens to a drug from the time it is taken until it is finally eliminated from the body. This is often referred to, rather dramatically, as the fate of a drug.

In the body, the drug is subject to four basic processes:

- ◆ **Absorption.** The movement of a drug from the site at which it is given to the blood.

- ◆ **Distribution.** The movement of a drug from the blood to its target site(s) where it works.

- ◆ **Metabolism.** Chemical changes in the drug.

- ◆ **Elimination.** Removal of the drug from the body.

The study of these four processes, which are sometimes referred to by the acronym ADME, is collectively called pharmacokinetics. We take a closer look at these processes in the following sections, beginning with the first stage of the process: absorption.

Drug Absorption

Absorption is the transfer of a drug from where it has entered the body into the bloodstream. Not all drugs must be absorbed before they work. For instance, anti-acne creams and dandruff shampoos are applied to and work on the skin and hair. These topical drugs don't need to be absorbed. Drugs taken to treat diarrhea or gas don't enter the blood, instead remaining and working in the intestines.

But most common prescription medicines—for high blood pressure, diabetes, osteoarthritis, coughs, and colds, to name just a few—must first get into the blood and be carried to some distant target site.

Oral or Injection?

After deciding which medicine to use to treat a medical condition, the doctor must decide how it should be given. The most common choices are by mouth (orally) or by injection (parenterally). As with most choices in life, there are advantages and disadvantages to each.

For patients being treated at home, the decision is easy. Oral administration is generally preferred because it is the simplest, least expensive, and most convenient option. You simply pop the tablet in your mouth and wash it down with a swig of liquid. You don't need the assistance of a professional caregiver to administer the drug.

Like foods, drugs taken by mouth are primarily absorbed from the small intestine. The faster the drug is absorbed, the faster it can get to work. Oral drugs generally begin to act within 30 to 60 minutes of being ingested. In an emergency situation where an immediate drug effect is essential, oral drugs don't work fast enough. Some drugs, such as insulin, are not absorbed at all or are not effective when taken by mouth and must be injected.

In a hospital setting, medicines are frequently given by injection. Trained personnel are available to administer drugs into the veins (intravenously), into muscles (intramuscularly), or under the skin (subcutaneously).

The following table gives you a quick summary of the ways drugs are given (a.k.a. routes of drug administration), with their advantages and disadvantages or limitations.

Common Routes of Drug Administration

Route	Where Administered	Advantages	Possible Disadvantages	Examples
Topical	On skin or mucous membrane	Drug effects localized to site of administration	Possible absorption into blood; irritation or allergy	Ointments, creams, eye and nose drops, vaginal jellies, and rings
Systemic	Distributed in the body in bloodstream to a distant site			
Oral	Taken by mouth and absorbed mainly from small intestines	Safest Most convenient Most economical	Irritating: nausea and vomiting Broken down by intestinal enzymes Food interferes with absorption Uncooperative patient	Ibuprofen tablets/caplets Cough and cold syrups

continues

Common Routes of Drug Administration

Route	Where Administered	Advantages	Possible Disadvantages	Examples
Sublingual	Placed under the tongue	Bypasses liver breakdown before entering systemic circulation Rapid onset	Few drugs suitable	Nitroglycerin sublingual tablet
Rectal	Placed into lower rectum as a suppository	Useful for vomiting or unconscious patient Bypasses liver metabolism before entering systemic circulation	Irregular, incomplete absorption Irritation to rectal mucosa Inconvenient	Anti-vomiting suppositories Aspirin suppositories
Transdermal	Patch placed on skin for systemic drug administration	Simple application; no stomach upset	Few drugs suitable	Nicotine patch Estradiol transdermal system
Inhalation	Gaseous and volatile drugs are inhaled and absorbed through alveoli (fine divisions of lung)	Very rapid drug absorption into blood Pulmonary disease (as asthma): drug at site of action	Poor/irregular regulation of dosage Inconvenient	Albuterol aerosol Halothane
Injection (parenteral)				
Subcutaneous (hypodermic)	Into or under skin	Slow, even, and prolonged effects Implantation pellets (act for months)	Only useful for nonirritating drugs Painful	Insulin Testosterone pellets
Intramuscular	Deep into muscle	Aqueous; rapid absorption Oil: Slow, even absorption; long duration of action Useful for poorly soluble drugs	Injection into blood vessel Painful	Procaine Penicillin G

Route	Where Administered	Advantages	Possible Disadvantages	Examples
Intravenous	Directly into vein	Bypasses absorption Immediate onset Exact/entire dose enters blood Irritating solutions can be used Large volumes can be injected	Irreversible once administered Potentially dangerous High cost Difficult to administer (requires trained personnel) Danger of infection or embolism (blood clot in blood vessel)	Norepinephrine Midazolam Doxycycline

Doses can be more exactly and reliably given by injection. Drugs can be delivered into the blood more rapidly and start working faster. When steady drug levels must be maintained over long periods of time (as antibiotics) or large volumes of fluids need to be given, drugs can be given intravenously.

Dosage Forms

After deciding how the medicine will be administered, you or your health-care provider (depending on whether you're taking a prescription or OTC drug) decide on an appropriate dosage form. This is medical jargon for how the medicine is taken (e.g., a tablet taken by mouth or a cream applied to the skin). Before talking about the various dosage forms, let's start at square one and consider why dosage forms are needed. Why not just give the pure active medicine? Because we usually take tablets, let's use them as an example.

Warning!

When drugs are injected, in particular intravenously injected medicines, they can't be retrieved. This is a major problem if a medication error has been made or if the patient experiences an undesirable response to the medicine. In addition, intramuscular injections can be painful or cause injury at the site of injection.

Suppose you have a headache and decide to take 325 mg of Tylenol (acetaminophen). Assuming you had acetaminophen in bulk, how would you weigh out 325 mg accurately? It would be pretty hard, when you consider that there are 30,000 mg in 1 ounce. Not much to weigh. How about weighing out a 0.1 mg dose of Synthroid (levothyroxine) to stimulate your sluggish thyroid function? A tablet provides you with an accurate dose in a convenient form that can be easily taken.

If your 0.1 mg Synthroid tablet only contained the active drug, you would be barely able to see it much less handle it. Therefore, the tablet also contains inactive materials to give it bulk so that you can pick it up.

Other medically inactive ingredients may be contained in oral dosage forms to maintain their stability, mask an unpleasant taste, provide color, and control the speed and length of time the medicine works.

The following table lists some common dosage forms that are used for one or more routes of administration.

Common Dosage Forms

Route of Administration	Dosage Form
Oral	Tablet, capsule, caplet, solution, suspension, elixir syrup
Injection (parenteral)	Suspension, solution
Topical	Ointment, cream, lotion, patch
Rectal/vaginal	Solution, ointment, suppository

In order to decide on an appropriate dosage form, your physician must know the basic functions different dosage forms serve. Similarly, when you select an OTC form off the shelf at your pharmacy, you should be aware of the purpose of the dosage form you're considering. Here's a breakdown of dosage forms and their functions:

◆ **Tablets.** The most common drug dosage form, tablets can be swallowed, chewed, or placed under the tongue (taken sublingually). Tablets often have a distinctive size, shape, and color, and are labeled with letters or numbers for purposes of identification. Some tablets are scored with a groove, permitting them to be broken so that a fraction of a dose can be taken.

◆ **Capsules.** Oblong dosage forms in which the active drug(s) and medically inactive materials are enclosed in a soft or hard gelatin shell. The shells are often fused to prevent tampering. They often have a distinctive size, shape, and color, and are labeled with letters or numbers for identification purposes. When compared with tablets, capsules are easier to swallow and their medicinal contents are more rapidly absorbed.

◆ **Caplets.** Capsule-shaped, coated tablets that are easier to swallow than tablets.

◆ **Modified-release tablets or capsules.** Dosage forms in which the medicine is released over extended periods of time. These medications are commonly identified using such abbreviations as SR (sustained-release), SA (sustained-action), ER (extended-release), and TR (timed-release). Modified-release products should never be chewed, crushed, or broken into smaller pieces. The products will not act as intended, and it can be potentially harmful.

◆ **Suspensions.** Preparations in which finely divided drug particles are suspended in a liquid, which is often water. Because the particles tend to settle out on standing, suspensions must be shaken well before using. Suspensions permit the administration of large amounts of the drug to be easily taken in amounts that would be too large if contained in a tablet or capsule.

◆ **Solutions.** Clear preparations in which the drug is dissolved in a liquid, often water.

◆ **Elixirs.** Clear preparations in which the drug is dissolved in a sweetened or flavored alcohol-water mixture.

◆ **Syrups.** Clear preparations in which the drug is dissolved in a concentrated sugar solution.

◆ **Suppositories.** Solid bodies of different sizes and shapes intended to be inserted into a body orifice (e.g., rectum, vagina, urethra), where they soften and release their medication. Medicines contained in suppositories can have local or systemic (whole body) effects.

◆ **Ointments.** Drug is contained in a greasy base. They leave an oily coat on the skin, don't wash off as easily, and are longer acting than creams and lotions.

◆ **Creams.** Drug is contained in an oil and water base. Although shorter acting, creams are often preferred because they are less greasy than ointments. They usually disappear when rubbed into the skin.

◆ **Lotions.** Shorter acting liquid suspensions of drugs that are not greasy and may be easily spread over large areas of skin.

◆ **Patches (transdermal drug delivery system).** The drug, which is in a patch, is released and absorbed through the skin into the bloodstream. Such drugs include scopolamine (motion sickness), female hormones (contraceptive, hormone replacement therapy), and nicotine (smoking cessation).

Drug Distribution

After the drug has been absorbed or intravenously injected directly into the blood, it makes its way to the intended site(s) of action. (You should not assume that all, or even most, of the drug reaches its intended target site. Large portions of the dose taken may be chemically broken down, causing a loss of effectiveness, or the drug may be eliminated from the body before ever reaching its target.)

Some drugs are distributed to virtually all parts of the body, whereas others only selectively travel. For instance, the brain is off-limits to many drugs taken orally.

Warning!

The placenta serves the developing fetus as a multipurpose breathing, digestive, and elimination organ. With the exception of very large drug molecules (e.g., proteins), most drugs taken by pregnant women rapidly pass to her fetus.

As a consequence, medicines safe for the mother may cause profound adverse effects to her fetus. During the first trimester of pregnancy, the fetus is particularly susceptible to physical deformities caused by some drugs (e.g., thalidomide and the anti-acne drug isotretinoin [Accutane]). Pregnant women should assume that any drug they take may be potentially harmful to the fetus. They should only take those drugs a doctor considers essential.

Drug Metabolism

Now that the drug has been distributed in the blood throughout the body, is this foreign chemical doomed to sail eternally in your blood like the legendary ship *The Flying Dutchman?* Thankfully, no. *Drug metabolism* prevents our bodies from becoming junkyards for all the drugs we have taken.

def•i•ni•tion

Drug metabolism (which is also called drug biotransformation) refers to chemical changes to the drug. Enzymes, which are the body's natural catalysts, are essential for these chemical reactions to occur. Drug metabolizing enzymes (a.k.a. cytochrome P450 enzymes) are found in the liver, the body's major organ for the metabolism of drugs. Metabolism also takes place to a lesser extent in the blood and the intestines.

Because drug-metabolizing enzymes are located in the liver, individuals with impaired liver function may not be able to adequately metabolize drugs, making them less active in the body. As a consequence, the levels of drug build up in the body creating an overdose. This can result in toxicity and even death.

A variety of medications and dietary substances can increase the activity of these drug-metabolizing enzymes (a process called enzyme induction) or decrease their activity (called enzyme inhibition). As discussed in Chapter 3, enzyme induction and inhibition underlie many drug-drug interactions. Use of a new drug may increase or decrease the effectiveness or toxicity of another drug you have been taking.

The changed or metabolized chemical is called a metabolite. As a result of metabolism …

- The metabolite is converted to a chemical more easily eliminated from the body, in particular, in the urine. If metabolism does not occur normally, drugs accumulate in the body.

- The drug may lose some or even all of its medicinal value.

- The drug may be converted from an inactive compound (called a prodrug) to a medically active metabolite.

- The metabolite may cause adverse or toxic effects.

Did You Know That …?

Drug metabolism explains, in part, why some of us are naturally extremely sensitive to medicines, whereas others are extremely resistant. Hypersensitive individuals metabolize and inactivate medicines slowly, leading to drug buildup. Drug-resistant individuals, by contrast, metabolize drugs more rapidly than normal, and don't derive the full benefit from them.

Drug Elimination

Drugs and their metabolites are primarily eliminated from the body by the kidneys in the urine. In young infants and seniors, kidneys function less effectively. Individuals with impaired kidney function, resulting from age or disease, may not be able to adequately eliminate drugs, making them more susceptible to drug-caused toxicity.

Drugs may also be eliminated in exhaled breath, in the feces, and in sweat. Some drugs are also eliminated in breast milk (for instance, lithium for bipolar disorder).

Nursing mothers should either not use such drugs or take drug doses immediately after breast-feeding.

Where and How Medicines Work

Thus far, we have followed drugs in their travels around the body. Let's now talk about *where* drugs work and *how* they work to produce their beneficial (and adverse) effects.

Medical conditions result from abnormalities in the chemistry or function of the body. Most medicines work by counteracting these abnormalities, acting on receptors and on enzymes. Other drugs, such as antibiotics and other chemotherapeutic agents, act directly on foreign invading organisms.

Drug Receptors

Many commonly used drugs work by acting on specific proteins located on cell membranes or within the cell. These are called *drug receptor* sites. To help get a mental picture of a receptor, imagine a lock. To open the lock, we need a key. For our purposes, it helps to think of the drug as the key.

Very few keys can fit the keyhole, and still far fewer can actually turn the tumblers and open the lock. Some drugs fit, and interact with, the receptor to cause a response. This response might be opening airways closed during an asthmatic attack or lowering blood pressure. We'll call drugs that produce such responses *agonists*.

def•i•ni•tion

A **drug receptor** is that specific region of the cell with which a chemical interacts to produce its effects. This chemical may be naturally occurring (endogenous) or laboratory-made (e.g., a drug). An **agonist** interacts with the receptor to cause an effect. An **antagonist** interacts with the receptor to prevent the neurotransmitter from causing an effect.

On the other hand, suppose we have a second key that also fits the keyhole but that doesn't open the lock. As long as this key is in the keyhole, it blocks the keyhole, and the agonist can't work. We'll call this second key, or drug, an *antagonist*.

Many naturally occurring chemicals in the body function as agonists. Some of these chemicals, called neurotransmitters, are responsible for carrying messages from one cell to another. They also carry messages from nerves to involuntary muscles, glands, and the heart. Neurotransmitters work by interacting with specific receptor sites.

Some drug agonists closely resemble neurotransmitters, act at the same receptors, and cause effects that resemble neurotransmitters. Other drugs—the antagonists—block receptor sites and prevent neurotransmitters from interacting with them.

Defects in neurotransmitters are involved in a variety of diseases. These include Alzheimer's disease, schizophrenia, depression, myasthenia gravis, and stroke.

Receptor sites are named according to the neurotransmitter with which they naturally interact. So acetylcholine interacts with cholinergic receptors, histamine with histaminergic receptors, noradrenaline (also called norepinephrine) with adrenergic receptors. Drugs that interact with the acetylcholine receptor are referred as cholinergic agonists and cholinergic antagonists (or blocking agents).

Did You Know That ...?

Receptor types have subtypes—think of them as first cousins—each with different functions. For example, adrenergic receptors are of two primary subtypes: alpha-adrenergic and beta-adrenergic receptors. Beta-blocker drugs, such as propranolol (Inderal), are antagonists of norepinephrine at beta-adrenergic receptors.

Histamine's two primary receptor subtypes are H-1 and H-2. H-1 antagonists (a.k.a. antihistamines), such as fexofenadine (Allegra), are used to treat allergic conditions. H-2 antagonists, such as ranitidine (Zantac), are used for ulcers and heartburn.

Some drugs interact with only one receptor type, whereas others are less discriminating and interact with multiple receptor types. If a drug interacts with only one receptor site, it will produce far fewer effects (both good and bad) than a drug that acts at multiple receptor sites. Drugs interacting with multiple receptors, such as chlorpromazine (Thorazine), cause a wide array of side effects. Pharmaceutical companies are continually working to develop new drugs that are more selective in their effects.

Warning!

No medicine produces one and only one effect! In my discussion of the use of medicines to treat various medical conditions in Part 2, you'll see that almost all drugs cause some undesirable side effects or adverse effects. These vary in severity from being rather trivial to, in rare instances, potentially life-threatening.

Drug Effects on Enzymes

If we want to synthesize new compounds in a chemistry laboratory, we often need to heat chemicals to very high temperatures, add strong acids or bases, or patiently wait for hours or even days. The body is in a constant state of building up and breaking down chemicals that are essential for life. It cannot withstand extreme changes in temperature or acid-base balance, and we often need those essential chemicals *now*. To speed up these reactions, the body uses protein catalysts, called enzymes.

A number of drugs act by interfering with, or inhibiting, enzymes that are responsible for the breakdown and inactivation of neurotransmitters. Some of these medicines are used for the treatment of glaucoma, depression, and Alzheimer's disease.

Antibiotics and Other Chemotherapeutic Agents

Thus far, I have talked about drugs that work by changing the body's function. Some medications, such as antibiotics, change the function of invading foreign organisms such as bacteria, viruses, and parasites, and cause their death.

How Much and for How Long

Dose determines how strong the drug effects will be and how long it will work. Let's now turn our attention to doses and how fast and how long drugs work.

How Much of the Drug

Too much medicine may be harmful, and too little won't do the job.

Very generally speaking, the more drug you take (i.e., the higher the dose), the greater will be the drug effect and the longer the drug will work. But wait—there are exceptions.

A basic difference between OTC and prescription drugs is the margin between doses that are safe and those that can cause adverse effects. OTC drugs typically have a much wider margin of safety.

The OTC drug label provides dosage guidance information based on the age of the user. These are average doses, and they may be too high for some users and inadequate for others.

A doctor's dosage recommendation for a prescription medicine is also based on the age of the patient. For many potent drugs—in which there is a relatively small differ-

ence between a safe dose and one that can produce major adverse effects—the dose may also be based on body weight and whether the patient has a history of liver or kidney disease. In such cases, your doctor and pharmacist should emphasize the need to take just the right dose and at the appropriate time interval between doses.

If your doctor has prescribed one tablet every six hours, what happens if you, on your own, decide to take two tablets every six hours? It's hard to predict, but all possibilities are on the table. Nothing may happen, or you might experience significant adverse effects. Or you might derive greater benefit from the drug but also have side effects that were absent or only modest at the prescribed dose. These side effects may offset the benefits of the drug or prove to be so troublesome that you stop taking the drug.

> **Did You Know That …?**
>
> One of homeopathic medicine's basic principles states that the more a drug is diluted, the more powerful it becomes. This concept is precisely opposite to the teachings of traditional medicine. For more on homeopathy, see Chapter 1.

> **Warning!**
>
> All drugs are potentially dangerous. When sufficiently high doses of even the safest drugs are taken, adverse effects can occur. Conversely, if low enough doses of even highly poisonous drugs are taken, they may not produce adverse effects.

How Long Drugs Work

Some drugs work rapidly, whereas others act for long periods of time. TV ads for drugs that relieve stomach distress associated with peptic ulcers attempt to capitalize upon these differences when promoting their products. Victims of osteoarthritis are told that only one of the sponsor's product need be taken every 12 hours, whereas two of the competitor's drug must be taken every 4 hours to relieve pain.

Are these differences important? It depends on your medical condition. If you need relief from an occasional but intense headache, you want a drug that acts *now*. If treating a chronic condition, you would probably prefer a drug that acts for an extended period of time rather than a drug that requires multiple doses during the course of a day.

To an increasing extent, drugs are appearing on the market that act for longer periods and that require fewer daily doses. Fosamax (alendronate) can be taken once a day or once a week to prevent osteoporosis. Both are equally effective and cost the same. You can take hormones by mouth every day or apply a patch weekly and get equivalent degrees of contraceptive protection.

Some of the factors that modify how rapidly and for how long a drug works include …

◆ How the drug is given, e.g., intravenously, under the tongue, or inhaled versus orally, which effects the speed at which the drug reaches its target site of action.

◆ Whether the drug is in solution or is a solid (e.g., a tablet).

◆ The dose of the drug taken. Higher doses usually act faster and for longer periods of time.

◆ Whether the medicine is a modified-release product that extends effects over longer time periods.

◆ How rapidly the drug is metabolized and eliminated from the body, which may be affected by liver or kidney diseases.

The Least You Need to Know

◆ Pharmacokinetics includes the processes of absorption, distribution, metabolism, and elimination (ADME) of drugs.

◆ The speed and extent to which drugs are absorbed depend on how they are taken and the dosage form used to deliver the active medicine.

◆ Drug metabolism by the liver causes chemical changes in the drug (a.k.a. metabolite) that usually increase its elimination from the body by the kidneys.

◆ Both drug agonists and antagonists interact with receptors, but only agonists are able to produce an effect.

◆ Neurotransmitters (e.g., acetylcholine, dopamine, serotonin) carry messages from nerves to involuntary muscles, the heart, and glands.

◆ In general, the higher the dose, the greater the effects and the longer the drug works.

All People Are Not Created Equal

In This Chapter

- ◆ Learning why some of us are very sensitive to medicines, whereas others are hardly affected
- ◆ Understanding why pregnant women shouldn't use drugs
- ◆ Administering drugs to children and older people
- ◆ Getting the scoop on the positive and negative consequences of combining different drugs

Although there are "usual" doses for medicines, don't assume that all people respond to drugs in the "usual" way. Some of us seem to be very sensitive to the medicines we take, whereas others are only minimally affected. Making matters even more confusing, sometimes the same drug can have greater or lesser effects in the same individual.

In this chapter, I talk about some of the real-life factors that might cause differences in how people respond to medicines. Some of these influences—such as age, genetic makeup, and medical condition—are beyond our control.

Why We Respond Differently: An Overview

People don't all respond in a like manner to medicines for a wide variety of reasons. In this chapter, I talk about such factors as these:

- Age

- Body weight

- Genetic influences

- How the drug is given or taken (the route of administration) and dosage form used

- Time of drug administration, in particular, how your meals and the presence of foods influence drug response

- Diseases or other medical conditions

- Drug history, i.e., other drugs being taken

These seemingly different factors are linked to the pharmacokinetic processes (ADME) described in Chapter 2.

Let's take a closer look at each of these factors.

Age

From a drug perspective, the "usual patient" is typically between 12 to 65 years old, in reasonable health, and of average weight. Individuals outside this range—infants and pre-teenage children at one end and seniors at the other—are thought to be more sensitive to the effects of medicines. We generally deal with their greater sensitivity by reducing the usual dose. In many cases, all adults in reasonable health receive the same dose, regardless of age.

In this section, we talk about why infants and the elderly might be more sensitive to drugs. We then take a look at potential problems for fetuses and nursing infants when pregnant women take drugs.

Infants and Young Children

Over the years, many formulas have been devised to calculate doses for infants and young children as a fraction of the adult dose. These so-called "rules" are based on age, body weight, or body surface area—calculated based on height and weight—and are intended to be only approximations. They continue to be used widely because no perfect method for calculating young people's doses has been devised.

The problem with these formulas is that they are based on the erroneous assumption that infants and young children are miniature adults. This problem was highlighted when the antibiotic chloramphenicol (Chloromycetin) was found to cause deaths in many very young infants being treated for infectious diseases. Based on the body weights of the infants, the doses used appeared to be quite reasonable.

 Warning!

In the absence of medical supervision, medications should not be given to children less than 2 years of age. What may be a very reasonable dose for a 3-year-old child may be unreasonably high for a 1-year-old infant.

What happened, then? We now know that infants, and especially newborns, have poorly developed drug metabolizing enzymes in their young livers, and that their kidneys are unable to excrete drugs efficiently. Drug levels of the antibiotic built up in the body and toxicity resulted.

Elderly

Although many of us might take exception, gerontologists have traditionally considered 65 to be the start of the "elderly" years. People over 85 are now defined as "very old," and this is the fastest-growing age group in North America. The use of medications by the elderly presents special problems because of the number of different drugs they use and the nature of the medical conditions for which they are being treated.

The over-65 group represents only 12 percent of all Americans, and yet they take 25 percent of all prescriptions. Ambulatory elderly persons generally take three to four prescription and OTC medications a day. Nursing home residents take some seven medications daily. We don't have an accurate count of the alternative medicines that many seniors are likely taking, including dietary supplements, herbal products, and homeopathic remedies. As discussed later in this chapter, the use of multiple drugs increases the risk of drug-drug interactions.

As an inevitable consequence of the aging process, our bodies' organs become less efficient doing their vital jobs. This includes the heart's ability to pump blood, the capacity of the kidneys to filter and collect urine, and the efficiency of the liver to metabolize drugs.

The bottom line: in the elderly, drug-elimination processes are reduced, and drugs remain in the body for longer periods of time. This may result in "usual adult doses" causing an intensified medical effect, for longer periods of time, as well as increase in their potential for drug toxicity. Just as adjustments in doses are made for infants, the dose of many drugs must be reduced for the elderly.

Less well studied are changes in drug sensitivity that are independent of pharmacokinetic influences. Seniors appear to be more sensitive to the behavioral effects of Valium-related benzodiazepines, the pain-killing effects of opioids (a.k.a. narcotics), and the blood-thinning effects of warfarin and heparin. In contrast, they show reduced sensitivity to some drugs that affect the heart and blood pressure.

Developing Fetuses

Because most drugs cross the placenta, pregnant women must be extremely careful when selecting and taking medications. The potential problems drugs might cause a fetus include …

- **Physical abnormalities (also called teratogenic effects).** These abnormalities most commonly occur when the pregnant woman takes the offending drug during the first trimester of pregnancy. This problem has been documented with many drugs including thalidomide, the anti-acne drug isotretinoin (Accutane), and alcoholic beverages, which can cause fetal alcohol syndrome.

- **Physical dependence and a withdrawal syndrome.** These problems are seen in newborns after extended periods of maternal use of heroin, methadone, and related opioids, as well as after binge drinking alcohol.

- **Premature labor.** May be caused by the use of harsh laxatives, such as castor oil.

- **A range of exaggerated effects in the newborn that are also seen in the mother.** Examples include depression of the baby's thyroid gland function after the pregnant woman has taken the antithyroid drug propylthiouracil or excessive drowsiness and breathing difficulties in the newborn after Mom is given morphine to reduce pain during labor.

Pregnant women should critically consider the potential risks of any drug use. The *FDA Pregnancy Categories* is the most reliable (and conservative) source of information. For each drug, the risk is summarized in a five-point scale, with each category described in the table. Information on specific drugs appears in drug package information inserts and other drug information references. Women should also seek such information from their doctor or pharmacist.

FDA Pregnancy Categories

Category	What This Means
A	Adequate number of good studies have been conducted in pregnant women and have not shown any risk to the fetus in any phase of pregnancy.
B	No evidence of harm to the fetus has been seen in animal studies, but an adequate number of good studies have not been conducted in pregnant women. Or Animal studies have shown harm to the fetus but an adequate number of good studies in pregnant women have not shown any risk to the fetus in any phase of pregnancy.
C	Animal studies have shown harm to the fetus but an adequate number of good studies have not been conducted in pregnant women. Or No animal studies have been conducted, and there are not an adequate number of good studies in pregnant women.
D	An adequate number of good studies in pregnant women have demonstrated a risk to the fetus. However, the benefits of the medicine may outweigh the potential risk to the fetus. For example, the drug may be if needed in a life-threatening condition or a serious disease for which safer drugs cannot be used or are ineffective.
X	An adequate number of good studies in animals or pregnant women have clearly demonstrated a positive risk to the fetus. The medicine must not be used in women who are or who may become pregnant.

Nursing Infants

Most medicines taken by the mother may be passed to her nursing infant in breast milk, although few such drugs cause adverse effects to the infant. Some exceptions include opioids, which may cause infant drowsiness, and tetracycline antibiotics, which may cause staining of young teeth.

For each medicine, nursing mothers should check with their doctor or pharmacist to determine whether it's safe for her and her baby.

It may not be possible or even reasonable for nursing mothers to avoid medications. However, timing when the medication is taken can significantly reduce how much of the drug gets passed to the infant. Taking drugs 30 to 60 minutes prior to feeding produces *maximum* drug concentrations in the milk. Instead, mothers should take drugs 15 minutes after nursing or 3 to 4 hours before the next feeding.

Body Weight

Placing a teaspoonful of sugar in a demitasse cup versus a coffee mug results in a considerable difference in the concentration of sugar in each beverage. Similarly, compare giving 100 mg of drug to a 100 lb. man versus someone who weighs 200 lbs. There will be significant differences in the drug levels in the blood and ultimately at the drug's target site.

Drug dosage is not generally adjusted for OTC drugs or for those prescription drugs in which there is a wide margin between safe therapeutic doses and those doses that cause toxicity. By contrast, anticancer drugs and some antibiotics medicines have a narrow margin of safety. That is, doses only slightly greater than those used for therapeutic purposes are capable of causing toxic effects. In such cases, dosage is more critically calculated on the basis of body weight or body surface area.

Genetic Influences

Biologically speaking, all people are not created equal. Genetic factors may influence our response to drugs. This is termed pharmacogenetics. As a consequence of our genetic makeup, some of us may respond to a greater or lesser degree than the average.

A small proportion of individuals may have highly unusual, so-called idiosyncratic, reactions to drugs. These reactions may not only be more or less of a normal response, but also different from normal. These differences have also been attributed to genetic influences.

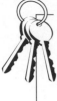

Did You Know That …? _____

The Human Genome Project, completed in 2000, estimated that each human has some 30,000 genes, and that humans share 99.9 percent of the same gene pool. This has led some to question whether racial identity is a biologically valid notion.

Only 1 out of every 1,000 genes accounts for the differences among us, and this includes our different responses to drugs.

Drug Metabolism

The best examples of genetic influences that account for differences in drug response and toxicity come from variations in drug metabolizing enzymes. Let's look at isoniazid (INH) and alcohol.

INH is used worldwide for the treatment of tuberculosis. Half the white people and half the black people in the United States rapidly metabolize INH and the other half metabolize it slowly. The percentage of slow metabolizers is markedly different in other ethnic groups: Native Americans, 21 percent; Japanese, 13 percent; and Eskimos, 5 percent. Slow metabolizers have genetically determined, reduced amounts of a specific drug metabolizing enzyme. Such individuals are more likely to experience side effects involving their nerves. Some groups of fast metabolizers are more prone to liver toxicity.

Genetic influences also account for why Asians are much more sensitive to alcoholic beverages than are whites. They show flushing of the face, heart palpitations, and a more rapid heartbeat. These differences result from genetically determined differences in the buildup of acetaldehyde, an alcohol metabolite.

Target Sensitivity

In Chapter 2, we talked about drug responses that result from the effects of a drug at its target site. Receptors and enzymes are among the most important of these targets and may be subject to genetic influences, which accounts for racial differences in drug response.

Compared to white patients, Asians often require lower doses or have side effects at lower doses of some drugs, including medicines used to treat bipolar disorder, depression, and schizophrenia. Blacks, Chinese, and whites have been found to respond differently to various categories of drugs used for high blood pressure.

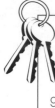

Did You Know That ...? _____

The Food and Drug Administration (FDA), for the first time in 2005, approved a medication specifically for a racial group. Whereas clinical studies failed to show its effectiveness in the general population, BiDil (a combination of isosorbide dinintrate and hydralazine) was approved for the treatment of heart failure in African Americans, a group particularly prone to this condition. The FDA said that the approval was "a step toward the promise of personalized medicine," a concept we return to in Chapter 4.

Route of Administration and Dosage Forms

The route of drug administration and the dosage form used directly influence how rapidly and to what extent a drug is absorbed, distributed, metabolized, and eliminated (Chapter 2). These, in turn, affect the intensity with which the drug works.

Time of Drug Administration and Meals

Many of us know that imbibing the same amount of alcohol has a more rapid and pronounced effect before a meal than after one. Likewise, food can reduce the speed and extent to which other drugs are absorbed after being taken by mouth. As the result of these drug-food interactions, the start of drug effects may be delayed, and less of the drug may reach its target site, thereby reducing the magnitude of the drug's effects.

Maximizing Your Medicine

Remembering to take multiple drugs at different times of day can be confusing and difficult. If this is a problem for you, work with your doctor or pharmacist to find the most convenient dosing schedule for taking your drugs—one that you can remember and that won't interfere with your daily activities. The use of pill boxes that separate medications by the time of day they are to be taken may also be helpful in staying on schedule.

Milk is often, but unwisely, taken with tetracycline to reduce intestinal upset. Although milk does reduce nausea, the calcium in milk also decreases the amount of tetracycline absorbed. This lowers antibiotic blood levels and reduces its antibacterial effectiveness.

Fosamax (alendronate), used for the prevention and treatment of osteoporosis in postmenopausal women, is very poorly absorbed by mouth. It must be taken at least 30 minutes before the first food, drink, or medication of the day is swallowed, and can only be taken with water.

Far more dramatic are the life-threatening drug-food interactions involving monoamine oxidase inhibitors (MAOIs), used for depression. These drugs interfere with the ability of the enzyme MAO to break down norepinephrine and serotonin, neurotransmitters involved in influencing mood.

MAO also rapidly breaks down tyramine, a natural chemical present in a wide range of food and drinks. These include aged cheeses, Chianti wine, broad beans, chicken liver, pickled herring, pepperoni, and salami. Tyramine is not broken down when taking MAOIs. Rather it builds up and stimulates the release of norepinephrine. This can potentially result in severe headaches, very marked elevations in blood pressure (a.k.a. hypertensive crisis), bleeding in the brain, and even death.

Disease State

Disease may modify the patient's response to medicines, most often how the body handles drugs. Diarrhea speeds the passage of drugs through the gastrointestinal tract, reducing its opportunity to be absorbed.

Liver diseases, such as cirrhosis or hepatitis, reduce the body's ability to metabolize drugs. Patients with diseases that impair liver or kidney function may be more susceptible to drug-induced toxicity unless adjustments in dosage are made.

Some drugs only work when a medical condition is present. Aspirin and acetaminophen reduce elevated body temperature but do not reduce normal temperature.

Drug History

How we respond to a new prescription may be modified by our prior use of that medication or another drug we are taking. This altered response may be an effect that is greater or less than the normal effect. Let's now talk about tolerance, cumulative effects, and drug-drug interactions.

Tolerance

Tolerance refers to a progressive decline in the normal drug response after repeated doses have been taken. This is often seen in those taking sleep-producing drugs or who are suffering from chronic pain (as terminal cancer) and are using pain-killing opioids (narcotics).

It's often the case that doses that once provided relief become less effective over time. To counteract tolerance, higher doses must be taken or doses must be used at more frequent intervals.

In the past, many well-meaning doctors were overly obsessed with the fear of causing a narcotic-dependent state (i.e., addiction) in terminally ill patients and did not prescribe sufficiently high doses of these drugs to adequately reduce pain. Happily, this philosophy has changed. Doctors have an obligation to prescribe drugs to make their patients pain-free or, at least, relatively so. To forestall the development of tolerance to opioids, doctors typically delay prescribing the heaviest drugs until the milder drugs are no long effective in providing pain relief. We should also note that tolerance also develops to some (but not all) of the undesirable and toxic effects of opioids.

Cumulative Effects

The results of tolerance and cumulative effects are the flip sides of one another. When tolerance occurs, repeated doses cause less effect. When cumulative effects occur, repeated doses cause greater effects. The effects we are referring to may be good (desirable) or bad (undesirable).

After multiple doses of a drug are given and the desired blood level of drug has been reached, the amount of new drug taken into the body (i.e., the dose) should equal the amount of drug leaving. Cumulative effects result when drug intake exceeds the rate at which the drug is being metabolized and inactivated. As drug blood levels increase, so does the risk of toxicity.

Cumulative effects can also result from the inability of the body to effectively eliminate the drug or its metabolites. I've already talked about the kidney as the most important organ involved in drug elimination. In some cases, it may be the only organ responsible for the removal of drugs from the body.

The kidney is of particular importance for aminoglycoside antibiotics, such as gentamicin, that are not metabolized but are only eliminated in the urine. Although these drugs can be lifesaving for the treatment of certain very serious infections, they have a very narrow margin of safety and can produce severe kidney toxicity and hearing loss. In such cases, timing is everything. The time required to reduce body levels of aminoglycosides by 50 percent is 2 hours for patients with normal kidney function and about 50 hours for those with severe kidney failure. Doses or the interval between successive doses must be adjusted for patients with kidney problems.

Drug-Drug Interactions

When you are taking two or more drugs at a time, there is the possibility that these drugs will interact with one another. The more drugs that are taken, the greater the odds this will occur. Such drug-drug interactions may benefit the patient or cause harm.

Few individuals take one and only one medication at a time. As mentioned earlier, seniors commonly take multiple prescription and nonprescription medications to manage their chronic diseases. Patients with heart disease, high blood pressure, cancer, and AIDS routinely take more than one drug to treat each of these conditions.

The effects of one medicine may be modified by the prior or concurrent administration of another drug. These effects may be greater or less than that anticipated. In selected cases, these drug interactions may even be desirable.

Warning!

If you take more than one drug, the potential exists for a drug-drug interaction. With each additional drug, this potential increases significantly. Whenever you get a new drug—prescription, OTC, or herbal—always ask your pharmacist if it interacts with any other drug you are taking. If you drink, ask if the drug can safely be taken with alcohol.

As we shall see, drug-drug interactions may produce greater effects (i.e., additive effects) or reduce the effects of the other (i.e., antagonistic effects).

Additive Effects

An additive effect occurs when the combined effect of multiple drugs is equivalent to or even greater than the sum of their independent effects. The most common examples occur when depressant drugs—such as antihistamines or medications used for insomnia, anxiety, schizophrenia, or depression—are used in combination with one another or with alcohol.

Viagra and related drugs used to treat erectile dysfunction may lower blood pressure somewhat. When used in combination with nitroglycerin and nitrates to treat angina or when used with some adrenergic antagonists (as Hytrin, Cardura) to treat enlarged prostate, blood pressure can drop to dangerously low levels.

Antagonistic Effects

Antagonism may occur when one drug reduces the effect of another drug. Different processes may account for drug antagonism.

Dispositional (a.k.a. pharmacokinetic) antagonism takes place when one drug reduces the amount of another drug at its target site. This commonly results from changes in absorption or metabolism.

In our discussion of meals earlier in this chapter, we indicated that calcium in milk interferes with the absorption of tetracycline antibiotics. Calcium is also present in some commonly used antacids (such as Tums) and may act similarly if taken with tetracycline antibiotics.

In Chapter 2, we talked about cytochrome P450 drug metabolizing enzymes and how the activity of these liver enzymes could be increased, a process called enzyme induction. As a result of enzyme induction, drugs are broken down and inactivated more rapidly, making them less effective as medications. Enzyme induction is a common cause of drug-drug interactions.

Here's a list of some common enzyme inducers:

Alcohol

Carbamazepine (Tegretol)

Omeprazole (Prilosec, Losec)

Phenobarbital

Rifampin (Rifadin)

St. John's wort

Smoking

Did You Know That …?

Repeated use of some drugs results in tolerance to their own effects. Regular cigarette smoking increases the metabolism of nicotine. This is thought to account for the absence of nausea, flushing, and other unpleasant nicotine effects experienced by the neophyte smoker.

Herbal drugs are generally promoted as being safe and effective substitutes for traditional medications. One of the most widely used herbal products is St. John's wort, which has been found to be effective for mild to moderate depression. It is also an enzyme inducer capable of reducing the blood levels and therapeutic effects of blood thinners, oral contraceptives, and drugs for heart disease and AIDS.

We talked about drug effects resulting from their interaction with receptors in Chapter 2. Agonists interact with receptors to produce an effect, while in the presence of an antagonist, the agonist effect is reduced or even totally prevented. Consider the consequences of receiving prescriptions for the beta-adrenergic agonist albuterol (Proventil) for asthma and the beta-adrenergic antagonist propranolol (Inderal) for high blood pressure or other heart diseases. Both act at the same receptor site in opposite directions, resulting in the patient's asthma worsening!

Not all antagonism is undesirable. Morphine, heroin, and other opioids can depress breathing with fatal consequences. Naloxone (Narcan), a highly specific opioid antagonist, reverses this depressed breathing and is used as an antidote in opioid poisoning.

Beneficial Drug Combinations

Sometimes it is better to use multiple drugs, rather than a single drug, to treat a medical condition. Here are some situations when combinations of drugs are effective:

◆ Drugs A and B may act in different ways to produce an overall equivalent beneficial effect. Lower doses of each drug may reduce the incidence and severity of adverse effects produced by each individual drug. For instance, Acetaminophen or aspirin is frequently used in combination with codeine for relief of pain.

◆ Drug B itself may have no direct effect on the condition but may enhance the beneficial effects of A by favorably modifying its pharmacokinetic profile. In the combination product Sinemet (levodopa + carbidopa) for the treatment of Parkinson's disease, carbidopa prevents the breakdown of the neurotransmitter levodopa outside the brain.

◆ Drug B may be used to prevent or reduce the undesirable side effects caused by A.

◆ There may be cost savings associated with using lower doses of B, a very expensive drug.

The Least You Need to Know

◆ Most of our individual responses to drugs have been attributed to differences in such pharmacokinetic factors as drug metabolism and elimination.

◆ Infants and young children do not have fully developed systems for drug metabolism and elimination, making them more susceptible to drug toxicity.

◆ Because many drugs pass directly from mother to fetus, pregnant women should take only essential drugs that have been approved by a physician.

◆ Most genetically determined differences in drug response have been attributed to differences in metabolism and target site sensitivity.

◆ The risk of drug interactions increases with the number of prescription, OTC, and herbal drugs taken.

◆ Drug-drug interactions resulting from drugs used in combination may result in effects that are greater or less than the effects produced by the individual drugs.

Chapter 4

Is My Medicine Safe and Does It Work?

In This Chapter

♦ Learning the difference between a perfectly safe drug and one that is relatively safe

♦ Understanding that sugar pills sometimes make you feel better

♦ Understanding why FDA-approved drugs are sometimes pulled from the market

♦ Appreciating why there is a great time delay between the time a drug is discovered and the time you can get it on a prescription

Hardly a day passes without a newspaper or TV report proclaiming the discovery of a new lifesaving or life-changing drug. Just as often, or so it seems, we learn about a widely used drug that has been linked to blindness, liver toxicity, or increased risk of heart attack or stroke.

How do you make sense of the news we hear in the media?

In this chapter, we first look at the drug development process—that is, how drugs are evaluated in animals and humans. We shall see that evaluation of drugs in humans may be complicated by placebo (a.k.a. sugar pill) effects.

After the drug sponsor (e.g., manufacturer) has accumulated mountains of data supporting the safety and effectiveness of the new wonder drug, it submits the data to the Food and Drug Administration (FDA) for approval to market.

But after a drug gets on the market, its success is not assured. Unexpected adverse effects may become evident over time, which may lead to restrictions on its use or even to its unceremonious withdrawal from the market.

Drug Development Process: An Overview

A tortuous journey exists between the time a chemical is first found to have some potential value in animal studies and the time the general public can take it to treat a medical condition. Fewer than 1 out of every 1,000 chemicals tested are ever given to a human subject. Only one out five chemicals tested in humans ever appear on the market.

The pharmaceutical industry is among the most profitable of all on Wall Street with annual double-digit profits. Blockbuster drugs—and there are more than 50 of them— have annual sales that exceed $1 billion. The cost of your prescriptions is high—very high. But so is the cost of new drug development, in the billion-dollar range for each new drug and requiring more than 10 years of evaluation.

These high profits are balanced by high risks. Today's very successful drugs may find themselves sharing the market or even being replaced by new drugs tomorrow. These new drugs may work better in a larger number of patients, be safer, more convenient or easier to take, or may be more effectively marketed. Patents may expire, resulting in a loss of market exclusivity. The appearance of a life-threatening adverse reaction or an increased risk of causing a serious condition may result in its abrupt withdrawal from the market.

How do we know that our medicine is safe and really works? To answer this question, let's trace the drug evaluation process in animals and humans.

Animal Studies (Preclinical Studies)

Millions of chemicals are prepared in the laboratory with only a mere handful ever becoming medicines. Researchers perform studies, called preclinical studies, in laboratory animals to discover those relatively rare chemicals that can be used to treat various medical conditions.

Some animal studies serve as models for a specific human condition or disease. In others, search for a drug effect that might prove useful for treating several diseases that have a common link.

Suppose a chemical passes this first hurdle. It works in preclinical studies. Researchers then must ask a number of questions. Does it work without causing toxicity after a single dose or after multiple doses are given for several weeks to several years? What is its margin of safety—that is, the difference between doses that produce desirable effects and those that cause toxicity or other adverse effects? If the spread is too narrow, scientists will move on to another test compound.

Does the test compound produce adverse effects to different organs or body systems—liver, blood, kidneys, reproductive system—but only after it has been given for extended periods of time? These studies predict adverse effects that might occur in humans who must take medicines for a lifetime for chronic diseases, such as diabetes, high blood pressure, and osteoporosis.

In other words, animal studies provide detailed information about a promising compound's safe and toxic doses, potential adverse effects, and data concerning its pharmacokinetics.

Preclinical testing takes from two to six and a half years to complete.

Most chemicals tested must be discarded because they either lack sufficient potential or are too toxic. Others lack the properties that will make them suitable to be administered as medicines.

Human Studies (Clinical Studies)

Before testing a compound in humans, a process called clinical studies, the FDA must give its stamp of approval. The FDA looks at the safety of the compound based on the results of animal studies. It scrutinizes the proposed tests designed to evaluate its safety and effectiveness in humans and the precautions used to protect the study participants. If approved, the sponsor conducts a three-phase evaluation over an average period of some seven years.

Did You Know That ...?

Test subjects must willingly, and without direct or indirect coercion, provide their informed consent to participate in a drug trial. They must be told, in simple English, that they are participating in a medical experiment, and that there are a number of known or potential risks associated with taking the drug. Children, the intellectually disabled, and prisoners are not generally able to provide appropriate informed consent.

Phase 1

In phase 1, studies are conducted to determine safe doses and possible side effects in 20 to 100 disease-free individuals. Researchers determine the levels of the drug in the blood after different doses are given. Information about the metabolism and elimination of the drug are also obtained.

Phase 2

Having established safe doses in phase 1, phase 2 involves giving the test drug to several hundred patients who actually suffer from the condition the drug is intended to treat. The results of these studies provide the first clues as to whether the drug will be of value for the treatment of disease in humans.

In phase 2, great attention is focused upon the appearance of undesirable side effects. Some can be predicted in advance, based on the nature of the drug. In other cases, the adverse effects may be unpredictable, unanticipated, and severe.

If the drug proves to be relatively safe and provides benefit to the test subjects with the condition, researchers move on to phase 3.

Phase 3

This final phase, taking three to four years, critically determines whether the drug actually benefits the medical condition and causes adverse effects. Certain undesirable effects may only be evident when the drug is used for extended periods of time in large numbers of subjects.

def•i•ni•tion

The term **placebo** is from the Latin "I shall please." Placebos look like real drugs, but contain only inactive ingredients. Classic examples of a placebo include a sugar pill; a bitter tasting, liquid solution taken by mouth; or injection of a salt solution.

Carefully controlled clinical trials are the most expensive and time-consuming stage in drug evaluation. As we shall talk about below, these trials involve comparing the desirable and undesirable (i.e., side effects) of the test drug with a *placebo* (sugar pill) control in several hundred to several thousand subjects with the disease or condition.

Phase 4

A drug continues to be evaluated for adverse drug reactions even after it has been approved for marketing and is being used for the treatment of a medical condition. At this time, and after the drug has been used in a large number of individuals, unusual adverse effects might become evident. In some cases, drugs must be removed from the market. We will return to Phase 4 (post-marketing drug surveillance) in a later section of this chapter.

Placebos and Drug Effects

We know that health and disease are strongly influenced by psychological factors, and that the power of suggestion may be as effective as an active drug in treating disease. Might these subjective factors account for the positive results seen in phase 2?

Are placebos effective for the treatment of diseases and other medical conditions? Absolutely! Their effectiveness has been repeatedly demonstrated for the relief of pain, insomnia, depression, high blood pressure, headache, seasickness, anxiety, the common cold, and schizophrenia, among many other conditions. About one in three test subjects or real patients typically improve after receiving placebos. Just like real medicines, they are also capable of causing side effects.

Placebos are not uniformly effective. They are more likely to provide benefit when the therapy is intended to change behavior or mood or to alter a subjective sensation, such as pain or nausea. They are much less effective improving the joints of patients with rheumatoid arthritis or improving widespread cancers or chronic conditions that have periods of remission.

A French proverb tells us that "The presence of the doctor is the beginning of the cure." One of the most important elements of successful drug treatment is the feeling of confidence you have in your doctor. By writing a prescription, your doctor is at least very tacitly implying that the drug will benefit your condition.

If your doctor emphatically tells you that the prescribed medicine will improve your condition, you will be very receptive to taking it and will plan to get better. By contrast, suppose your doctor merely suggests that the drug might help, and then adds, "but then maybe it won't." Here, you may be less convinced about the drug's virtues.

Eliminating the Placebo Effect from Clinical Trials

In the phase 2 clinical trials, only the test drug was given to subjects with the disorder. If positive results were seen, the drug will surely be effective in phase 3. But wait, you say. Perhaps those favorable effects were really a placebo response. Maybe so, and it's something that needs to be checked out by comparing the test drug with a placebo control. Researchers have several ways to test for this.

One simple way might involve the doctor-investigator dividing the total subjects in half: one group gets the drug, while the other the placebo. Subjects don't know whether they are receiving a drug or placebo, but the doctor does. This is called a single-blind study.

After the treatment period has ended, the subjects are evaluated, and improvement is assessed in each treatment group. In these studies, the test drug often proves to be better. Why? The doctor knows who is receiving the active drug. Subconscious bias might creep in at the time the drug or placebo is given or when interpreting the results of the trial.

Warning!

In some situations it may be inappropriate or unethical to compare the test drug with a placebo. When the medical condition is life-threatening, a previously established effective drug, and not a placebo, should be used as a control.

The much-preferred approach in phase 3 studies is to randomly assign subjects to receive either the test drug or placebo. Neither the doctor nor the subjects know which treatment is being given. In this so-called double-blind study, the element of bias is eliminated or at least minimized. Statistical analyses are used to determine whether the test-drug improvement (if any) was real or occurred only by chance.

Drug Approval Process

The FDA is responsible for overseeing the evaluation of drugs in the United States and for granting approval prior to their being placed on the market. Their decision is based on evidence provided by the sponsor (i.e., drug manufacturer) that the prescription or OTC drug is safe and effective. The FDA's approval process is the most rigorous worldwide and has long served as the "gold standard."

The drug sponsor submits very extensive documentation supporting its claims for drug effectiveness and safety to the FDA. It's not unusual for the FDA to require additional evidence or documentation. The FDA might also require the manufacturer to revise its claims of effectiveness or cautions associated with the drug's use.

In the case of controversial drugs, FDA approval or disapproval—which may take a year or longer after initial documentation has been submitted—will bring forth its critics. The sponsor and its supporters will likely argue that the FDA's demands for proof of safety and effectiveness are un-reasonably excessive. They result in inordinate delays that are keeping valuable drugs off the market and unavailable to treat countless of Americans who are needlessly suffering and dying. Drug safety groups, by contrast, will argue that the FDA has overlooked or minimized potentially dangerous side effects or weak evidence establishing effectiveness. They will argue for additional patient trials and might even claim that the FDA decision has been influenced by political considerations.

What kind of adverse effects—risks—are reasonable for a drug to be approved? There is no simple "one-size-fits-all" answer. The risks must be balanced against its benefits and the condition that is being treated.

Did You Know That ...?

In response to industrial, consumer, and political pressure, the Dietary Supplement Health and Education Act (DSHEA) was enacted by Congress in 1994. Dietary supplements were classified as foods and not medicines and are not subject to FDA requirements for drug approval.

Suppose the new drug is intended to treat a rather simple, non-life-threatening disorder, for which there are many good, safe drugs available. Few, if any serious side effects would be acceptable. But what if the disease is a grave one, with an ominous prognosis, and for which there are few reasonably effective, but not very safe, medicines? Here, any new drug, even one with weighty side effects, might be as good as existing drugs and may be even better.

Raising the Standards

Life was much easier for drug manufacturers some 100 years ago. If they wanted to claim that their medicine cured diabetes, heart disease, baldness, impotency, female problems, and consumption and was completely safe, they simply did so. Such claims were boldly proclaimed on the medicine bottle label or in their newspaper ads. No trials were conducted. Evidence supporting claims were based on testimonials provided by doctors or satisfied users.

How could our forebears have been so gullible to believe these outrageous claims? Until the late nineteenth century, scientists, doctors, and, of course, the general public had little understanding of what caused disease.

Good health was believed to depend on a balance among the different parts of the body. This balance was between the flow in of nutrients and flow out of excrements (feces, urine, menstrual flow, sweat). Consistent with this belief was the view that medicines were needed

Did You Know That ...?

During the early days, doctors used purging, puking, bloodletting, and blistering to reestablish balance in the body. From the nineteenth century until the early 1970s, cathartics were the most popular category of drugs found in patent medicines—drugs that reestablished the balance by cleaning the bowels.

to treat symptoms by reestablishing a healthy balance, not by correcting the underlying cause of those symptoms.

The authority of the FDA and laws enacted in response to drug disasters have evolved slowly to protect us against unsafe and ineffective medicines. They have progressed from:

◆ Prohibiting false statements (misbranding) (1906).

◆ Requiring proof of safety prior to their marketing (1938).

◆ Requiring proof of drug effectiveness (1962).

Post-Approval Evaluation

Phase 3 clinical trials are meticulously managed by the sponsor, usually the drug manufacturer. Potential subjects for drug trials are carefully selected (or excluded) based on predetermined criteria. The clinical investigators control the doses of the test drug taken, ensure that the drug is in fact taken and when it is taken, and know whether any other drugs are being used.

Did You Know That ...?

The FDA has no authority over how doctors practice medicine, including how they prescribe drugs. After a drug has been approved for a specified medical condition, doctors are legally able to prescribe it for any condition. It is estimated that 40 percent of all prescriptions are written for "off-label," non-FDA-approved uses.

By contrast, after the drug has been approved, all bets are off with respect to how, for what, and to whom the drug is prescribed. In this "real-world" environment, and only after the drug has been taken by tens or hundreds of thousands of patients, can the true benefits and actual risks of the medicine be assessed.

Warnings and Withdrawals

During phase 4, called post-marketing drug surveillance, the drug sponsor is required to provide the FDA with any reports of adverse drug reactions. Doctors and pharmacists may also do so, but on a voluntarily basis. Only some 10 percent of all reactions are ever reported. Depending on the nature or frequency of these adverse effects, and whether they outweigh the drug's potential benefits, the FDA can order the sponsor to increase the warnings contained in the prescribing information or demand removal of the drug from the market.

Serious adverse drug reactions may only be fully recognized years after a drug has been marketed. In the 25-year period between 1975 to 1999, 548 new drugs were approved and marketed. Of these, 16 were subsequently withdrawn from the market and 40 received a *black box warning*.

def•i•ni•tion

A **black box warning** sounds ominous—and it is. These represent the most serious warnings placed on prescribing information for prescription drugs. These warnings highlight special problems relating to drug safety, particularly those leading to deaths or serious injury. Recent examples include antidepressants promoting suicidal thoughts in adolescents and children and the strong abuse potential of OxyContin.

According to an article in the *Journal of American Medical Association*, K.E. Lesser and colleagues found that half of the 16 drugs withdrawn were pulled within the first 2 years. But only half of the serious adverse drug reactions were discovered within seven years after the drug had been marketed. The most common of these included liver, blood, and cardiovascular toxicity, and serious risks when used during pregnancy.

In recent years, a number of high-profile, widely used, and effective medications have been withdrawn from the market after causing fatalities. These include …

- Baycol, a cholesterol-lowering drug, which caused muscle toxicity.

- Bextra and Vioxx, painkillers for osteoarthritis, which caused increased risk of stroke and heart attack.

- Fen-Phen, an appetite suppressant, which caused heart and lung toxicity.

- Propulsid, a nighttime heartburn treatment, which caused abnormal heart rhythms.

- Rezulin, an anti-diabetic drug, which caused liver toxicity.

- Seldane, an antihistamine for allergies, which caused heart toxicity.

 Warning!

Although many people take great pride in wearing the latest fashions and owning the newest automobiles, being prescribed the newest drugs might not be wise or safe. Your doctor should probably avoid using the latest drugs when older, equally effective drugs are available. There is great wisdom in an old adage that advises doctors to be "neither the first to use a new drug nor the last to discard the old."

Why weren't these adverse effects detected during phase 3 clinical trials? To answer this question, we must look at the number of subjects participating in a clinical trial. If testing a common condition, such as osteoarthritis, high blood pressure, or insomnia, it is relatively easy to find plenty of subjects. However, finding a sufficient number of willing subjects for rare diseases that only affect a few thousand people a year can be a major problem.

The second issue relates to the incidence of side effects. If the phase 3 study involves 2,000 subjects, it is easy to detect an unusual side effect that occurs in 1 percent (or 20) of the subjects. But what if the side effect is rather rare and occurs in only 1 of every 5,000 subjects? It would be very unlikely to be seen in a trial of only 2,000 subjects. After the drug is approved and is used by hundreds of thousands of patients, the number of affected people will be greatly increased.

Selective Data Reporting

When doctors are trying to select the best medicines for their patients, they read reports of clinical trials that appear in distinguished journals. Published studies describing the effectiveness of a drug are also an important tool used for marketing purposes. These reports have long been assumed to be honestly and objectively written and to include both positive and negative results about the drug studied.

In 2004, a number of antidepressant-making drug companies were accused of selectively releasing information and publishing studies about their drugs that only showed their positive aspects. They concealed other results—those that failed to show their drugs to be better than placebos or that some antidepressants increased the incidence of suicidal thoughts of children and teenagers.

Did You Know That ...?

One of the basic principles of the scientific method is to look at all the results of a study and then draw conclusions based on an evaluation of the results. It's not appropriate (or ethical) for scientists to cherry-pick—that is, include only favorable results, while purposely discarding unfavorable or negative ones.

Similarly, it was uncovered in 2005 that companies hid other clinical trial results that indicated that their COX-2 inhibitor painkillers might increase the risk of stroke and heart attack.

Doctors and patients were appalled and furious. They argue that it is much more difficult for a company to hide the results of a clinical drug trial if it announces, in advance, that it is conducting such a study and are informed of what the study is trying to determine and how many patients are in the study. That way, if a study starts with 2,000 subjects, and the published results only account for 1,000, consumers will know to ask what happened to the others.

Not all clinical trials are conducted to assess drug safety. Many evaluate drug effectiveness for the treatment of conditions and often to compare their effectiveness with other drugs. Sales of prescription drugs require convincing doctors and the public that their medicine is better (i.e., safer and more effective) than competing drugs. Doctors and pharmacists are receiving increased instruction on how to better analyze and interpret the results of clinical trials to permit them to draw their own conclusions.

> **Maximizing Your Medicine**
>
> In 2005, the National Institutes of Health set up a user-friendly website, www.clinicaltrials.gov, that tracks many clinical studies. Some companies have been more forthcoming with information than others. You might want to log on to check what's new with any diseases or drugs you're tracking.

The Least You Need to Know

- ◆ The development of medicines that save lives and improve the quality of our lives is very expensive but can be very profitable.

- ◆ The FDA evaluates the results of animal (preclinical studies) and human (clinical) studies to determine the safety, effectiveness, and labeling prior to approving prescription and drugs for marketing.

- ◆ Phase 3 human studies use double-blind, placebo controls to evaluate the effectiveness of test drugs.

- ◆ Phase 4 studies (post-marketing surveillance) are intended to detect adverse effects after the drug is used in real-life conditions in large numbers of patients.

- ◆ The selective disclosure of information on marketed drugs has undermined the confidence of the medical community and public in the integrity of some pharmaceutical companies.

Chapter 5

The Patient–Health-Care Professional Partnership

In This Chapter

- ◆ Fielding your own health-care team
- ◆ Finding out about the prescription medicines you are taking
- ◆ Understanding the importance of following treatment instructions

In this chapter, we give you the tools you need to be an active participant in your health-care treatment. Part of being an active participant involves asking your doctor questions about the prescription medicines you are taking.

As a key member of the team, with the most at stake, you'll be expected to share some of the responsibility by following your doctor's instructions. We wrap up this chapter by talking about the potential health consequences if you don't.

You and Your Health-Care Team

To assist you in your efforts to regain or maintain good health, you need health-care professionals working with you as members of your team.

Your winning team has three members, each having a critical role: your doctor, your pharmacist, and you. It's up to you to select the team. Success is based on the premise that your doctor and pharmacist are working cooperatively with you to devise a treatment plan that effectively manages your medical condition. You must not only be confident that the prescribed medications will work but must also be willing and able to take them as intended.

Let's take a look at what you should expect of each team member.

Your Doctor

You may be seeing several doctors who are specialists and experts in a given organ or part of the body (e.g., heart, eyes) or in a medical condition (diabetes, cancer). Each doctor likely treats your condition without regard to your other health problems and without communicating with the other doctors you are seeing.

These individuals were selected based on their expertise and not necessarily their "warm and fuzzy" bedside manner or their ability to communicate with you.

It's essential, however, that you find a single doctor who is fully aware of all your health conditions and who receives progress reports from each of the specialists after your visits. This coordinating doctor is likely a general-practice doctor or one specializing in general medicine. This highly competent individual can translate and effectively communicate the specialists' reports to you.

You should feel comfortable talking to such a doctor, with whom you can share your inner feelings about your health. Moreover, this doctor is someone who can tell you as much, or as little, as you want to know about your condition.

Your Pharmacist

You may come to the pharmacy with multiple prescriptions, written by different doctors, each of whom is oblivious to all your other prescriptions. In some cases, one medicine may antagonize another. Perhaps more than one medicine is really the same drug or is doing the same thing. Making matters even worse, if these prescriptions have been filled at more than one pharmacy, these problems might go undetected until an actual concern arises.

You should select a single pharmacy, and better yet, a single pharmacist, to keep track of all your medications and any possible interactions between and among them. When you have a new prescription filled, your prescription medication history appears on the pharmacist's computer screen. These records might also contain information about your medical conditions.

Your pharmacist can use this information to work with your doctor to select the best medications that fit your needs. This pharmacist can also serve as your advocate with your insurance carrier, attempting to reconcile the medication prescribed with those on the carrier's list of approved drugs. The pharmacist also can recommend that your doctor prescribe a more affordable substitute for a high-price, brand-name product.

Most important, the pharmacist you select should have the time, interest, and ability to clearly explain to you how to most effectively use the drug. In addition, you should be made aware of the precautions associated with its use, common side effects, and tips on how they can be minimized. And you should expect answers to any other questions you may have about the drug.

You, the Patient

To become an effective team member, you must take active responsibility for your own health. If you don't take primary responsibility for your health, then who will? You need to be informed about your medical condition and the drugs you are taking. At the very least, you should be acquainted with some of the essentials.

When partnering with your doctor and pharmacist, you should be seeking information about your illnesses and the medications that are being considered for your use and that have been prescribed. This is particularly important for drugs that you will be taking for extended periods of time.

 Warning!

This book is intended to provide you with basic information about drugs used to treat a variety of medical conditions. As we talk about in detail in Chapter 6, facts about your specific medicines can be obtained from your health-care provider, prescription package inserts, and Internet websites. Make sure that the information you consult on the Internet website is factual and not an infomercial.

It's not essential that you get all the facts every time you get a new prescription. Realistically, no one can assimilate and process all this complex information in one sitting. And some facts are more pertinent for certain medicines than others.

Wherever you get your information, it needs to be communicated in clear and understandable language, using words and concepts that you understand. If your health-care professionals are using jargon, obtuse medical terminology, multisyllabic jaw-breaking drug names, or other words you don't know, ask what they mean or what they are talking about. There's no such thing as a dumb question. And don't be afraid to ask someone to repeat information if you've forgotten it or aren't sure you heard it correctly.

Maximizing Your Medicine

Ask your pharmacist for printed material, such as a prescription package insert or, better yet, specific material about the medication written in patient (consumer) language. These materials can be used to supplement what your doctor and pharmacist have told you, as well as remind you of important information while you are taking the drug.

You should at least know the brand and generic names of your medications, their strengths, how they are administered, why they are prescribed, what they will do, and what risks they pose.

It's often a good idea to be accompanied by a spouse or other family member, friend, or caregiver. They may get more or different perspectives on the information than you.

If your doctor or pharmacist doesn't have the time or patience to speak to you, find someone who does. During the time allocated for your visit, you are the most important patient the health-care provider has.

The Savvy Patient

Let's start by considering the facts every savvy patient should be aware of. This includes information about your condition and the medications you'll be taking.

Understanding Your Medical Condition

Before talking about medicines, you should know some basics about your medical condition.

A good place to start would be its name—both its common and its official name. Questions to ask include the following:

◆ What's the nature of this condition and what caused it?

◆ Was I born with it?

◆ Was it the result of a germ or my lifestyle? Or is it an inevitable consequence of aging? (On the bright side, think of the alternative to aging.)

Based on the nature of the medical condition and your age and health, you might want to hear the *prognosis*. By modifying lifestyle or by faithfully taking the prescribed medication, is it realistic to hope that the condition can be cured, improved, or stabilized, and get no worse? For other conditions, it is clear that the medication won't change the outcome. They can only ease pain and prevent suffering or slow the speed of decline. It's important that you know what to expect from your medication.

A menu of treatment options might be available for some conditions. These might include dietary restrictions, physical therapy, surgery, radiation therapy, medications, or watchful waiting. The options presented will be influenced by your condition and the type of doctor you're seeing. If your doctor only presents a single option, ask if other options exist. Find out about the advantages and disadvantages of each treatment option. If you don't feel comfortable with the proposed option, get a second opinion.

Warning!

How much information should you find out? That really depends on you. Some of us want to become "experts" on all aspects of our medical condition and the drugs we are taking. Others, frankly, would prefer not to know too much. That's your call, and your medical team needs to respect that decision.

def•i•ni•tion

Prognosis refers to a forecast of the patient's prospects for recovery or improvement and is based on the usual course of the disease and the patient's particular condition. Since it is only a very well-informed guess, it could be very accurate or far from the mark.

Ask questions, do your own research, and get answers! The reference librarian at your local community health library should be the first person you contact to get started.

Making Sense of Your Medications

From here on, we'll assume that drugs are a primary option to treat your medical condition.

The first thing you should do after your doctor prescribes a medication is get the trade name and generic name of the drug(s) being prescribed. Many drug names even sound the same to health-care professionals, so ask them to spell it for you.

Multiple drugs are usually available to treat a condition. Why then, did the doctor select this drug? Is it the "tried-and-true" long-established drug of choice, used by doctors nationwide? Maybe it's a just-introduced drug claimed (at least by its manufacturer) to be a major medical breakthrough?

Maximizing Your Medicine

Drugs are marketed by their trade name. The most actively marketed drugs are new ones that are only available as trade-name products, and for which there are no generic equivalent products. Such drugs are typically the most expensive. If you are paying for the medicine in whole or in part, make sure your doctor can justify prescribing the more expensive trade-name medication.

If a trade-name product has been selected, find out from your doctor or pharmacist whether there are any equally effective, but less expensive generic or nongeneric drug alternatives available. Perhaps there are less expensive, but effective, nonprescription (OTC) drugs.

Not all insurance plans cover all drugs. Have your health-care provider determine whether your plan will cover your new prescription. If not, perhaps an equivalent drug can be substituted. (For more money saving tips, see Chapter 6.)

Knowing What to Expect

Having decided on the drug, let's now turn our attention to finding out more about the drug, what kind of drug it is, and what it's supposed to do.

Some drugs are able to cure medical conditions; others can make you feel better by relieving the symptoms; whereas still others prevent the condition from getting worse. Find out how long you'll need to continue taking the drug—for 10 days until the infection is cured, for months until the condition has stabilized and gotten better, or for a lifetime to manage a chronic condition?

Before you start taking the medication, get an idea how long it will take before the drug begins to work, and how long before it produces it greatest benefits. You may control diarrhea after only one or two doses, but lifting your spirits in depression may require two to four weeks. If benefits are not seen within the approximate time indicated, maybe you need a different dose or another drug.

Within a class of drugs that appears to be very similar, some individual drugs may be more effective and cause fewer side effects for some people but not for others. We can't predict in advance. Trial and error may be needed to find the best one for you.

Some medical conditions, such as high cholesterol, don't exhibit any symptoms but nevertheless are still there. The drug may be working, but because you don't have any symptoms, you may not know it. Medical exams or lab tests may be needed to assess the drug's effectiveness.

Some drugs are initially effective but, when used for more extended periods of time, lose their effectiveness. This may occur when an infectious disease or cancer is treated over a period of months. If so, find out how you or your doctor will know when the medical plan needs a change.

Understanding All Precautions

A doctor's choice of drugs is sometimes influenced by other conditions, including the following:

- **Pregnancy.** Many doctors believe that to protect the developing baby, only truly essential drugs should be taken when pregnant. Some drugs can be used with caution during pregnancy, whereas others should not and must not be taken. If you are a sexually active woman of childbearing age, it is essential that you ask whether you can continue to take your medication if you become pregnant or if you plan to become pregnant. For some conditions, the drug can continue to be given, but its dosage must be adjusted.

- **Impairment of function.** Before taking the first dose, find out whether this medication might interfere with your ability to drive safely or operate potentially dangerous machinery. If possible, take your first dose at home. If it makes you feel ill, drowsy, or otherwise impairs you, you will be in a safe place.

- **Allergic reactions.** Tell your doctor and pharmacist if you've experienced any allergic reactions or other unusual responses to a drug you've taken in the past. This information should be included in your medical and medication record. Depending on the drug and the nature of this unfavorable response, it might be wise to avoid taking related drugs.

- **Alcohol.** A number of drugs increase the intoxicating and depressing effects of alcohol. Conversely, alcohol can antagonize or intensify the effects of other drugs. If you are a social drinker, find out whether it's safe to drink when taking a new medication.

- **Drug interactions.** If you go to the same pharmacy to fill all your prescriptions, they can readily tell you whether your new medication will interact with any others you are taking, and also whether there any drugs you should avoid taking or take only with caution. Don't limit your list to prescription drugs; also consider nonprescription drugs, dietary supplements and other natural drugs, and foods.

♦ **Addiction risk.** Individuals with a history of addiction to drugs or alcohol have a greater risk of becoming dependent on drugs that modify behavior. Examples include narcotics (opiates) used to relieve pain and drugs used to treat insomnia and relieve anxiety. Persons with such a history should find out whether such a risk exists for this drug.

Being Aware of Potential Side Effects

All drugs, to a greater or lesser extent, produce side effects. Although it's far too confusing and overwhelming to get a list of all of these, you should be aware of the most common ones. Some may persist for as long as you take the medication, whereas others become less or more troublesome over time. Your doctor or pharmacist might be able to provide you with some tips about how these side effects can be reduced.

Some side effects are troublesome and unpleasant. Others, while occurring less often, are potentially dangerous. Your doctor and pharmacist should warn you about these. If they appear, you should stop taking the drug and immediately contact your doctor. Such effects may be early signs of very severe problems.

Sometimes it's not safe to suddenly stop using your medication after it has been taken regularly for several weeks. If you do so, a sudden worsening of the condition or signs of drug withdrawal may occur.

Taking and Handling the Drug

Let's now think about the drugs and how they are used correctly. Remember, even if the best medicine is prescribed for your condition, it won't work as it should if you don't take the drug as was intended.

♦ **Tablet swallowing.** If you have difficulty swallowing tablets, ask your pharmacist or doctor whether the same drug is available as a liquid. Sometimes the tablet can be broken or mashed into smaller pieces and taken mixed in soft food, such as applesauce.

Do not assume that all tablets can be broken, crushed, or chewed. Many long-acting products won't release their drug properly if broken.

♦ **Medication schedules.** Some drug-taking schedules are virtually impossible to follow, no matter how hard you try. Too many different drugs are being taken at different times throughout the day, before meals, after meals, and at bedtime. This problem can be compounded if you have atypical work hours. Explain this to your health-care professional, and perhaps they can work with you to simplify your drug-taking schedule.

See whether your medicine needs to be taken in a special way or before, with, or after meals, with milk, water, or soda. When and how it is taken may have an effect on whether it upsets your stomach or alters its absorption into the blood. For some drugs, how and when it is taken makes a big difference.

◆ **Inhalers.** There are right (effective) ways of using inhalers and there are wrong (ineffective) ways. Work with your health-care provider to learn the right way before you begin to use it. This is particularly important if you're using an anti-asthma drug to stop an attack in progress.

◆ **Missed doses.** Find out what to do if you miss a dose. Should you double the next dose or skip the missed dose and go back to the regular dosing schedule at the usual time?

◆ **Drug storage.** Find out whether any liquid medicine needs to be shaken before a dose is measured out and whether the drug needs to be refrigerated before or after it has been opened.

◆ **Expiration dates.** Determine whether this drug will still work and remain safe to use after its expiration date. If it is effective after the expiration date, for how long after this date?

Taking the Next Step

Your doctor should have a backup plan in case his or her first choice of drug doesn't work as prescribed. Options include increasing the dose, adding another drug to the mix, or try an altogether new drug.

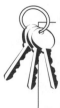

Did You Know That ...?

Who is the best source of all this information? It depends on what you're trying to find out. The doctor's specialty is disease and medical conditions, while the pharmacist concentrates on drugs. Sometimes it doesn't hurt to ask them both the same question. Ideally, you'll get the same answer. Often two explanations of the same facts, said somewhat differently, can make it more understandable.

Taking Your Medicine as Directed

Compliance, in the world of medicine, means taking your medicine and following the directions as you've been advised to do. In an ideal world, your doctor, pharmacist, and you are actively working together as a team to develop an effective medication plan that you can and will follow to the letter.

Sounds reasonable, doesn't it? Unfortunately, in most cases, the health-care provider prepares a plan without consulting the patient to see if it will work. The result, all too often, may be noncompliance.

Whether on purpose or by accident, noncompliance may lead to an unsuccessful treatment.

Maximizing Your Medicine

Many individuals on modest incomes must make very difficult choices on how to spend their limited funds. Sometimes, they decide that they can't afford all of their medicines. In Chapter 6, we grapple with some strategies for cost cutting on medications.

What might happen if you don't take your medication as prescribed? Lots of things. The condition might not be cured nor its symptoms relieved. Your condition may worsen. Hospitalization may be required, as may additional doctor visits and more diagnostic tests.

Although in most cases your recovery may be simply delayed because of noncompliance, in extreme cases your condition may worsen to the point where the damage cannot be reversed. In glaucoma, for example, failure to control eye pressure can lead to permanent blindness.

What Are Your Responsibilities?

Although many of us can and do take our drugs as directed, others need help. Maybe you can't keep track of the many drugs you need throughout the day. Maybe the problem is opening the medicine bottle or reading its label.

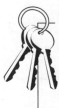

Did You Know That ...?

The elderly, individuals over 65, represent 12.4 percent of the population of the United States, yet they consume 34 percent of the total prescription drug expenses. They have some 20 prescriptions filled per year and account for a disproportionately large percentage of the total hospitalizations and deaths caused by adverse drug reactions.

If you are the patient or a caregiver, work with your health-care providers to over-come or minimize problems that may interfere with your successful use of the medications. The following strategies can help you deal with these issues:

♦ **Medication issues.** The size, shape, taste, or smell of a medication may discourage or prevent you from taking your medicines. Changing the dosage form from a solid to a liquid, breaking tablets into smaller pieces, mashing a tablet into a soft food, or masking the taste or smell might help.

Check with your pharmacist whether it's okay to break up your solid medication. In addition, your pharmacist can often be of great assistance in transforming the medication into a palatable form that can be more readily taken.

♦ **Side effects.** Side effects often discourage us from using drugs. Work with your doctor and pharmacist for ways to reduce them. If these side effects prove excessively troublesome, ask your pharmacist whether an alternative drug, without these effects, can be substituted.

♦ **Seeing and hearing.** If you have difficulty reading your prescription label, written instructions, or drug-related information, ask your pharmacist to use a larger size of print type. If you have a hearing loss, ask your pharmacist or doctor to speak louder or repeat the information; also ask them to provide all instructions in written form.

♦ **Medication containers.** Medications are routinely placed in childproof containers. This has significantly cut down on accidental medication poisoning by children under 5. But if you have problems opening such containers, ask your pharmacist to use nonchildproof or easy-to-open medication containers.

♦ **Memory aids.** A number of different memory aids are available that can help remind you to take your medication. These include reminder cards placed around the house, a visual or audible signal from the medication container, or a simple medication checklist on a calendar. Sometimes the services of a caregiver may be needed.

Maximizing Your Medicine

It is far more difficult to keep taking medication as directed when it's being used to treat a chronic illness for a lifetime, for preventive purposes, or for a condition that does not have any obvious symptoms. When the medication causes side effects, this further discourages people from taking their medicine. You may need periodic reminders of the health consequences of the condition, if untreated.

◆ **Medication plan.** When taking several drugs a day, it's easy to accidentally skip some of the doses. Work with your doctor and pharmacist to reduce the number of times you need to take your medications each day. If they are available, consider the use of long-acting, once-daily medications.

Warning!

When individuals live alone and are socially isolated, it's very common for them to become depressed. They often have little desire to care for themselves and are less likely to take medication. Family members or friends need to keep after them to ensure that they continue to take their drugs. Simply accepting their word that they have taken their drugs, in the absence of verification, may not suffice.

◆ **Health-care provider interactions.** Providers may fail to give adequate information or instructions. Some of these communication deficiencies may result from the harried provider trying to stay on schedule in the face of an increasing workload. Sometimes, hearing or cognitive problems may interfere with the capture and processing of information. A caregiver or family member should also attend these meetings to assist in getting the necessary information.

You may lack confidence in the provider's competence or concern for your well-being. If this is a valid concern, seek a new health-care provider.

Diagnosing your medical condition is only the first step in improving your health. A treatment plan must be developed, which may involve the use of a drug. We've talked about the fact that in order for that drug to help, the medicine should be taken as directed. You must actively participate, with your doctor and pharmacist, in devising a treatment plan that will work best for you.

The Least You Need to Know

◆ Doctors, pharmacists, and patients should work together to select medications and develop effective medication plans that promote patient compliance.

◆ Examples of medication noncompliance include failure to fill the prescription, failure to take the medication as prescribed, and prematurely stopping the medication.

◆ Noncompliance can have various negative health consequences and may even require stronger, potentially more dangerous drugs.

◆ When dealing with a health-care provider, you should seek basic information regarding the medical condition; the choice of medications; what medication benefits can be expected; how to handle and take the drug; precautions associated with its use; and common side effects.

Chapter 6

Medication Information Sources and Money Savers

In This Chapter

◆ Finding reliable information about your prescription medicines

◆ Locating reasonably priced, reliable sources for your drugs

◆ Taking a hard look at online pharmacies

◆ Saving money on your prescriptions

There's no shortage of information about drugs. Most of it appears on TV and in the print media. Some of this information is newsworthy, others are slick ads. If you're looking for more depth and objective information, this chapter gives you some places to start looking.

We also talk about where you can buy your prescription medicines. There are a number of sources out there, some emphasizing service and convenience, others sacrificing service for savings. As they say on TV, "It's your money, your choice."

Finally, if you or a family member is eligible for the Medicare Part D Prescription Drug Program, you're probably pretty confused. You've got a lot of company. We try to make some sense of a bewilderingly complex program.

Where to Go for Drug Info

Suppose you have a medical condition that is treated with a medication. You very wisely consult this book for an overview of the condition and the kinds of medications that are used to treat it. This information has whetted your appetite for more detailed materials. Where should you go from here?

Before checking one or more of the various sources, here are some things to think about:

♦ **Level of technical detail.** Most of the prescription drug information found in textbooks and scientific journals is intended for highly trained health-care professionals and are filled with technical jargon and concepts. Unless you're prepared to wade through a lot of difficult material, you'll likely want something written specifically for the lay consumer.

♦ **Accuracy and objectivity.** Most of the information found in textbooks and journals has been reviewed by a third party for, among other things, accuracy and objectivity. Such checks are sometimes absent in consumer materials. Here, the author or source is not providing general drug information but rather trying to sell a concept or, more often, a product or service. Try to discover the identity of the source, and where the source gets the information. Is a balanced viewpoint presented or does it just extol the virtues of the product or service?

♦ **Learning styles.** How do you prefer getting your information? By reading, talking directly to an expert, navigating from website to website, or some combination of these sources?

♦ **Ease of getting information.** The mass media is easy to get your hands on. You can subscribe to magazines that focus on medicines and health topics of interest to you without ever having to leave your home. Your pharmacist is readily available down the street. Some good, more detailed sources will require a trip to your local public library or to a more distant medical or pharmacy school library.

Let's now consider the various sources of information about medicines and their advantages and limitations.

Books and Review Articles

Books and articles written for health-care professionals generally contain and reflect the mainstream thinking on a medical condition or medicine. The information may be based on Food and Drug Administration–approved statements and should be balanced and objective.

Some books are more general, whereas others focus on a particular medical condition, and to a lesser extent, the drugs used to manage that condition. Several comprehensive prescription medicine-oriented books include the *American Hospital Formulary Service*, *Drug Facts and Comparisons*, *Goodman and Gilman's Pharmacological Basis of Therapeutics*, *Martindale: The Complete Drug Reference*, and *Physician's Desk Reference*.

These sources are highly technical in nature and may be quite difficult to wade through. They are strong on information and short on readability and an engaging writing style.

The most up-to-date information on drugs appears in research articles and case reports in journals such as the *Journal of the American Medical Association* and the *New England Journal of Medicine*. Excellent and authoritative reviews on medicines appear in *The Medical Letter on Drugs and Therapeutics*.

A few of these sources may be found in well-stocked public libraries, and all should be on the shelves (usually the reserved shelves) of community health libraries, affiliated with hospitals, or a medical school or pharmacy school library. Ask the reference librarian for help locating topic-specific review articles in journals.

A number of consumer-focused general medical reference books are available in print, on compact discs, or online through the Internet. Many of these clearly written and information-packed books might make valuable additions to your home library.

Consumer-oriented books and magazine articles commonly focus on a medical condition and the drugs used to treat it. Many have a strong viewpoint on its management, not infrequently advocating an alternative treatment approach. Because there's no guarantee that these books are reviewed by unbiased individuals, always carefully check the credentials of the author. Look for balance in their discussion of the treatments.

Clearly and objectively written articles about drugs used to treat various medical conditions appear in the *Consumer Reports Best Buy Drugs* series. In addition, *AARP The Magazine* often publishes articles on drugs and how to pay for them.

TV and Print Media

When we talk about TV and print media, it is important to distinguish between news pieces and direct-to-consumer ads and other infomercials.

News pieces present the most up-to-date information and feature the latest dramatic breakthroughs. They are typically based on the results found in a relatively small number of subjects and, very often, not subject to the scrutiny of outside reviewers. Initial optimism and hope run high, but later studies may sometimes fail to substantiate the early, highly enthusiastic findings.

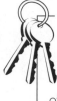

Did You Know That ...?

In a recent provocative article in the *Journal of the American Medical Association*, J. P. A. Ioannidis found that the results of one third of all highly cited clinical research articles were either contradicted or substantially weakened in later, more comprehensive studies.

Direct-to-consumer (DTC) ads on TV and in the print media are purportedly intended to make consumers aware of medical conditions and the new prescription medicines that are available to treat these conditions.

Plain and simple, they are commercials intended to get you to persuade your physician to write prescriptions for these often quite expensive brand-name medications. Have these ads been effective in selling the drugs? Absolutely! Consumers, of course, are footing the bill for these ads, which costs $4 billion each year. Are there equally effective, less-expensive, alternative brand-name or generic equivalents? Often yes.

These TV ads usually over-emphasize or glamorize the positive aspects of the medications. Side effects or cautionary material is too often concealed in miniscule print or in voiceovers presented at three times faster than normal speech in a soothing voice.

Websites

The Internet is a seemingly endless resource for information on prescription drugs, but because anyone can publish anything on the Web, it's easy to overlook the fact that these sites may be providing misleading or even downright inaccurate information.

Did You Know That ...?

Two of the most comprehensive and objective medical information sources are the National Library of Medicine's MEDLINE-Plus (www.medlineplus.gov) and the U.S. Department of Health and Human Services' Healthfinder (www.healthfinder.gov).

If you get started by putting a key word(s) into a search engine such as Google or Yahoo!, you'll likely get many hits. Now your challenge is to try to assess the reliability of the website of interest. Here are a few points you should think about.

Whose site is it and why are they paying to run it? Check the end of the web address. If it ends with ...

- ◆ **gov,** then it's a federal government-sponsored group.

- ◆ **edu,** then it's an educational institution

◆ **org,** it's a noncommercial organization such as scientific or health professional group (e.g., familydoctor.org) or a nonprofit organization focused on a particular medical condition (cancer.org).

◆ **com,** then it is commercial organization, such as a pharmaceutical company or hospital. Although such sites may provide excellent and highly reliable information, their primary aim is usually to sell a product or a service.

Information about the sponsor of the site and its purpose may be found on the site's "About This Site" link. A noncommercial site may provide information obtained from a commercial source or might be receiving sponsorship from such a source. If so, this should be noted.

The information presented should be based on fact and documented by references in the professional literature or by links to reliable and objective websites. Is an author with professional qualifications identified or is a "satisfied customer" the source of the information? Be particularly skeptical of claims touting an "amazing breakthrough" or a "secret ingredient" that "cures" an otherwise fatal disease.

In addition, all drug-related information should be current and updated on a regular basis. The date of the latest review of the material should be posted.

Health-Care Providers

The simplest, least complicated and, for many, most immediate source of medication information is your doctor or pharmacist. You simply pick up your phone or pay them a visit.

These professionals know you and have access to your health and medication records. The answers to your questions will be tailored to your health and personal needs.

Although they should be able to answer common questions right away, health-care doctors and pharmacists are not encyclopedic drug information services and might not be able to answer all of your questions on the spot. However, they should be willing to get you the answers you need in a timely fashion. Other sources include the pharmaceutical manufacturer and the Food and Drug Administration (www.fda.gov or 1-888-463-6332).

Where to Buy Your Drugs

Prescription drugs can be purchased at three types of retail outlets: a retail pharmacy, a mail-order pharmacy, or an Internet pharmacy. Let's look at each and, based on your needs and preferences, decide which is best for you.

Retail Pharmacies

Retail pharmacies need no introduction. There is at least one in almost every town. In some communities, two or three occupy a single intersection.

For all but the most homebound individuals, your retail pharmacy is the most convenient site to have your prescriptions filled, and filled while you wait. Any problems with your medication can be resolved on the spot, in consultation with your pharmacist, who will also provide you with verbal and written information on your prescriptions.

Mail-Order Pharmacies

Unlike retail pharmacies, mail-order pharmacies are primarily involved with dispensing prescriptions. Their interactions with you are never live, only via the phone. They are either associated with "bricks-and-mortar" chains or health plans.

Warning!

If you're getting your prescriptions filled at both a retail pharmacy and a mail-order site not associated with the same retail pharmacy, the medication record sets at both will be incomplete. Pharmacists will be unable to detect drug-related problems arising from medications obtained from the other pharmacy.

Your prescription is delivered to your mailbox, usually within 14 days after ordering it. Clearly, this delivery time lapse, which may be longer during vacation periods, is not suitable when you need your drugs immediately. Rather, it is primarily intended to supply long-term maintenance medication needs and refills. It is particularly convenient if you are homebound or live far away from a retail pharmacy.

Many insurance plans encourage your use of mail-order pharmacies. As incentives, they might lower your co-pay fee and extend to 90 days, from 30 days, the supply of medication you can get at one time with a co-pay.

Internet Pharmacies

Internet pharmacies are the most variable source of medication. The quality of their products and services range from excellent to deplorable. Some are owned and operated by pharmacy chains located in the United States and Canada, whereas others are operated by individuals located at sites and in countries determined only with great difficulty.

Purchase of drugs from Internet sources appeals to worldwide buyers and to homebound individuals who find it difficult to travel to a pharmacy. They offer 24-hour shopping and privacy in purchasing medications.

There are a number of very highly reputable Internet drug providers, many of which are located in the United States and Canada. The National Association of Boards of Pharmacy, working with state and provincial boards of pharmacy, grants a Verified Internet Pharmacy Practice Sites (VIPPS) seal to those Internet pharmacies that meet the standards of the state (in the United States) or province (in Canada) in which they dispense medications. Such sites post a U.S. or Canadian address and phone number, and a pharmacist is available to answer your questions.

Maximizing Your Medicine

Pharmacists and pharmacies are licensed by boards of pharmacy in individual states and provinces. The National Association of Boards of Pharmacy (NABP) has pharmacy board members in the 50 states and the 8 provinces of Canada. If you're going to purchase medications from Internet pharmacies, only buy from those that have a VIPPS seal on their website.

Before your prescription order can be processed by a VIPPS site, you'll need a valid doctor's prescription, which must be verified by a doctor working for the Internet pharmacy.

Some other non-VIPPS Internet sites are used by buyers seeking "bargains" or to obtain potent drugs without a prescription for nonmedical purposes. Drugs can generally be purchased by completing a superficial health questionnaire and without seeing a doctor.

You may encounter several problems when obtaining drugs from non-VIPPS Internet sources: the drugs may be counterfeit, outdated, or may not contain the ingredients or strengths specified on the label. Sometimes the drug container has no label or identifying information. There is no indication in what part of the world the medications were made. In some cases, the drugs are found to be contaminated with harmful substances or arrive broken.

Drug orders have been placed, paid for, but not received. Because you don't know where your medicines are coming from, you have no recourse in dealing with your non-VIPPS Internet medicine provider.

Money-Saving Tips

No matter where you get your prescription drugs, they are going to put a dent in your budget. In this section, we talk about some of the different approaches you might consider when trying to trim your prescription medicine expenses. These include the use of generic equivalent products, pharmaceutical manufacturer discount drug cards and other assistance programs, the Medicare Part D Prescription Drug Program, and tablet splitting.

Generic vs. Trade-Name Drugs

Throughout this book, we talked about the cost savings associated with the use of generic product equivalents. Brand names and their generic product equivalents are equally safe, effective, pure, and stable. Often, generics are manufactured by brand-name pharmaceutical companies. The major difference for you: generic products may cost from 30 to 80 percent less than their brand-name counterpart.

Did You Know That ...?

According to information provided by the National Association of Chain Drug Stores, in 2004, the average price of a brand-name prescription drug was $96.01, whereas the average price of a generic prescription drug was $28.74—a difference of 70 percent!

Maximizing Your Medicine

AARP found that over the 12-month period ending March 2005, the price of 195 brand-name drugs most commonly used by elderly Americans increased in price an average of 6.6 percent. By contrast, 75 of the most commonly used generic drugs increased, on average, only 0.7 percent. The inflation rate during the same period, measured by the Consumer Price Index (CPI), increased 3 percent.

Newly introduced drugs enjoy patent protection and market exclusivity, and are only available by brand name. This generally translates into a higher price. Being new doesn't necessarily mean safer or more effective for you. Older products, available as generics, may be just as good.

Don't assume that brand-name drugs are always more expensive. Consider the results of a 2005 *Consumer Reports* price analysis comparing U.S. and Canadian Internet pharmacies. The five best-selling brand-name drugs were much less expensive from Canadian sources.

By contrast, the prices of the five most frequently dispensed generic drugs were considerably less from the American Internets when compared with Canadian sources. These lower prices result from the vigorous competition among generic drug sources in the United States.

There is a take-home lesson from these and similar studies. For the same drug, the least expensive are American-source generics, followed by Canadian generics, and then Canadian-source brand-name products and, most expensive, American brand-name drugs.

Drug Samples and Discount Drug Cards

Pharmaceutical companies give free drug samples to doctors for use by their patients. These samples are intended to allow the patient to try out the medication and determine its effectiveness and side effects. The obvious hope is that patients will get started on these more expensive drugs and continue to use them.

Many doctors give these same samples to patients who would otherwise find it difficult, if not impossible, to purchase them on their own. Don't be shy about asking your doctor if they have such free samples for you. Free samples, however, can't be counted on if you're going to use the drug over an extended period of time.

Maximizing Your Medicine

The Partnership for Prescription Assistance (PPA) coordinates the distribution of free medications to eligible persons, based on their age, income, and other government assistance. PPA provides a single access point to more than 275 public and private programs, including 150 drug-sponsored programs, and links to Medicare and other government programs. Contact PPA by phone at (1-888-477-2669) or www.pparx.org.

A number of pharmaceutical companies provide discount drug cards to consumers to enable them to get their prescription medicines (made by that manufacturer) at discounts ranging from 15 to 40 percent.

The eligibility requirements for these discount cards varies among companies. They are generally intended for individuals who do not have health insurance or who don't qualify for government assistance programs. Some of these programs and the Medicare Prescription Drug Discount Card will disappear by 2006 when the Medicare Part D Prescription Drug Program begins. Check with your pharmacist about such programs.

Medicare Part D Prescription Drug Program

Medicare is a government health insurance program covering individuals over 65 and the disabled. In January 2006, the Medicare program was expanded to include, for the first time, a prescription drug benefit.

The program is voluntary and available from and administered by private health insurers. In theory, the insurers will be able to negotiate lower prices from pharmaceutical manufacturers, which are supposed to result in lower prices for both you and the taxpayers. (Many outside observers believe that the major beneficiaries of the program will be the private health insurers and the pharmaceutical manufacturers.)

So far this program has been confusing even to the "well informed." At its simplest level, there is a minimum "standard benefit" (based on 2006 dollars) that must be included in all private plans:

◆ You pay an annual out-of-pocket deductible of $250 for your prescription medications.

◆ To participate, you pay monthly premiums, which average about $32. (This amount may be higher or lower depending on the private plan you select and the region of the country in which you reside).

◆ You must pay a 25 percent co-pay for your prescription expenses up to $2,250 (or about $552 for the first $2,250 in drug bills). The insurer pays the balance.

◆ After you have incurred $3,600 in out-of-pocket expenses or a total of $5,100 in total prescription expenses (including your monthly premiums), the insurer pays 95 percent of your remaining annual drug costs. You pay either a 5 percent co-pay or $2 for a generic drug and $5 for any other drug, whichever is higher.

Note that there is no program coverage between $2,251 and $3,600 out of pocket expenses, the so-called "doughnut hole." You are responsible for 100 percent of the drug expenses in this gap.

Maximizing Your Medicine

Individual plans may choose to cover some drugs, but not others. Plans must include at least one drug for each disease category. But are these drugs the ones that you are using?

For you, the most important consideration may be the drugs that are covered in a given plan. However, the list of covered drugs may change at any time during the year, although you can only change plans once a year.

That's the basics. But differences among the various plans are many, including the following:

◆ Annual deductibles that may range from $0 to $250.

◆ Lower co-pays and coverage of the normally excluded gap.

◆ Monthly premium range $2 up to $80. As with all other insurance plans, this amount depends on the coverage you select.

◆ Whether your local pharmacy will be participating in that specific plan or will you be obligated to use a mail-order pharmacy.

◆ Whether the plan covers the drugs you are using.

Part D prescription benefits are very generous for low-income beneficiaries. These are defined as persons having an annual income of less than $6,000 (in 2006) for an individual or less than $9,000 for a couple. Such beneficiaries would receive full low-income subsidies and pay no monthly premiums or deductibles nor be subject to the gap in coverage. Individuals and couples with annual incomes of less than $10,000 and $20,000, respectively, are eligible for partial low-income subsidies.

> **Maximizing Your Medicine**
>
> Medicare-eligible individuals with high drug expenses will benefit significantly from this program, but will it help you? For expert, more comprehensive, and personalized information, you should contact the Centers for Medicare and Medicaid Services at www.medicare.gov or call toll-free 1-800-633-4227.

Tablet Splitting

Very often, there are relatively little differences in price between different strengths of the same medication. In some cases, the prices may be exactly the same. Suppose you take a 10 mg tablet of a medication, and it comes from the same manufacturer in both 10 mg and 20 mg tablet strengths. If your doctor gave you a prescription for 20 mg tablets, and you split them in half, you could potentially save a bundle—on average 23 to 50 percent per tablet.

For obvious reasons, your insurance company thinks it's a great idea, and they encourage you to split tablets. Some health-care professionals are less enthusiastic. Before you run out to buy a *tablet-splitter*, let's talk about this a little more.

> **def•i•ni•tion**
>
> A **tablet-splitter** (a.k.a. tablet-cutter) is a device that can hold the tablet in place while a steel blade can be lowered to cut the tablet into two pieces that are (ideally) the same size.

If the tablet is scored (i.e., it has a groove down the center), it's suitable for and intended to be split. However, not all tablets should be split. For instance, extended-release drugs should never be split. Their effectiveness as long-acting products may be reduced. Other tablets are coated to protect your stomach or mouth from upset or irritation or to mask a very unpleasant drug taste.

If the tablet is not accurately split in half, neither of the two pieces will have the same amount of medicine. One piece will be too low in dosage, the other too high. Depending on the medication, small differences may or may not be significant.

If the idea of tablet splitting appeals to you, first speak to your doctor and pharmacist as to whether it is appropriate for one or more of your medications and take the time to calculate your anticipated cost savings. Tablet-splitters are relatively easy to use, even with many unscored tablets, and can be purchased at your pharmacy for around $10 or less.

The Least You Need to Know

♦ Depending on your learning style and personal preferences, sources of prescription medication information include books, Internet websites, and your health-care professionals.

♦ Before relying on Internet websites, check on their sponsorship (i.e., who's paying their bills), and whether the information they provide is factual and current.

♦ Depending on your preferences and those imposed by your insurer, medications can be obtained from retail, mail-order, and Internet pharmacies.

♦ Before ordering your prescription medicines from an Internet pharmacy, make sure that their website displays a VIPPS seal.

♦ Cost savings averaging 30 to 80 percent can be achieved by using generic product equivalents of trade-name medications.

♦ Comparing Canadian and American Internet pharmacies, trade-name products, on average, cost less from Canadian sources, whereas generic products, on average, are more expensive in Canada.

♦ The voluntary Medicare Part D Prescription Drug Program, effective in January 2006, has the potential to save considerable amounts for Medicare-eligible beneficiaries with high drug expenses.

Part 2

Directory of Medical Conditions and Their Drug Treatment

Part 1 gave you a good, general understanding about drugs. Now, you're ready to get more specific.

Part 2 deals with many common medical conditions and the important classes of drugs used to treat them. These medical conditions are arranged alphabetically or can be readily found in the very comprehensive index at the book's end. Since each of these conditions is independent and self-contained, you can read them in any order you want to. Go to it!

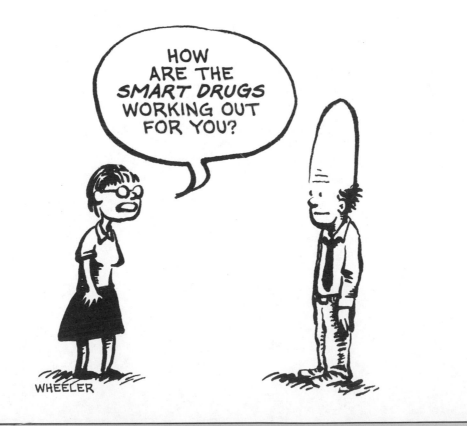

Acne

Acne afflicts 80 percent of us from the years of puberty to our mid-20s, when it usually disappears. It is a chronic skin disorder in which blackheads, pimples, or cysts may appear on the face, neck, shoulders, chest, and back.

At puberty, boys and girls experience increased secretion of the male hormone testosterone. Testosterone stimulates the flow of oils from the sebaceous glands, through pores, up to the surface of the skin. If these pores become blocked, the normally present bacterium aggressively multiply, causing inflammation and infection, which we recognize as a pimple.

Anti-Acne Drugs: An Overview

The first choice for acne treatment is benzoyl peroxide, an OTC drug applied to the skin. If this drug fails, a prescription drug will be required.

The two major groups of prescription anti-acne medicines are the antibiotics and the vitamin A–like drugs.

Antibiotics: Bacteria Killers

It is always preferable to direct drugs to their intended targets rather than let them wander freely about the body where they can cause undesirable effects. That is why the preferred treatment of acne is to apply antibiotics directly to the skin. The most commonly used prescription topical antibiotics are clindamycin and erythromycin, which are often used in combination with benzoyl peroxide.

Oral antibiotics of the tetracycline and erythromycin families are reserved for severe cases of acne. These drugs, given over periods of months and even years, suppress the growth of bad bacteria and prevent acne from reappearing.

Each antibiotic produces its own side effects and precautions. For example, erythromycin upsets the stomach; tetracycline and doxycycline increase the sensitivity of the skin to sunburn; in addition, tetracycline cannot be taken by pregnant women because it may discolor the teeth of their newborns, nor should it be taken with meals.

OTC Alternatives

Benzoyl peroxide is the most effective and widely used OTC drug for the treatment of acne. It is sold under a number of trade names (e.g., Clean & Clear, Clearasil, Oxy Balance) and is available for application to the skin in lotions, gels, creams, and soaps. In addition to killing bacteria, it also unplugs pores and increases peeling. People with sensitive skin may experience burning, blistering, or swelling. If so, try the lower concentrations or use less often.

Vitamin A–Like Drugs: Unclog Pores

Tretinoin and a group of newer derivatives of vitamin A (called retinoids) unclog pores when they are applied to the skin. For the first few weeks of tretinoin use, the skin becomes irritated, making it look worse than ever. Be patient. Thereafter, the acne begins to improve, and dark spots, caused by old acne, may also begin to lighten.

Most vitamin A–like products increase the sensitivity of the skin to sunburn. Users are warned to wear protective clothing and also apply a sunscreen with a SPF (sun protection factor) of 15 or greater.

As a last option, the vitamin A–like medicine isotretinoin (Accutane) (never to be confused with tretinoin) is used to treat—and often cure—very severe cases of acne. It is taken by mouth for periods of 15 to 20 weeks. Before using isotretinoin the patient should carefully consider its risks and discuss them with a doctor. Although all drug use involves weighing benefits versus risks, it is of particular importance for this drug.

 Did You Know That ...?

Tretinoin is also used to reduce fine wrinkles, roughness, liver spots, and age spots on the face. Prior to running out and buying this prescription cream (sold as Renova), you should note that it does not correct deep wrinkles, repair skin damaged by the sun, or restore the structure of the skin to its former, more youthful appearance.

Potential benefits come at a high price, because isotretinoin produces a high incidence of side effects, some quite serious. These include dryness of the skin, nose, and mouth; nosebleeds; and pain, tenderness, or stiffness of muscles, bones, and joints. Its use has been linked to depression.

Blood levels of fat (triglycerides) and cholesterol should be checked periodically as these can be raised by isotretinoin.

Isotretinoin must never be used during pregnancy.

Warning!

Women who are pregnant, or who may become pregnant, must never use isotretinoin. Use by pregnant women, for even short periods of time, carries an extremely high risk of causing multiple defects to the developing fetus.

Before taking this drug, tests are performed to make absolutely sure the woman is not pregnant. The woman must adopt a reliable method of contraception from the period one month before starting use through one month after drug therapy stops.

The Least You Need to Know

◆ Drug treatment of acne is determined by its severity.

◆ Mild cases are treated by applying benzoyl peroxide (an OTC drug), antibacterial antibiotics, or vitamin A–like drugs (as tretinoin) to the skin, which unplug pores.

◆ Users of topical vitamin A–like drugs must protect themselves against increased sensitivity to sun by wearing protective clothing and using sunscreens.

◆ For severe cases, antibiotics are taken by mouth for months or years.

◆ For the most severe cases, isotretinoin is highly effective, but its use may cause major side effects and, if taken during pregnancy, birth defects may occur in the fetus.

Drugs Used to Treat Acne

Generic Name	Trade Name(s)	How Taken	Generic Available
Antibiotics			
Azithromycin	Zithromax	Mouth	Yes
Clindamycin	Cleocin	Skin	Yes
Clindamycin	BenzaClin	Skin	Yes
Doxycycline	Vibramycin, Vibra-Tabs	Mouth	Yes
Erythromycin	Emgel, Eryderm	Skin	Yes

continues

Drugs Used to Treat Acne   (continued)

Generic Name	Trade Name(s)	How Taken	Generic Available
Erythromycin + benzoyl peroxide	Benzamycin	Skin	Yes
Minocycline	Minocin	Mouth	Yes
Tetracycline	Achromycin V, Sumycin	Mouth	Yes
Vitamin A–Like Drugs			
Acitretin	Soriatane	Mouth	No
Adapalene	Differin	Skin	No
Isotretinoin	Accutane	Mouth	No
Tazarotene	Tazorac	Skin	No
Tretinoin	Avita Retin-A	Skin	Yes

AIDS/HIV

Acquired immunodeficiency syndrome (AIDS) is a viral infection caused by the human immunodeficiency virus (HIV). The virus kills protective cells of the human immune defense system. In the absence of treatment, the patient becomes vulnerable and falls prey to potentially fatal cancer and infections caused by bacteria, fungi, and other viruses. With the appearance of at least one of these infections, the individual is given the diagnosis AIDS.

Did You Know That ...?

There are two types of HIV (human immunodeficiency virus): HIV-1 and HIV-2. HIV-1 is found worldwide, including North America and western Europe. HIV-2 is present mainly in western Africa. In this chapter, when we use the term HIV, we are referring to both types.

In the United States, some 850,000 to 950,000 people have HIV, with an additional 40,000 people being diagnosed each year. Worldwide, 35 to 45 million people are infected, with 60 to 70 percent of those people living in sub-Saharan Africa. It is the fourth leading cause of death in the world.

HIV symptoms are diverse. There is often weight loss, feelings of fatigue, fever, diarrhea, and swollen lymph nodes. Fungal infections of the mouth appear as normal defense mechanisms fail.

In the absence of effective anti-HIV drug treatment, the health of the AIDS patient generally deteriorates rapidly, with a fatal outcome within two years. Available drugs do not cure the disease but can bring it under control and permit the patient to resume a reasonable quality of life.

HIV Transmission

Spreading the HIV virus requires the exchange of infected body fluids such as blood, semen, vaginal secretions, and breast milk. In North America, Europe, and Australia, the HIV virus is primarily transferred by male homosexual intercourse and illicit drug use by abusers sharing infected needles that contain any amount of tainted blood. Heterosexual intercourse has become an increasingly important mode of transmission as well and is the primary mode of spreading the virus in Africa, Asia, and the Caribbean.

HIV transmission occurs in one of three ways:

- ◆ **Sexual activity.** Such as vaginal or anal intercourse.

- ◆ **Exposure to contaminated blood.** Drug abusers using contaminated needles or, far less commonly, in blood products.

- ◆ **Perinatal infection.** Newborns become infected during delivery or by ingesting HIV-contaminated breast milk.

HIV Reproduction

As is the case with all other viruses, HIV lacks the enzymes and other metabolic machinery needed to multiply (replicate). Viruses live and replicate by usurping the metabolic machinery found in living cells. In the process, the virus kills the cells it infects.

HIV's target in humans is the CD4-receptor on T lymphocytes (also called CD4 T cells), a kind of white blood cell. The T cell is a major player in the body's immune defense system and has a critical role in protecting us from foreign invaders.

Let's briefly talk about the HIV life cycle to understand how drugs work.

HIV Life Cycle

After entering the body, the HIV virus binds to the CD4 receptor located on the surface of a T lymphocyte cell. To reproduce, the virus assumes control of the metabolic processes of the cell. The HIV first inserts its RNA—its genetic code—into the cell. (Some anti-HIV drugs can prevent the virus from entering the lymphocyte cell.)

Viral RNA is then converted to DNA, which enters the cell's nucleus. In this form, the virus is able to reproduce itself. The enzyme reverse transcriptase is essential for the formation of DNA. (Reverse transcriptase inhibitors, such as zidovudine [AZT], inhibit this enzyme.)

Did You Know That ...?

Viruses consist of DNA or RNA (genetic information) wrapped in a protein coat. HIV enters the cell as RNA. It makes a copy of DNA, which enters the cell's nucleus and directs viral replication. It acts backward (a.k.a. "retro") to that of normal human cell reproduction. Hence, it is called a retrovirus, and anti-HIV drugs are antiretroviral.

The new virus buds off from the cell. It undergoes chemical changes that transform it into a mature and infectious HIV virus. (This transformation requires protease, an enzyme blocked by protease inhibitors, such as saquinavir.)

As the virus takes over and then kills lymphocytes, the immune system becomes ineffective. The HIV-infected person is defenseless to combat infections that in healthy individuals are not a problem. Two such conditions, among many others, are a fungal infection of the lungs (Pneumocystis carinii pneumonia) and a cancer of the skin and mouth (Kaposi's sarcoma).

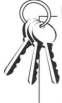

Did You Know That ...?

In healthy individuals, CD4 T cell counts number 800 to 1,300 cells per microliter. When the cell count falls below 200 per microliter, the HIV-infected person cannot combat common infections caused by bacteria, fungi, and other viruses and certain cancers. When at least one such infection develops or T cells are less than 200, the diagnosis of AIDS is rendered.

Anti-HIV Drugs: An Overview

AIDS treatment typically involves the simultaneous use of three or four drugs drawn from several anti-HIV drug classes. Combinations are given to aggressively prevent virus reproduction and reduce the risk of developing drug-resistant viral strains.

Prior to the availability of these drugs, the health of HIV-infected patients deteriorated rapidly, often with a fatal outcome. Available medicines don't cure HIV infections, but they can keep the infection in check.

Drugs have transformed AIDS from a debilitating and often fatal disease to a chronic but stable condition in which the patient is able to live many years and maintain a productive quality of life.

Many significant challenges remain in the successful treatment of HIV infections, including the following:

♦ Drug dosing is highly complicated and difficult to follow because multiple anti-HIV drugs must be taken many times throughout the day. Additional drugs may be required to treat other infections that have developed in the susceptible patient.

♦ Anti-HIV drugs cause major adverse side effects and toxicity and interact with many other drugs. The patient should tell their doctor and pharmacist about any other drugs they are taking.

◆ These drugs are very expensive, often prohibitively so.

◆ Patients must remain highly motivated. If they discontinue taking their anti-HIV medicines or fail to take their medicine as directed for a lifetime, viral resistance develops, virus levels increase, and disease symptoms recur.

Based on how they work, there are three major classes of anti-HIV medicines: reverse transcriptase inhibitors, protease inhibitors, and entry blockers.

Reverse Transcriptase Inhibitors

Reverse transcriptase inhibitors such as AZT prevent the conversion of viral RNA to DNA.

There are two types of reverse transcriptase inhibitors—NRTIs and NNRTIs—and several may be taken at once.

Side effects vary considerably among NRTIs but often include liver toxicity, nausea, vomiting, abdominal pain, diarrhea, and skin rashes.

With NNRTIs, skin rashes are rare, but potentially fatal; other side effects include headaches and behavioral disturbances. Many drug-drug interactions can occur.

Protease Inhibitors

Protease inhibitors such as saquinavir prevent the immature newly formed virus from maturing and becoming infective. These very powerful drugs are an integral component of AIDS treatment and are routinely combined with NRTIs or NNRTIs.

Note the ending "navir" in their generic names.

All protease inhibitors cause nausea, vomiting, diarrhea, and increases in blood levels of cholesterol and glucose (a problem for diabetics). With long-term use, fat may be redistributed to the abdominal area, breasts, and back of the neck.

These medicines interact with many drugs, interfering with their effects.

Maximizing Your Medicine

Nausea is generally most severe during the first 4 to 6 weeks a new anti-AIDS drug is taken. Thereafter, the nausea often decreases or even disappears. A number of anti-nausea drugs are available that might help. These include prochlorperazine (Compazine) and perphenazine (Trilafon). Two of the newest and most effective drugs are granisetron (Kytril) and ondansteron (Zofran). Dronabinol (Marinol), the behaviorally active chemical in marijuana, may also be useful.

Entry Blockers

Entry blockers prevent the virus from entering the lymphocyte cell. This is the latest class of anti-HIV drugs. Unlike most other anti-HIV drugs, Fuzeon must be given by injection, twice daily under the skin.

Almost all patients experience pain, itching, swelling, and cysts at the site of injection. Other common effects include diarrhea, nausea, and feelings of fatigue.

The Least You Need to Know

- ◆ AIDS is caused by HIV, a virus.

- ◆ When taken as directed, anti-HIV medicines have transformed AIDS from an invariably fatal disease to a chronic and stable disorder in which the patient can maintain a reasonable quality of life.

- ◆ HIV attacks and kills lymphocytes (a type of white blood cell), which play a major role in the normal immune defense mechanisms of the body.

- ◆ Anti-HIV therapy usually involves taking multiple drugs to block the replication of viruses and reduce the risk of the development of drug-resistant strains.

- ◆ Anti-HIV drugs, which must be taken as directed for a lifetime, are expensive, cause numerous adverse effects, and interact with many drugs.

Drugs Used for Treatment of HIV/AIDS

Generic Name	Other Designations	Trade Name	Generic Available
Reverse Transcriptase Inhibitors			
NRTIs			
Abacavir	ABC	Ziagen	No
Didanosine	ddI	Videx	No
Emtricitabine		Emtriva	
Lamivudine	3TC	Epivir	No
Stavudine	d4T	Zerit	No
Tenofovir		Viread	No
Zalcitabine	ddC	Hivid	No
Zidovudine	Azidothymidine, AZT, ZDV	Retrovir	Yes
NNRTIs			
Delavirdine		Rescriptor	No
Efavirenz		Sustiva	No
Nevirapine		Viramune	No
Protease Inhibitors ("navir")			
Amprenavir		Agenerase	No
Atazanavir		Reyataz	No
Fosamprenavir		Lexiva	No
Indinavir		Crixivan	No
Lopinavir + Ritonavir		Kaletra	No
Nelfinavir		Viracept	No
Ritonavir		Norvir	No
Saquinavir		Fortovase, Invirase	No
Entry Blockers			
Enfuvirtide		Fuzeon	No

Airborne Allergies

Among the most common of all chronic conditions, airborne allergies (technically called allergic rhinitis) affect 20 to 30 percent of all adults and 40 percent of children.

Common symptoms include a running and stuffed nose, sneezing, and tearing, as well as itching of the nose, throat, and eyes. In severe cases, the sufferer may experience general feelings of fatigue, interference with thinking and sleeping, and nervousness and depression. These symptoms can interfere with work and other daily activities.

Airborne allergies can be seasonal (hay fever) or perennial (year-round). Hay fever typically appears in spring or fall when pollens (most commonly ragweed and grass) are in the air and plants are blooming. The perennial variety is caused by animal dander, molds, or house dust mites. The seasonal condition is more common, although some people suffer from both.

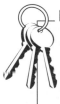

Did You Know That ...?

Allergies are hypersensitivity reactions of the immune system to specific and normally harmless substances, called allergens. These include pollen, animal dander, mites, drugs, and food. Exposure to the allergen stimulates formation of antibodies. Subsequent exposures to the allergen release chemical triggers (histamine, leukotrienes, prostaglandins), which are responsible for allergy symptoms.

Three approaches can be taken to dealing with airborne allergies:

◆ **Prevention** by avoiding contact with the allergen. This is the best approach, although it's not always possible.

◆ **Allergy shots** (immunotherapy) which are slow in working, expensive, effective in preventing the symptoms or reducing their severity in only some patients, and potentially dangerous. Because of their potential dangers, these shots should only be given in a doctor's office.

◆ **Treatment of the symptoms** (with antihistamines, decongestants, or nasal steroids) or preventing symptoms from occurring (cromolyn).

Antihistamines

Antihistamines, used alone or in combination with decongestants, are the most commonly used medicines for airborne allergies. Histamine is an important trigger of allergy. Antihistamines (a.k.a. H1 antagonists) block histamine at its receptor site, reducing (but not eliminating) the symptoms.

Allergy sufferers have a wide variety of oral antihistamines to select from—some are OTC, others require a prescription. Antihistamines are classified as being either sedating (called first-generation antihistamines) or nonsedating (called second-generation antihistamines).

Sedating Antihistamines

First-generation antihistamines were developed more than 50 years ago. These drugs produce varying degrees of sedation; some, such as diphenhydramine, produce very pronounced sedation. They also cause *atropine-like side effects*, which contributes to their reducing running noses and tearing.

def•i•ni•tion

Atropine-like side effects are the side effects caused by atropine and other anticholinergic drugs and some antihistamines. To a greater or lesser extent, these effects include dry mouth, blurred vision, difficulty in urinating, and an increased heart rate.

The sedating effects may be beneficial when the symptoms of allergy interfere with sleep, but such effects are troublesome when they cause daytime sedation or impair mental or physical performance.

Excessive and potentially dangerous drowsiness may occur when these drugs are used with alcohol, and anxiety-relieving, sleep-promoting, and other depressant medicines.

OTC Alternatives

Among the many sedating OTC antihistamines are chlorpheniramine (Chlor-Trimeton), clemastine (Tavist, Antihist), diphenhydramine (Benadryl), and phenindamine (Nolahist). Loratidine (Claritin) is a nonsedating antihistamine. All are available as generic products, and many come in combination with decongestants, whose product names often end in "-D."

Warning! _____

Atropine-like (called anticholinergic) side effects are commonly seen with many anti-histamines and some drugs for depression and psychosis. These effects may worsen other medical conditions, including glaucoma (blurred vision), enlarged prostate gland (difficulty in urination), and heart disease (increased heart rate). Other atropine-like effects include dry mouth, constipation, and drowsiness.

Nonsedating Antihistamines

Second-generation antihistamines are nonsedating because they don't enter the brain. In addition, they don't cause atropine-like side effects. These newer drugs are no more effective for airborne allergies than their sedating cousins.

What's the downside of these widely used drugs? They are very expensive. Consider costs for a 30-day supply:

OTC sedating, $5 or less

OTC nonsedating, $20 to 25

Prescription nonsedating trade-named brands, more than $70

Nasal Antihistamines

Azelastine (Astelin) is a prescription antihistamine nasal spray. It provides relief of nasal stuffiness and itching and running noses in mild-to-moderate hay fever. This product causes fewer atropine-like effects but may cause drowsiness, sedation, headache, and a bitter taste. Sedation, drowsiness, and headache are the most common side effects.

Decongestants

Decongestants are available for nasal application (spray and drops) and by mouth. These OTC products provide rapid relief of running nose and nasal congestion.

Nasal products should not be used for longer than three to five consecutive days because they may produce "rebound congestion"—i.e., the beneficial effects wear off more rapidly and even greater congestion occurs. This problem is far easier to prevent than to correct.

> ## OTC Alternatives
>
> Topical decongestants include naphazoline (Privine), oxymetazoline (Afrin, Dristan), phenylephrine (Neo-Synephrine, Vicks Sinex), and xylometazoline (Otrivan). Common side effects include nasal burning, stinging, and dryness. Pseudoephedrine (Sudafed) is an oral decongestant that can increase blood pressure and heart rate and potentially cause stroke.

Nasal Steroids

When used as nasal sprays, steroids are highly effective for the relief of sneezing, running nose, itching, and nasal congestion. Nasal steroids (called corticosteroids) are more effective than oral antihistamines for both seasonal and perennial airborne allergies. They act in many ways, including reducing the release of chemical triggers of an allergy.

Unlike antihistamines and decongestants, which provide very rapid relief of symptoms, nasal steroids must be used one or more times daily for several days before benefits are seen. Maximum improvement requires several weeks of daily usage. Antihistamines can be taken with nasal steroids to produce rapid relief of symptoms. Patients should avoid sneezing or blowing their noses for 10 minutes after using.

Very small amounts of steroids taken intranasally enter the blood and affect other parts of the body. Since little of these drugs enter the blood stream, side effects are minimal and include sneezing, stinging, and headache.

> ## OTC Alternatives
>
> Cromolyn (Nasalcrom), administered as a nasal spray, is used to both prevent and treat airborne allergies. It works by interfering with the release of chemicals that trigger allergies. This drug is considered safe and can be used during pregnancy. It must be taken four times daily for two to four weeks before maximum benefits are seen for sneezing, nasal itching, and running nose.

The Least You Need to Know

◆ Medicines are effective for the treatment of symptoms caused by both seasonal airborne allergies (hay fever) and perennial airborne allergies.

◆ If the sedative and atropine-like side effects of older antihistamines are not a problem, they are at least as effective and far less expensive than the newer nonsedating antihistamines.

◆ Decongestants and antihistamines, as OTC products, produce rapid relief of symptoms of airborne allergies.

◆ Nasal steroids are considered safe and are the most effective medicines available for the treatment of seasonal and perennial airborne allergies.

Drugs Used for Airborne Allergies

Generic Name	Trade Name	Generic Available
Sedating (First-Generation) Antihistamines		
Azatadine	Optimine	No
Dexchlorpheniramine	Polaramine	Yes
Hydroxyzine	Atarax, Vistaril	Yes
Tripelennamine	PBZ	Yes
Nonsedating (Second-Generation) Antihistamines		
Cetirizine	Zyrtec	No
Desloratadine (OTC: Canada)	Clarinex	No
Fexofenadine (OTC: Canada)	Allegra	No
Steroids		
Beclomethasone	Beconase AQ	No
Budesonide	Rhinocort Aqua	No
Flunisolide	Nasarel	Yes
Fluticasone	Flonase	No
Mometasone	Nasonex	No
Triamcinolone	Nasacort AQ	No

Alzheimer's Disease

Alzheimer's disease (AD) affects some 4 million Americans, 1 in 10 over 65. What are the signs of its presence?

AD typically progresses slowly and insidiously over a period of years. Early on, there is a loss of memory for recent events, persons, or places; difficulty in finding the right word to express thoughts; and anxiety or depression.

Over months to years, basic coping mechanisms become less satisfactory and, in time, fail. People with AD progressively lose the ability to interact socially, care for themselves, think and reason (cognition), and speak. Ultimately, they deteriorate into a vegetative state.

During its early stages, testing can lead to a probable diagnosis of AD. Based on the presence of some signs and the absence of others, a tentative diagnosis can be made with less than a 10 percent chance of error. The diagnosis can only be confirmed with an autopsy of the brain revealing degeneration and the presence of telltale abnormal structures, which interfere with communication between nerves.

There appear to be genetic influences in AD. Some genes types are linked to its earlier appearance, whereas other gene types protect against its occurrence.

AD-Treating Drugs: An Overview

In Chapter 2, we discussed the role of chemical messengers, called neurotransmitters, which permit nerve cells to communicate with one another. Among the most important messengers are acetylcholine and glutamate. Medicines modifying their effects are used for AD treatment.

Early studies using cholesterol-lowering statin drugs, nonsteroidal anti-inflammatory drugs (NSAIDs) such as ibuprofen, and the herbal ginko biloba, for AD treatment have generated great interest.

Acetylcholine-Preserving Drugs

Acetylcholine is thought to play an important role in thinking and memory. Significant losses of acetylcholine are seen in the brain of AD individuals.

A number of AD medicines, called cholinesterase inhibitors, protect acetylcholine by preventing its breakdown by an enzyme. These drugs, all taken by mouth, are used for mild-to-moderate stages of AD. Two such drugs are donepezil and rivastigmine, and they help about half the patients. These expensive drugs can't reverse the symptoms of AD, nor do they stop its progression. Rather, they modestly delay the loss of cognition and the appearance of other symptoms. Even these benefits are limited; they continue for only a limited period of time and only work in some patients. They may also control such behavioral signs of AD as wandering, anxiety, and depression.

Common side effects of cholinesterase inhibitors include nausea, vomiting, diarrhea, and insomnia.

Glutamate Blockers

Glutamate is the primary chemical messenger that increases brain activity. When too much glutamate is released, it destroys nerves, which may be responsible for AD as well as stroke symptoms.

Memantine, a new drug, blocks glutamate at its target site. Used for the treatment of moderate to severe AD, it appears to delay the loss of cognition. Memantine use permits patients to successfully perform daily functions for a longer period before declining.

Memantine is a well-tolerated drug that may cause dizziness, headache, constipation, and confusion.

Potential Treatments

As our population ages, there is an increasing need to find more effective and safer drugs that will reverse AD symptoms or at least stop or slow its progression. Clinical trials have involved many drugs, including cholesterol-lowering statins, nonsteroidal anti-inflammatory drugs (NSAIDs), ginko biloba, and estrogens:

◆ **Cholesterol-lowering statins.** A relationship may exist between cholesterol levels and the risk of developing AD. The cholesterol-lowering statins pravastatin (Pravachol) and lovastin (Mevinolin) may provide some benefit to patients with mild-to-moderate stages of AD.

◆ **Nonsteroidal anti-inflammatory drugs (NSAIDs).** Inflammation may contribute to brain damage in AD. Studies in the Netherlands found that persons taking a variety of NSAIDs had a lower risk of AD. It is unclear if they are useful for the treatment of AD.

◆ **Ginko biloba.** Mixed results have been seen with the herbal product ginko for the treatment of AD.

◆ **Estrogens.** The female hormone estrogen was long believed to reduce the risk or slowed the progression of AD. Instead, women taking estrogen in hormone-replacement therapy, over many years, have been shown to have double the risk of developing AD.

The Least You Need to Know

◆ Effective treatment of AD does not exist at present, but this is a very active area of research.

◆ Acetylcholine-protecting (cholinesterase inhibitor) drugs may provide modest benefit in slowing the progression of AD in a patient in mild to moderate stages.

◆ Glutamate blockers have promise in treating moderate to severe stage patients.

Drugs Used for the Treatment of Alzheimer's Disease

Generic Name	Trade Name	Generic Available
Acetylcholine-Protecting Drugs		
Donepezil	Aricept	No
Galantamine	Razadyne (formerly Reminyl)	No
Rivastigmine	Exelon	No
Tacrine	Cognex	No
Glutamate Blocker		
Memantine	Namenda	No

Anemias

Red blood cells (RBCs) carry hemoglobin, and hemoglobin carries oxygen from the lungs to the tissues of the body. When the number of RBCs is low, there is a reduction in the amount of oxygen carried, and anemia results.

Early signs of anemia include feelings of fatigue, weakness, difficulty in breathing after exertion, and loss of skin color. As the anemic condition worsens, fainting, dizziness, a rapid heartbeat, and shortness of breath are experienced.

Red Blood Cells and Anemias

To better understand the most common types of anemia, we need to first talk about RBCs (which are also called erythrocytes) and hemoglobin.

RBCs begin to develop in the bone marrow, where they pick up hemoglobin, and then enter and mature in the blood. To mature and function normally, the following factors must be present:

- EPO (erythropoietin), a hormone, is needed to stimulate RBC production.

- Iron is needed for hemoglobin manufacture.

- Vitamin B_{12} and folic acid are needed for the RBC to mature normally.

Anemias are caused by too-rapid loss or too-slow manufacture of RBCs. They also can result from obvious or obscure bleeding related to accidents, surgeries, or diseases. Here we focus on three common types of anemias, which can be treated with medicines: iron-deficiency anemia, vitamin-deficiency anemia, and anemia caused by kidney failure.

Iron-Deficiency Anemia

Iron deficiency most commonly occurs when demands for iron exceed its intake. To be more specific, iron-deficiency anemia can be caused by inadequate dietary intake, inadequate gastrointestinal absorption, increased iron demand (like in pregnancy), or blood loss (menstruation).

Treatment consists of providing iron supplements. In most cases, OTC oral products can be used.

OTC Alternatives

Oral iron, or ferrous, salts are available, each containing a different amount of iron. Ferrous sulfate is the most commonly used and least-expensive form of iron, and it is also the kind that the body absorbs best. Ferrous fumarate and ferrous gluconate are also available. All iron supplements should be taken on an empty stomach (or, if needed, with crackers) one to two hours before meals. Iron supplements often cause constipation. If so, this problem can be relieved with a stool softener.

Keep all iron supplements out of the reach of children. Iron is a major cause of fatal poisoning in children under six.

For individuals who can't absorb iron by mouth or who can't or won't take oral iron, injectable products are available. Injectables are no more effective than oral dosage forms and are potentially far more dangerous.

Three injectable irons are available in the United States. The most commonly used is iron dextran, which can be injected into veins, which is preferred, or into muscles.

Rare but potentially fatal allergic reactions may occur after injection. A small test dose must be injected prior to the full dose, and resuscitation treatment must be readily at hand.

Sodium ferric gluconate and iron sucrose are used to treat iron deficiency anemia in patients undergoing kidney dialysis and who are receiving epoetin (EPO).

 Did You Know That ...?

Iron-deficiency anemia is the most common nutritional deficiency worldwide, in both the developed and developing world, and affects more than 500 million individuals.

Vitamin-Deficiency Anemia

Vitamin B_{12} and folic acid are needed for the normal maturation of RBCs. In the absence of either, RBCs fail to properly mature. They grow too large, assume abnormal shapes, and live short lives. These abnormal RBCs are called megaloblasts, and the condition is megaloblastic anemia.

Vitamin B$_{12}$ Deficiency and Treatment

B$_{12}$ deficiency usually results from its inadequate absorption. In addition to causing megaloblastic anemia, vitamin B$_{12}$ deficiency leads to nerve disorders.

Vitamin B$_{12}$ deficiency is treated with cyanocobalamin, a purified form of vitamin B$_{12}$. It can be taken by mouth, injection, or intranasally. The oral form is not suitable for individuals who cannot absorb vitamin B$_{12}$.

Cyanocobalamin is a relatively safe drug whose use must be continued for a lifetime.

Did You Know That ...?

Folic acid deficiency early in pregnancy can cause spinal cord defects (spina bifida) in the fetus. All women of child-bearing age, before pregnancy has occurred, should ensure that they maintain an adequate folate intake of 0.4 mg daily. This can be obtained from their diet or vitamin supplements.

Folic Acid Deficiency and Treatment

Folic acid deficiency is commonly seen in chronic alcoholics and also results from inadequate vitamin absorption. Such deficiency can result in megaloblastic anemia.

Megaloblastic anemia, associated with folic acid deficiency, can be treated with vitamin supplementation, provided by tablets (OTC and prescription) or injection. Folic acid is considered very safe.

Daily doses of folic acid greater than 1 mg can mask a vitamin B$_{12}$ deficiency and permit irreversible damage to the nervous system to continue. Because of the risk, people taking folic acid must also take B$_{12}$.

Anemia in Kidney Failure

Erythropoietin, or EPO, stimulates the bone marrow to produce RBCs. Patients with chronic kidney failure almost always develop anemia because their kidneys are unable to secrete this hormone.

Epoetin alpha (the laboratory version of EPO), by injection, is used for anemia associated with chronic kidney failure in patients prior to and after they receive dialysis.

The most important side effect associated with epoetin alpha is an increase in blood pressure.

The Least You Need to Know

◆ Iron-deficiency anemia is treated with oral or injectable iron supplements.

◆ Vitamin-deficiency (megaloblastic) anemia results from deficiencies of vitamin B_{12} or folic acid.

◆ Anemia associated with chronic kidney failure is treated with EPO (erythropoietin; epoetin alpha).

Drugs Used for Treatment of Anemias

Generic Name	Trade Name	Generic Available
Injectable Iron Preparations		
Iron dextran	DexFerrum, InFeD	No
Iron sucrose	Venofer	No
Sodium ferric gluconate complex	Ferrlecit	No
Vitamin B$_{12}$ (Cyanocobalamin)		
Oral forms		Yes
Intranasal	Nascobal	No
Injections		
Cyanocobalamin	Crystamine, Cyomin, Crysti 1000, Rubesol-1000	Yes
Hydroxocobalamin	Hydro-Crysti-12, LA-12	Yes
Folic Acid		
Oral		Yes
Injection	Folvite	Yes
Epoetin alpha	Erythropoietin (EPO), Epogen, Procrit	No

Anxiety

When faced with threatening or stressful situations, it is normal to have emotional, behavioral, or bodily responses. When such responses are extreme and long lasting, or are inappropriate for the situation, they may interfere with our everyday normal life and activities. Anxiety disorders may affect 10 to 25 percent of us during our lifetime.

The Many Faces of Anxiety

All anxiety disorders are not the same. Some may involve excessive worrying about things that matter, as well as the small stuff. Others may involve sudden panic attacks or unrealistic fears (phobias). And still others may involve compulsively repeating an action for no apparent reason (obsessive-compulsive disorder) or reliving, in the mind, a combat situation, sexual assault, or other traumatic event that was once experienced for real.

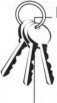

Did You Know That ...?

Most individuals with obsessive-compulsive disorder (OCD) intentionally repeat rituals to control what they perceive to be a danger or risk.

Humorous characters experiencing OCDs have been portrayed in the movies (*As Good As It Gets,* for example) and on TV (*Monk*). The classic character is Lady Macbeth (with her compulsive need to wash blood from her hands).

Some anti-anxiety medicines relieve these symptoms, others don't. Often behavioral therapy may be required to chase away these demons. Two commonly prescribed anti-anxiety medications are the Valium-related class of drugs called benzodiazepines and the drug buspirone (BuSpar). Antidepressants are also sometimes used for the treatment of anxiety disorders.

Benzodiazepines

About a dozen benzodiazepines are marketed in the United States and Canada, the best known being diazepam (Valium). Their differences are primarily based on how long it takes them to begin to act and how long they remain effective.

The benzodiazepine class of drugs is used to treat a wide variety of medical disorders. These include anxiety, insomnia, spastic muscle disorders, and seizure disorders. Some of these drugs are used to treat all or most of these disorders, whereas others are used more selectively.

Ideally, drugs for treating anxiety disorders should calm you down but not knock you out. You want to be able to think clearly and drive safely. You cannot do these things if the drug makes you sleepy. Unfortunately, benzodiazepines cause some degree of drowsiness and interference with physical performance.

Valium-related drugs are highly effective in relieving the symptoms of many anxiety disorders, often within hours after the first dose is taken. Alprazolam is useful for controlling panic reactions, but has a tendency to be abused.

Common side effects of benzodiazepines include drowsiness, dizziness, and impairment of driving.

Individuals who have a history of abusing alcohol or other drugs are the most likely candidates to also abuse benzodiazepines. Using these drugs, even at normal doses for periods of four to six weeks, can lead to dependence on them.

Taking benzodiazepines for several months and then suddenly not taking them can result in real signs of withdrawal. These include nervousness, sleep disturbances, and tremors. To avoid these problems, doses should be reduced gradually.

 Warning!

When taken alone, even in high doses, benzodiazepines are virtually "suicide-proof." However, their potential for harm is much greater when they are taken with alcohol or other drugs that produce reduced mental or physical functioning.

Benzodiazepines have been reported to cause fetal abnormalities when taken during the first trimester of pregnancy. These drugs should not be used during pregnancy or by nursing mothers.

Buspirone (BuSpar)

BuSpar is an effective drug for the treatment of anxiety. Unlike Valium-related drugs, it does not cause drowsiness, which may interfere with thinking or operating motor vehicles, nor is it subject to abuse.

BuSpar must be taken for about a week before its anti-anxiety effects begin. Therefore, it is not useful for individuals who need immediate relief.

Antidepressant Drugs

Antidepressants were first developed and used for the treatment of depression. This original name is now somewhat misleading and outdated, because some of these same medicines are used to treat anxiety and other medical disorders.

There are several classes of antidepressants. The most widely used are the selective serotonin-reuptake inhibitors (SSRIs) and include such common trade-name drugs as Lexapro, Prozac, Paxil, and Zoloft. These drugs are considered to be relatively safe, have few side effects, and are effective for a number of anxiety disorders, in particular, the long-term management of chronic anxiety. Unlike the benzodiazepines, the anti-anxiety effects of benzodiazepines may require two to four weeks of drug treatment.

Selected tricyclic antidepressants, in particular, venlafaxine (Effexor) and monoamine oxidase (MAO) inhibitors, are also used to treat anxiety but cause a wide range of troubling side effects. For a thorough discussion of these drugs or their names, see "Depression."

The Least You Need to Know

♦ Valium and other benzodiazepines are highly effective in rapidly relieving many anxiety symptoms. They cause a low degree of drowsiness and impairment of physical activities that require alertness.

♦ Regular benzodiazepine use may cause a drug-dependent state. In addition, they should never be taken with alcohol or during pregnancy.

♦ BuSpar effectively relieves anxiety only after it is taken for about a week. This drug does not cause sedation nor a dependent state.

♦ Antidepressants, such as the SSRIs (selective serotonin-reuptake inhibitors), are also useful for the relief of some anxiety disorders.

Drugs Used for Anxiety

Generic Name	Trade Name	Generic Available
Benzodiazepines		
Alprazolam	Xanax	Yes
Chlordiazepoxide	Librium	Yes
Clorazepate	Tranxene	Yes
Diazepam	Valium	Yes
Lorazepam	Ativan	Yes
Oxazepam	Serax	Yes
Non-Benzodiazepines		
Buspirone	BuSpar	No
Hydroxyzine	Atarax, Vistaril	Yes
Venlafaxine	Effexor	No
Selective Serotonin-Reuptake Inhibitors (SSRIs)		
Citalopram	Celexa	No
Duloxetine	Cymbalta	No
Escitalopram	Lexapro	No
Fluoxetine	Prozac, Sarafem	Yes
Fluvoxamine	Luvox	Yes
Paroxetine	Paxil	Yes
Sertraline	Zoloft	Yes

Asthma, Chronic Bronchitis, and Emphysema

These three breathing disorders are very common. Almost 20 million people in the United States have asthma. Emphysema and chronic bronchitis are the second-most-common medical conditions responsible for people stopping work and the fourth leading cause of death in the United States.

In asthma, the breathing tubes—called bronchi—temporarily narrow or collapse (*bronchoconstriction*). This reduces the flow of air into the lungs. Common asthma symptoms are wheezing, coughing, shortness of breath, and inflammation of the airways.

Unlike the temporary interference with airflow caused by asthma, in emphysema and chronic bronchitis airflow is persistently blocked. These latter breathing disorders are very descriptively and commonly called chronic obstructive pulmonary disease (COPD). The most common symptoms include cough, with phlegm, and shortness of breath. By far, the most important cause of COPD is cigarette smoking, although it can also be caused by exposure to chemical fumes, dust, and other air pollutants.

Asthma

Two types of medicines are used to treat asthma—those that stop asthma symptoms and those that prevent asthma symptoms from occurring in the first place. The choice depends on how severe the symptoms are and the frequency with which they occur.

Drugs that stop asthma symptoms by rapidly opening up airways are called bronchodilators. In asthma, inflammation swells the airways, which interferes with airflow. Anti-inflammatory drugs reduce this inflammation and are used to prevent attacks from occurring in the first place, or at least reduce the frequency with which they occur.

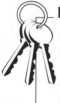

Did You Know That ...?

Steroids are the most commonly used anti-inflammatory drugs. In addition to being used for asthma, steroids are used for the treatment of dozens of different medical conditions, including severe allergies, skin and eye disorders, rheumatoid arthritis, hormone deficiencies, certain cancers, multiple sclerosis, and disorders of the blood and gastrointestinal tract.

Airway-Opening Drugs

To stop an attack after it has started, albuterol and similar quick-relief drugs are the fastest acting and most effective medicines available. They act by opening air passages that are narrowed as the result of asthma. Long-acting airway openers such as salmeterol and formoterol are used to prevent attacks.

Quick-relief airway openers are inhaled from a handheld *metered-dose inhaler* (MDI) or *nebulizer*. After being inhaled, welcome breathing relief starts within minutes and continues for three to six hours.

def•i•ni•tion

A **metered-dose inhaler** (MDI) is a small, handheld pressurized device. Each time the MDI is activated, it delivers a fine spray, which contains a premeasured dose of drug. A **nebulizer** has a rubber bulb that, when squeezed, delivers a mist of drug. Nebulizers are easier to learn to use than MDIs.

Maximizing Your Medicine

Medicines used for the treatment of asthma and COPD are commonly inhaled using either a metered-dose inhaler or a nebulizer. When used properly—which is the only way these devices will be of benefit—they rapidly deliver medication to the intended location in the airway tubes while minimizing their effects on other parts of the body.

Inhalers don't help much if they are not used correctly, and so users must be taught the skills needed to use them correctly. Work carefully with your health-care provider to learn and master the use of the inhaler *before* you need it most.

What can be done when asthma attacks occur frequently? Long-acting airway openers, such as salmeterol, are used to prevent attacks. After being inhaled, this drug opens airways for up to 12 hours. Because there is a considerable delay before it begins to work—about 20 minutes—this drug is of little value when frantically gasping for air.

Use cautiously if you have diabetes, overactive thyroid, heart disease, high blood pressure, or angina (chest pains).

Side effects are usually are minimal and include a rapid heartbeat, heart palpitations, and tremors.

Warning!

Airway-opening drugs should restore normal breathing within 20 minutes. If they don't, seek medical assistance immediately! Avoid the natural temptation to take higher doses or take doses more often than have been prescribed. Long-acting airway openers should never be used to replace the quick-acting inhalers!

Anti-Inflammatory Drugs

Steroids are the most important anti-inflammatory drugs used to prevent asthma symptoms and stop severe attacks.

Patients experiencing symptoms on a frequent basis commonly use inhaled steroids, such as beclomethasone, to prevent attacks. Inhaled steroids do not provide help in stopping an asthmatic attack when it is in progress because they cannot open narrowed airways. Inhaled steroids are sometimes used in combination with airway-opening drugs.

Inhaled steroids must be used every day, for up to four to six weeks, before early signs of improvement are seen. Such favorable signs include fewer episodes of breathing difficulties or less severe symptoms when they do occur. These drugs must be taken for several additional weeks before their maximum benefits kick in.

To treat severe cases of asthma that cannot be adequately controlled with safer drugs, steroids are taken by mouth. The beneficial effects produced by such oral steroids as prednisone are often nothing short of dramatic and may be even lifesaving. As good as they are, when oral steroids are used for long periods, at high doses, they may cause severe side effects. When the time comes to stop taking steroids, it must be done gradually.

When properly used, steroids can be lifesaving drugs. When improperly used, their adverse effects can affect organs throughout the body. In general, steroids should be taken at the lowest effective doses for the shortest period of time. Some major problems include …

 ◆ Adrenal insufficiency. High steroid doses cause the adrenal glands to shut down and become unable to release natural steroids when the body is confronted with stress.

 ◆ Bone loss, osteoporosis, and bone fractures.

 ◆ Increased susceptibility to infections.

- ◆ Loss of control of sugar levels in diabetics.

- ◆ Muscle weakness.

- ◆ Salt and water retention, causing high blood pressure.

- ◆ Suppression of growth in children.

- ◆ Behavioral and mood changes, such as depression or a high feeling (euphoria).

- ◆ Cataracts and glaucoma.

- ◆ Peptic ulcer disease.

Steroids should not be used by people with systemic fungal infections or those receiving live-virus vaccines.

Steroids should be used cautiously in children and pregnant or nursing women—also by people with high blood pressure, heart failure, kidney disease, peptic ulcers, diabetes, osteoporosis, and infections resistant to treatment.

Inhaled steroids are quite safe. Side effects include cough, dry mouth and throat, hoarseness, and thrush (a fungal infection of the mouth). To prevent thrush, patients should rinse their mouth with water after each use of a steroid inhaler.

Emphysema and Chronic Bronchitis (COPD)

Many of the same drugs used to treat asthma are also useful in relieving the shortness of breath seen in COPD. Unfortunately, none of the available medicines reverse existing lung damage and obstructed airflow.

Airway-Opening Drugs

Similar drugs are used to treat COPD as asthma and are inhaled using a metered-dose inhalator or nebulizer. Albuterol and other quick-relief drugs are used to relieve sudden shortness of breath in COPD and long-acting airway openers, such as salmeterol, are inhaled to prevent breathing difficulties.

Inhaled ipratropium taken alone or in combination with albuterol is often the first-drug choice used to prevent COPD attacks. Ipratropium is an atropine-like drug that may cause dry mouth and a headache. This drug should be used cautiously by individuals suffering from glaucoma or prostate enlargement.

> **Maximizing Your Medicine**
>
> Drugs used for the treatment of chronic obstructive pulmonary disease (COPD) can prevent the disorder from worsening and can improve breathing. Whereas these drugs are useful, the most important treatment is to stop smoking. As COPD progresses, shortness of breath becomes more extreme and is worsened by exposure to polluted air. Pneumonia or bronchitis cause flare-ups and are treated with antibiotics and may require that the patient be hospitalized.
>
> In advanced cases of COPD, oxygen therapy is often required. Homebound individuals can use electrically driven devices that concentrate oxygen from the air. Liquid (compressed) oxygen, contained in small portable tanks, can be used by individuals up and about and away from the house for periods of several hours at a time.

Anti-Inflammatory Drugs

When other drugs are not effective, inhaled steroids are used to reduce symptoms and prevent flare-ups. Unfortunately, they do not prevent loss of lung function. Oral steroids are used to stop flare-ups that are not controlled with safer drugs.

The Least You Need to Know

- ◆ Some medicines are used to treat the symptoms of asthma, whereas others prevent these symptoms from occurring. Sometimes better results are obtained when these drugs are used in combination. How the physician decides which approach is more appropriate depends on the symptoms.

- ◆ If asthma symptoms occur infrequently, there is no need to take medication each and every day.

- ◆ For fast relief of asthma symptoms, take a short-acting inhaled drug that opens airways.

- ◆ To prevent or control regularly occurring asthma symptoms, use inhaled steroids every day.

- ◆ To control asthma symptoms that occur every day, use both an inhaled steroid and a long-acting inhaled drug that opens airways.

- ◆ Drugs used for the treatment of emphysema and chronic bronchitis prevent the disease from worsening and can improve symptoms.

- ◆ The best treatment for COPD is to avoid smoking.

♦ In addition to drugs used for asthma, inhaled ipratropium is used to prevent COPD attacks.

♦ In advanced cases of COPD, oxygen therapy may be required.

Drugs for Asthma, Emphysema, and Chronic Bronchitis

Generic Name	Trade Name	Generic Available
Opens Airways		
Albuterol	Proventil, Ventolin	Yes
Formoterol	Foradil	No
Fluticasone/Salmeterol	Advair Diskus	No
Ipratropium	Atrovent	Yes
Levalbuterol	Xopenex	No
Salmeterol	Serevent	Yes
Terbutaline	Brethine, Bricanyl	Yes
Theophylline	Theo-Dur, Theovent, Uniphyl	Yes
Anti-Inflammatory		
Beclomethasone [Beclometasone]	Beclovent Vanceril	Yes
Budesonide	Pulmicort	Yes
Fluticasone	Flovent	No
Fluticasone/Salmeterol	Advair Diskus	No
Methylprednisolone	Medrol	Yes
Montelukast	Singulair	No
Prednisone	Deltasone, Meticorten	Yes
Zafirlukast	Accolate	No
Zileuton	Ziflo	No

Atherosclerosis

Atherosclerosis, often simply called hardening of the arteries, is responsible for more deaths in the United States and other developed countries than any other condition. Fatty materials deposit on the inner walls of blood vessels, interfering with or blocking the flow of blood. This can result in heart attack, stroke, or peripheral arterial disease, conditions discussed elsewhere in this book.

def•i•ni•tion

Atherosclerosis is a specific type of arteriosclerosis, more commonly known as hardening of the arteries. In arteriosclerosis, the walls of very small arteries become thicker, less elastic, and calcified, resulting in restricted blood flow. In atherosclerosis, fat deposits compound the thickening and hardening of arteries. Blood vessel inflammation and infection may contribute to the development of atherosclerosis.

The medical community has identified many well-established and important risk factors that promote the development of atherosclerosis. These include smoking, high blood levels of cholesterol, high blood pressure, diabetes, and obesity. Preventing or controlling these conditions can suppress or delay the worsening of atherosclerosis. We talk about the specific drug management of each of these conditions elsewhere in this book.

The Least You Need to Know

◆ In atherosclerosis, deposits of fats and the thickening and hardening of arteries restricts the flow of blood, which can lead to heart attack and stroke.

◆ Among the factors that increase the risk of developing atherosclerosis are smoking, elevated blood levels of cholesterol, high blood pressure, diabetes, and obesity.

Attention-Deficit/Hyperactivity Disorder (ADHD)

Attention-deficit/hyperactivity disorder (ADHD) is the most common behavioral disorder in children. It has three characteristic hallmarks: inattentiveness, excessive physical activity (hyperactivity), and impulsive behavior. The first signs are typically seen by the age of 3 but must be seen by 7. It may continue into the adolescent years and even during adulthood.

The reported prevalence of ADHD among school-age children varies considerably among sources, some estimating 3 to 5 percent, whereas others push the range to 4 to 12 percent. Some researchers have questioned whether ADHD is being overdiagnosed. It is generally agreed that it may be 4- to 8-fold more common in boys than girls. Both genetic and nongenetic factors appear to contribute to this condition.

Drug Treatment of ADHD: An Overview

The most effective treatment approaches combine behavioral measures with medication. ADHD drugs are classified as stimulants and nonstimulants.

Stimulants

Stimulants, such as methylphenidate and amphetamines, are the first drug choice for treating ADHD. They are very widely used and have proved effective in improving many of the ADHD symptoms in 70 to 95 percent of treated children.

Within 30 to 60 minutes after their oral administration, there is a reduction in physical movements and impulsive behavior and an increase in attention span. When given over an extended period of time, academic performance improves.

Did You Know That ...?

You might wonder how stimulants, which increase physical and mental activity in adults, calm children. The explanations offered—more accurately, the theories proposed—are complex and not very convincing. In short, it is not clear how they work in ADHD, but they do.

The drugs are not making kids any smarter but rather they are improving their focus on their schoolwork.

Methylphenidate is the most commonly used drug for ADHD. It is available in tablets that are taken two to three times daily and long-acting tablets taken only once daily. A methylphenidate-containing patch (Daytrana) is also available for once a day use by children 6 to 12.

Warning! _____

Methylphenidate in oral form (Methylin, Ritalin, Concerta) and amphetamine (Adderall), in rare circumstances when used for ADHD, may increase the risk of sudden death and cardiac arrest.

Common side effects of stimulants include reduced appetite, insomnia, irritability, and stomachache.

Growth may be suppressed or delayed when stimulants are used. This effect may result from the reduction in appetite.

Experts recommend drug-free periods, such as during weekends or school holidays. These breaks provide an opportunity to assess the benefits of treatment and for greater growth to occur. After stimulants are discontinued, children experience a growth spurt, and the final height attained at adulthood is not generally reduced.

Although methylphenidate and the amphetamines are subject to abuse by adolescents and adults, their abuse potential in children doesn't appear to be an important risk.

Nonstimulants

Nonstimulants used for ADHD include several antidepressants and atomoxetine. These drugs are backups when stimulants are not effective or cannot be taken.

Imipramine and desipramine, tricyclic antidepressants, must be given for two to four weeks before they provide benefits in ADHD. They primarily reduce excessive activity but do little to improve inattention or impulsive behavior. When used over a period of several months, they become less effective.

Warning! _____

In rare instances, atomoxetine has caused severe liver toxicity. Patients or their caregivers should immediately notify their doctors if they have itching, dark urine, yellow skin or eyes, tenderness in the upper right side of their abdomen, or flu-like symptoms.

When taken in excessive doses, tricyclics can produce adverse effects to the heart. However, they do not cause insomnia nor suppress growth.

Selective serotonin-reuptake inhibitors (SSRIs) do not appear to be effective for ADHD.

Atomoxetine (Strattera) is the first nonstimulant approved specifically for the treatment of ADHD. Benefits occur within two to four weeks after treatment begins. Early studies suggest that it may be as effective as the stimulant methylphenidate. Common side effects of atomoxetine include headache, insomnia, dry mouth, and nausea.

Drug-drug interaction: At least two weeks should pass after using a monoamine oxidase inhibitor (MAOI) and atomoxetine.

The Least You Need to Know

- Stimulants, such as methylphenidate and the amphetamines, are the most effective drugs for treating ADHD.

- Stimulants decrease excessive activity and impulsive behavior and increase attention span.

- Drug-free periods should be instituted for children receiving stimulants.

- Atomoxetine, a nonstimulant effective for ADHD, may, in rare instances, cause severe liver toxicity.

Drugs Used for Treatment of ADHD

Generic Name	Trade Name	Generic Available
Stimulants		
Amphetamine salts	Adderall	Yes
Dextroamphetamine	Dexedrine, Dextrostat	Yes
Dexmethylphenidate	Focalin	No
Methylphenidate	Ritalin, Methylin, Metadate	Yes
Long-acting methylphendiate	Concerta	Yes
	Daytrana (patch)	No
Nonstimulants		
Atomoxetine	Strattera	No
Bupropion	Wellbutrin	Yes
Desipramine	Norpramin, Pertofrane	Yes
Imipramine	Tofranil	Yes

Autism

Autism is a developmental condition, appearing in early childhood, in which there are deficiencies in social relationships, language skills, interpretation of the feelings and thoughts of others, and behavior and control of emotions. Compulsive and ritualistic routines are common; mental retardation (IQ less than 70) occurs in about 70 percent of afflicted children. Many theories have been offered as to its cause, but to date, none have been proven.

Treatment of Autism: An Overview

It is generally accepted that there is no single best treatment for all children with autism. Treatment approaches include behavioral modification, communication therapy, dietary changes, and drugs.

Drugs are used to control the symptoms seen in autism. They do not modify the underlying causes of this condition. Classes of drugs prescribed for autism include medicines primarily intended for the treatment of depression, psychoses, seizures, and attention-deficit/hyperactivity disorder.

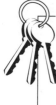

Did You Know That ...? _____

No drug has been approved by the Food and Drug Administration as safe and effective for the treatment of autism. However, drugs used for other conditions can be beneficial and are prescribed by doctors in what is called "off-label" use, i.e., for a condition that has not been approved by the FDA. "Off-label" drug prescribing is legal and is a common practice.

Antidepressant Drugs

Medications primarily intended to treat depression and obsessive-compulsive disorders (OCD) may reduce the repetitive actions and aggressive behavior seen in autism. Eye contact and social contact may also improve. These medications include antidepressants of the selective-serotonin reuptake inhibitor class (SSRI) and clomipramine.

Common side effects include headache, insomnia, dizziness, and drowsiness.

Antipsychotic Drugs

Antipsychotic medications have been used to lessen increased activity, aggressiveness, and other behavioral problems. In addition, these drugs may decrease the social withdrawal seen in autistic patients.

Common side effects include nervousness, drowsiness, dizziness, headache, restlessness, muscle stiffness, and tremors.

Did You Know That ...?

Risperidone is highly effective and widely used for psychotic disorders. It is often prescribed on an "off-label" basis for the treatment of autism. Citing safety concerns, in May 2005 the FDA rejected an application to market this drug for autism.

Antiseizure Drugs

Medications approved for epilepsy and other seizure conditions often reduce the frequency of seizures that occur in many autistic children. Such medication, however, does not eliminate seizure activity.

Side effects vary with the specific drugs used. The lowest effective doses should be used to avoid potentially severe adverse effects.

Attention-Deficit/Hyperactivity Drugs

Selective medications with stimulant properties, used for ADHD, such as methylphenidate (Ritalin), may also reduce the impulsive and excessive activity seen in autism.

Common side effects include insomnia, nervousness, loss of appetite, abdominal pains, and increases in blood pressure.

The Least You Need to Know

◆ There is no best single treatment for all children with autism, and no drug has been approved by the FDA for its treatment.

◆ Medications are used to reduce such autistic symptoms as repetitive and aggressive behaviors, social withdrawal, impulsive and excessive activity, and seizures.

Drugs for Treatment of Autism

Generic Name	Trade Name	Generic Available
Antidepressants		
Clomipramine	Anafranil	Yes
Fluoxetine	Prozac	Yes
Fluvoxamine	Luvox	Yes
Sertraline	Zoloft	Yes
Antipsychotics		
Olanzapine	Zyprexa	No
Risperidone	Risperdal	No
Ziprasidone	Geodon	No
Antiseizure Drugs		
Carbamazepine	Tegretol	Yes
Lamotrigine	Lamictal	No
Topiramate	Topamax	No
Valproic acid	Depakote	Yes
Anti-ADHD Drugs		
Amphetamine salt combination	Adderall	Yes
Detroamphetamine	Dexedrine, Dextrostat	Yes
Methylphenidate	Concerta, Methylin, Ritalin	Yes

Bacterial Infections

In this section, we talk about a number of conditions.

First, we briefly talk about bacteria—what they are and what kinds there are.

We then look at some different kinds of common infections caused by bacteria. These are ear infections, meningitis, pneumonia, skin infections, and urinary tract infections. As you scan the table of contents and index, you'll find that we devote additional sections to other, specific bacterial infections.

Finally, we look at medicines used to treat bacterial infections. As you'll see, these drugs are used for many different infections. This being the case, it makes sense for us to include them all in one place—here.

Bacteria

Bacteria are among the smallest and simplest living organisms. Each bacterium consists of only a single cell. It has all the metabolic machinery needed to maintain an independent existence, including the ability to reproduce. Unlike the cells of animals, the bacterial cell is surrounded by a rigid cell wall.

Our body harbors many different kinds of bacteria, but fortunately relatively few cause diseases. Most are harmless or coexist with us in a mutually beneficial relationship.

Did You Know That ...?

Peering under a microscope, we find that bacteria assume a number of different shapes:

- ◆ Spherical, called *cocci*
- ◆ Short-straight rods, referred to as *bacilli*
- ◆ Corkscrew or spiral shaped, termed *spirochetes*

Cocci are also named based on how they group: staphylococci are in grape-like clusters, whereas streptococci are in chains.

Dyes are needed to see bacteria under a microscope. The Gram stain—named after its discoverer, Hans Christian Joachim Gram—is the simplest and most widely used. Some bacteria pick up a purple stain and are classified as Gram-positive. Others don't, and these so-called Gram-negative bacteria assume a pink color.

Although interesting and aesthetically attractive, we talk about these stains because they provide a basis for classifying bacteria and for differentiating the sensitivity of bacteria to different antibacterial drugs.

Gram-positive bacteria and Gram-negative bacteria require different antibiotics to kill them. This results from differences in the chemistry of their cell walls. Resistance to antibacterial drugs—that is, their ability to become less susceptible to their effects—also develops more rapidly in Gram-negative microbes.

Bacterial Infections

Bacteria enter the body through any available opening. This includes the skin, lungs, mucous membranes (nose, mouth, vagina), and tracts (e.g., intestines, urinary system). Bacteria are carried in the air, food, feces, and through physical contact with infected individuals.

Body Defense Mechanisms

Exposure to disease-causing bacteria doesn't necessarily result in an infection. That result depends on the bacteria's ability to cause disease, called its virulence, and the *host's* ability to resist the infection by the following:

def•i•ni•tion

When talking about the disease, the patient is referred to as the **host.** An infection occurs when the microbe has set up house and multiplied within the host. When the host experiences injury as the result of the infection, it is called an infectious disease.

- Physical barriers, such as the skin and mucous membranes

- The hostile environment caused by stomach acid, urine, and vaginal secretions

- Antimicrobial factors present in tears and saliva

- Respiratory defenses, such as hair-like filters and coughing

- Immune defense mechanisms

Diagnosing Bacterial Infections

When seeing a sick patient, the doctor's first challenge is to determine whether the illness is an infectious disease.

Many infections are caused by a number of different types of bacteria and sometimes, by more than one bacteria at a time. These include those that are both Gram-positive and Gram-negative. In addition, some of these conditions also may be caused by viruses or fungi.

The patient's physical signs and symptoms plus the results of laboratory analyses are used to identify the microbe. When the cause of the infection has been identified, the doctor can then think about its treatment.

Of the hundreds of bacterial infections out there, in this section we talk about a few of the more common types, including the following:

◆ Ear infections

◆ Meningitis

◆ Pneumonia

◆ Skin infections

◆ Urinary tract infections

After considering each of these conditions, we then talk about the major classes of *antibacterial* drugs.

def•i•ni•tion

These medicines are variously called **antibiotics, antibacterial,** and **antimicrobial** drugs. Anti-biotic was once reserved for drugs obtained from microbes (such as penicillin). It is now used to refer to drugs used against all microbes (bacteria, viruses, and fungi).

Ear Infections

Middle ear infection, or *otitis media*, is extremely common in infants and children. By the age of 1 year, some three out of four children have had at least one episode. It is far less common in older children and adults. Why so?

One of the main reasons is the physical layout of the Eustachian tube, which connects the middle ear and the nose. In the young child, the tube is shorter, narrower, and more horizontal. This makes it easy for bacteria and viruses, present during a cold or nasal congestion, to travel from the nose to the middle ear.

Common symptoms of middle ear infections include ear pain, difficulty in sleeping, irritability, and fever. Some children respond by pulling on the ear. It is important to note that, even in the absence of treatment, the pain and fever are generally gone after two to three days. All the symptoms will be just a bad memory within seven days, although the ear should be checked by a physician to ensure that the infection is gone.

Causes and Treatment

Common causes of *otitis media* include *Streptococcus pneumoniae*, *Haemophilis influenzae*, and *Moraxella catarrhalis*, all Gram-positive bacteria. In passing, it is important to note that almost half of all cases are caused by or at least have viruses present. In these cases, an antibiotic is not necessary.

Treatment of *otitis media* has three objectives: (1) relieve pain (often with acetaminophen), (2) eliminate the infection, and (3) prevent complications.

Doctors don't have a single game plan for how they treat ear infections. Some prescribe antibiotics immediately. Others delay antibiotic use for two to three days when, in most cases, the condition will improve even in the absence of drugs. If the condition hasn't improved after a few days, they prescribe antibiotics.

Why do some doctors hold off on prescribing antibiotics? Doing so avoids exposing the child to antibiotic side effects and also saves money better spent elsewhere. But from a public health perspective, there is a more important reason. Limiting the use of antibiotics when they are not needed delays the development of bacterial resistance to these drugs. With resistance, the antibiotics become less effective. We talk much more about resistance later in this chapter.

Amoxicillin, a penicillin-like drug, is the first choice for treating most cases of middle-ear infections. It is highly effective when taken by mouth, quite safe, and inexpensive. If amoxicillin doesn't work, amoxicillin-clavulanate (Augmentin) or cefuroxime, a cephalosporin, are highly recommended backups.

For severe cases that don't improve with these drugs, or when young patients can't take drugs by mouth, ceftriaxone is used. The drug's main downside is that it must be given by intramuscular injection on three consecutive days.

Meningitis

The brain and spinal cord have a jelly-like consistency. They are protected from injury by bone—the skull and vertebrae—and are directly surrounded by three layers of tough connective tissue, which are called the meninges. Meningitis is the inflammation of the meninges.

Common symptoms include fever, severe headache, sensitivity to bright lights, sore neck, and abnormal responses to nerve testing. Lethargy and coma may be seen, as might seizures in children. Meningitis is a very serious infection and requires hospitalization.

Causes and Treatment

Meningitis is caused by both Gram-positive and Gram-negative bacteria. Almost half of all cases are caused by *Streptococcus pneumoniae*, followed by *Neisseria meningitis* and *Hemophilus influenzae*. A spinal tap is performed to check the fluid for the presence of bacteria. Less-common causes of meningitis are fungi (commonly seen in HIV/AIDS patients) and viruses. Delayed treatment may result in permanent brain damage, and death may occur within hours or days. Speed is of the essence when treating meningitis. Treatment must be initiated immediately, even before the exact cause of meningitis has been identified.

For patients between the ages of 1 month and 60 years, this initial treatment is usually cefotaxime or ceftriaxone + vancomycin. Both are given intravenously. After the microbial cause has been determined, adjustments may be made in the choice of the antibiotics. Depending on the patient response, antibiotic therapy may continue for 7 to 21 days.

Antibiotic treatment causes the bacteria to break up. These pieces may cause inflammation, swelling, and increased pressure. To prevent this problem, many doctors routinely give dexamethasone for four days to all young patients over 2 months of age. Such steroid therapy is initiated even prior to the start of antibiotics.

Maximizing Your Medicine

A vaccine is available to prevent both meningitis and pneumonia that are caused by *Hemophilus influenzae*. This vaccine is now strongly recommended as one of the basic childhood immunizations and is available as PedvaxHIB and ComVax. The first injection of the series is given at two months of age. The vaccine reduces the risk of disease by over 90 percent, and its side effects are mild and temporary.

Pneumonia

Pneumonia is the most common cause of death in the United States that is caused by an infectious disease. It is often a terminal illness in the elderly. The general term *pneumonia* includes all infections of the lung in which the microscopic air sacs are filled with fluid.

Common symptoms of pneumonia include the sudden appearance of fever, chills, and labored breathing, with shortness of breath, and a cough that brings up phlegm.

Causes and Treatment: An Overview

Pneumonia has many causes that include both Gram-positive and Gram-negative bacteria, as well as viruses and fungi. Chest x-rays are used to confirm a suspected diagnosis of pneumonia. Sputum (mucus from the respiratory tract) sometimes, but not always, provides the identity of the culprit microbe.

Antibiotics are generally started before the precise bacterial cause of the pneumonia has been determined. The antibiotic selected for initial use is generally one that is active against a wide range of bacteria, called a broad-spectrum antibiotic. Many such drugs (e.g., cephalosporins, penicillins) are available and effective for treating bacterial pneumonia.

Pneumonia may be picked up in the community or during a period of hospitalization.

Pneumococcal vaccine (Pneumovax 23, PnuiMmune 23) should be given in patients 65 or older that have a chronic disease (e.g. asthma, diabetes), or that live in nursing homes.

Community-Acquired Pneumonia

Streptococcus pneumoniae (a.k.a. *pneumococcus*), a Gram-positive bacterium, accounts for 70 percent of all bacterial causes of pneumonia in the United States. Other causes include *Hemophilis influenzae* and *Mycobacterium tuberculosis*.

Patients are generally treated orally with erythromycin-like or quinolone-class drugs.

Hospital-Acquired Pneumonia

It is not uncommon for patients to pick up pneumonia during the course of a hospitalization for other conditions. This most commonly occurs when the patient has been placed on a mechanical ventilator.

Hospital-acquired pneumonia is far more difficult to treat because the patient is often debilitated by another medical condition. Moreover, the Gram-positive and Gram-negative bacteria that cause pneumonia in this setting have often developed resistance to commonly used, and often safer, antibiotics. These include the Gram-positive bacterium *Staphlococcus aureus*.

Of the several Gram-negative microbes, the most common are *Klebsiella pneumoniae* and *Pseudomonas aeruginosa*. Infections caused by these microbes tend to progress rapidly, are very severe, and have a high death rate.

Hospital-acquired pneumonia is usually treated with combinations of antibiotics from the aminoglycoside, cephalosporin, quinolones, and penicillin classes.

Pneumonia in Infants and Children

In young patients, pneumonia is caused by both bacteria and viruses, with viruses being the more common cause. As mentioned previously, with the use of a vaccine to prevent *Hemophilus influenzae*, this microbe is no longer an important cause of pneumonia.

Skin Infections

Although our skin comes in regular contact with bacteria and other microbes, and these microbes live on our skin, we rarely develop skin infections. Susceptibility to bacterial skin infections increases as the result of injury to the skin; conditions such as HIV-AIDS, which reduce our immune defenses; and diabetes.

These infections are often on the skin surface and can be easily managed with an OTC antibiotic ointment. Others involving deep tissues and leading to body-wide infections may be life threatening.

OTC Alternatives

OTC first-aid antibiotics are available to treat minor cuts, wounds, scrapes, and burns. Among the ingredients found to be safe and effective after application to the skin are bacitracin, neomycin, polymyxin B, and tetracycline. Most products contain a combination of ingredients. If healing doesn't occur within five days, a doctor should be consulted.

Common bacterial skin infections include folliculitis, abscesses, and carbuncles; impetigo; cellulitis; and necrotizing cellulitis.

Folliculitis, Abscesses, and Carbuncles

All three skin conditions are pus-filled infections of the hair follicles that are commonly caused by *Staphyloccus aureus*, a Gram-positive microbe.

- **Folliculitis.** The infection remains on the skin surface. It is most often seen on the scalp, on the face of bearded men, on legs of women who shave, and on the eyelids in the form of a stye. The affected areas are reddened and may be only slightly tender and may itch.

- **Abscesses (also called boils, furuncles).** These are infections that travel down single hair follicles into deeper layers of the skin. The pus-filled lesion is deep, firm, red, and painful, and may rupture if not treated.

- **Carbuncles.** These are infections involving a number of hair follicles that are connected beneath the skin and that may spread to other tissues. They are commonly found on the back of the neck and on the upper regions of the back. The individual often has fever and chills and feels ill.

Folliculitis can be treated with warm compresses and, if necessary, the topical application of clindamycin, eythromycin (both available as generic products), or mupirocin. More severe cases of abscesses and carbuncles are treated with oral doses of clindamycin or dicloxacillin for 7 to 10 days.

Impetigo

Impetigo is a superficial skin infection caused by *Staphylococcus aureus* or *Staphylococcus pyogenes*. The lesions start as small red spots that expand into vesicles filled with an amber-colored fluid. After bursting, the discharge dries and forms a yellow crust. This itchy condition most commonly occurs in children. It may be spread by contact with the lesion to the individual or to others.

Impetigo can be treated topically with mupirocin or erythromycin. To prevent complications, such as cellulitis, more severe cases are treated with oral dicloxacillin or with cephalexin or cefadroxil. Penicillin- and cephalosporin-allergic individuals can be treated with clindamycin.

Cellulitis

Cellulitis is a potentially dangerous condition in which the infection can spread from under the skin into the bloodstream. Commonly seen on the legs, the lesions tend to be red and swollen, and are hot and painful. The individual often has fever, chills, and feels ill.

This condition can occur after a wound, superficial skin infection, or surgery. It sometimes arises in the absence of broken skin in individuals who have impaired immune function. Cellulitis is commonly caused by *Streptococcus*, *Staphylococcus aureus*, or *Staphylococcus pyogenes*, but it's not uncommon to be caused by multiple microbes.

Drug treatment is intended to rapidly eliminate the infection and prevent its spread to other parts of the body. The choice of antibiotics is based on the identified or suspected microbes. Depending on the severity of the condition, drugs may be given by mouth or intravenously.

The antibiotics given for cellulitis include the following:

- Penicillins, such as dicloxacillin, nafcillin

- Cephalosporins, such as cefaclor, cefuroxime, cefoxitin

- Aminoglycosides, such as gentamicin

- Quinolone, such as ciprofloxacin

Necrotizing Cellulitis

Popularized in the press as a "flesh-eating" disease, this rare condition starts off looking like cellulitis. Early on, the affected area is hot, swollen, red, and painful. Rapidly the area becomes purple and, as tissues die, they blacken. Patients experience fever, shock, a drop in blood pressure, and organs fail. Gas bubbles, called gas gangrene, may be present under the skin. In the absence of immediate treatment, the mortality rate ranges from 20 to 50 percent.

Treatment involves the surgical removal of dead tissues and the intravenous injection of multiple antibiotics that are capable of combating a wide range of different bacteria. These include the drugs used to treat cellulitis.

Urinary Tract Infections

The major function of our kidneys is to filter the blood and eliminate waste materials in the urine. Urine travels from the kidney to the bladder through a tube called the ureter. Urine is stored in the bladder before it is eliminated from the body, passing through the urethra.

Urinary tract infections (UTIs) are among the most common of all infections and may involve any of the organs of the urinary tract. These include infections of the kidney, bladder, and urethra.

By far the most common infections are caused by Gram-negative bacilli, most often by *Escherichia coli*. UTIs may also be caused by viruses and fungi. A number of classes of antibacterial drugs are used to treat UTIs. These include sulfa drugs, penicillins, cephalosporins, tetracyclines, quinolones, and carbapenems. These same medicines are used for infections in other parts of the body. Nitrofurantoin and other urinary tract antiseptics are only used for the treatment of UTIs. The drug chosen depends on the identity of the disease-causing bacteria.

Did You Know That ...?

The kidneys not only eliminate waste materials from the body—including drugs—they also play an important role in regulating blood pressure. The kidneys also secrete a hormone that stimulates the manufacture of red blood cells by the bone marrow and another that is involved in maintaining the health of bones.

Some medicines are used to treat UTIs and prevent recurrent infections, a common problem in women. Depending on the nature and severity of the UTI, oral treatment may be required for 3 to 14 days.

Kidney Infections

Kidney infections (sometimes called pyelonephritis) may result from bacteria arising from other parts of the body or by traveling up from the urethra. The risk of this latter cause increases when the normal outward flow of urine is blocked, as might occur during pregnancy.

Common symptoms of a kidney infection are chills, fever, lower-back pain, nausea, vomiting, and frequent and painful urination.

Mild-to-moderate cases are treated with drugs taken by mouth for 7 to 14 days. Severe cases require hospitalization and are treated with intravenous antibacterials for several days, followed by oral medication.

Bladder Infection

Bladder infections (also called cystitis) are usually seen in women of childbearing age and are often recurring. They are normally associated with sexual intercourse. Common symptoms include frequent urination, the urgent need to urinate, and a painful or burning sensation when urinating.

Acute cases are generally treated for three days with an oral antibacterial drug, although a single dose may be used. Some doctors prefer treating complicated cases for 7 to 10 days. Individuals with recurring bladder infections sometimes take low doses of nitrofurantoin or trimethoprim-sulfamethoxazole daily or several times weekly on an ongoing basis.

Urethral Infection

Infection of the urethra (a.k.a. urethritis) is most often seen in women and is a sexually transmitted disease. Common symptoms in women include the frequent and urgent need to urinate and a painful sensation when urinating. In addition to these symptoms, a discharge containing pus or mucus is often seen in men.

A number of different bacteria, as well as viruses and fungi, can cause these infections. Treatment is based on the identity of the microbe.

Antibacterial Drugs

More than six dozen different drugs are used to combat bacterial infections, and they fall into about 10 different classes. Each of these classes has its own distinct characteristics.

Selection of Antibacterial Drug

Your doctor takes the following factors into account when selecting an antibacterial drug for your infection:

- ◆ **Cause of infection.** On the basis of the patient's signs and symptoms and the results of laboratory tests, the doctor attempts to determine the cause of the infection. If the germ is a bacterium, which one? Because antibacterial drugs don't work against viruses, they shouldn't be prescribed.

- ◆ **Bacterial sensitivity to drug.** The doctor selects the drug class and the specific drug that works best against the bacteria. If multiple microbes are causing the infection, particularly a life-threatening infection, a combination of drugs may be needed.

Maximizing Your Medicine

Although experts generally discourage prescribing a combination of antibacterial medicines, there are important exceptions:

◆ When the specific cause of a life-threatening infection (such as meningitis) has not or cannot be determined

◆ To treat infections caused by multiple microbes

◆ To prevent the development of microbial resistance

◆ To reduce doses of each drug, and thereby reduce drug toxicity

---

◆ **Patient factors.** Use of some drugs during pregnancy or when nursing may expose the fetus or newborn to its potentially harmful effects. Patients allergic to one antibiotic will likely be also allergic to all other members of the same antibiotic class (such as to all penicillins). Moreover, they may also be allergic to closely related antibiotics (such as the cephalosporins). Some drugs are mainly eliminated from the body by the kidneys. This could be a problem for individuals with reduced kidney function.

Many of these drugs are very expensive. Check with your doctor or pharmacist to see whether the same or a comparable drug is available as a generically equivalent product.

◆ **How the drug is given.** When the patient is treated at home, an oral medicine is generally prescribed. If a severe infection requires hospitalization, the patient is often started on intravenous therapy for several days. After the infection is brought under control and the patient is "out of the woods," a longer period of oral drug use may follow.

Maximizing Your Medicine

The doctor prescribes an antibiotic for a time period sufficiently long (e.g., 7 to 10 days) to eradicate the microbe from the body and reduce the odds that microbial resistance will develop to the drug. If you stop taking the medicine when you feel better, but before the germs have been eradicated, you face the risk of a relapse, which may be far worse than the original infection.

Antibiotic Resistance

One of the greatest challenges facing doctors and their patients is the development of microbial resistance to antibiotics.

When we talk about resistance, we are interested in the development of resistance by microbes that were once sensitive to that antibiotic. With resistance, the drug becomes progressively less effective.

Higher doses must be used to fight the injection, which increases the patient's exposure to the adverse effects of the medicine. In time, the drug may fail to work at all. This may necessitate the use of more powerful, potentially harmful, and expensive alternatives.

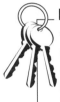

Did You Know That ...?

When exposed to an antibiotic, most susceptible microbes die, but a few survive. Resistance develops because advantageous genetic differences in the surviving microbes permit them to thrive and reproduce in an adverse environment (such as in the presence of an antibiotic). The development of microbial resistance exemplifies Darwin's law of natural selection—the survival of the fittest.

Classes of Antibacterial Medicines

In this section, we talk about the general properties of the most important classes of antibacterial medicines. These classes include aminoglycosides, carbapenems, cephalosporins, eythromycins, penicillins, quinolones, sulfas, tetracyclines, and the urinary tract antiseptics.

Antibacterial drugs work in several ways to combat microbes:

- ◆ Prevention of the manufacture of the cell wall of bacteria, a structure essential for its survival: penicillins, cephalosporins, carbapenems

- ◆ Interference with manufacture of proteins required for survival, growth, and reproduction: tetracyclines, erythromycins

- ◆ Interference with manufacture of DNA, needed for bacterial cell reproduction: quinolones

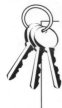

> **Did You Know That ...?**
>
> For an antimicrobial drug to be useful, it must be more harmful to the disease-causing microbe than the patient. This has been aptly called "selective toxicity." For this to occur, there must be some differences between the microbe and the patient. Penicillin, for example, prevents the manufacture of cell walls by bacteria. Animals lack cell walls and so are not harmed.

Aminoglycosides

Aminoglycosides, such as gentamicin, are antibiotics that work against only Gram-negative bacteria. Common examples of such bacteria include Escherichia coli and Psudomonas aeruginosa. These bacteria might be responsible for hospital-acquired pneumonia, cellulitis, and severe urinary tract infections.

Most generic aminoglycosides end in "mycin" or "micin."

Because aminoglycosides do not enter the blood after being taken by mouth, they must be given by intravenous or intramuscular injection. Their use is primarily limited to a hospital setting. Some are also applied topically to the eyes to treat conjunctivitis.

Aminoglycosides can cause significant toxicity to the kidneys and to the inner ear, causing permanent hearing loss and dizziness. The dosage must be reduced or doses must be given less frequently to patients with impaired kidney function.

The risk of kidney toxicity is increased when aminoglycosides are used with other drugs capable of causing kidney damage, such as amphotericin B, cephalosporins, polymyxins, and vancomycin.

The risk of damage to the inner ear is increased when used with ethacrynic acid.

Carbapenems

Imipenem and related carbapenems are active against a wide range of Gram-positive and Gram-negative bacteria that cause infections of the respiratory tract, urinary tract, abdominal area, bone, skin, and blood. They are particularly useful in treating serious infections that are caused by multiple microbes or where the specific microbe has not been identified.

Generic versions of carbapenems have names ending in "penem."

> **Warning!**
>
> Patients allergic to penicillins and cephalosporins may also be allergic to carbapenems.

These drugs do not enter the blood after being taken by mouth. Their use is primarily in a hospital setting because they must be given by intravenous or intramuscular injection.

Side effects are few and include nausea and vomiting. Seizures rarely occur.

Cephalosporins

Cephalosporins are the most widely used class of antibiotics. As a group, they are effective against a very wide range of Gram-positive and Gram-negative bacteria, cause relatively little toxicity, and can be given by mouth or injection.

Because these drugs are often given to children, palatable, fruit-flavored oral, liquid dosage forms are available.

Name hint: most generic names start with "cef" or "ceph."

Over the years, more than 20 cephalosporins have appeared on the market, and their activity against different microbes has expanded. These have been differentiated into one of four "generations," based on when they were introduced and their antimicrobial activity:

- **First generation (such as cephalothin).** Primarily active against Gram-positive bacteria (staphylococci, streptococci), with little activity against Gram-negative microbes. Common uses: skin infections and given prior to surgery to prevent infections.

- **Second generation (such as cefuroxime).** Primarily active against Gram-negative bacteria, with less effectiveness against Gram-positive microbes. Common uses: ear, sinus, respiratory tract, and abdominal infections.

- **Third generation (such as cefotaxime).** Highly active against Gram-negative bacteria but also effective against Gram-positive microbes. Useful in urinary tract infections.

- **Fourth generation (such as cefepime).** Even more highly active against Gram-negative bacteria but also effective against Gram-positive microbes.

The first- and second-generation drugs are typically backups to preferred drugs, whereas the third- and fourth-generation drugs are first-choice selections in some cases. Unlike first- and second-generation drugs, third- and fourth-generation drugs enter the nervous system and are effective against such infections as meningitis.

In general, cephalosporins are among the safest antimicrobial medicines, with diarrhea a common side effect.

Some people develop allergic reactions to cephalosporins, including a rash that develops after several days. Cephalosporins chemically resemble penicillin, and the rashes are similar to that produced by penicillin. If difficulties in breathing are experienced when taking these drugs, the doctor should be contacted immediately.

Warning!

About 10 percent of penicillin-allergic patients may also be allergic to cephalosporins. Individuals exhibiting mild penicillin-allergic reactions can probably use cephalosporins safely. Those with a history of severe penicillin-allergic reactions should never be given cephalosporins.

The effects of cephalosporins are prolonged by probenecid.

The specific cephalosporins—cefmetazole, cefoperazone, and cefotexan—produce significant alcohol intolerance. Alcohol should not be taken with these drugs. These same medicines increase bleeding tendencies, in particular, when they are used with blood thinners and nonsteroidal anti-inflammatory drugs (NSAIDs) such as aspirin.

Erythromycins

Erythromycin-like drugs (a.k.a. macrolides) act against the same types of bacteria as penicillin and are a safe alternative for patients who are allergic to penicillin. These include most Gram-positive and some Gram-negative bacteria. Erythromycins are used as the first-choice medicines for the treatment of such infectious diseases as whooping cough, diphtheria, and Legionnaire's disease.

Most generic erythromycin-like drugs have names ending in "mycin."

Erythromycins are best taken on an empty stomach (one hour before meals or two hours after) with a full glass of water.

Common side effects include indigestion, nausea, vomiting, and diarrhea. These adverse effects can be minimized by taking the drug with meals.

Individuals should notify their doctor if they have severe abdominal pain, yellow coloration of the eyes or skin, or dark urine. These are signs of drug-caused liver toxicity. Individuals with a history of liver disease should not take these drugs.

Penicillins

Penicillins were the first class of antibiotics to be discovered and continue to be among the most effective antibiotics and least toxic of all medicines.

The early penicillins were primarily active against Gram-positive cocci, such as Steptococci; these are called the "narrow-spectrum" penicillins. Derivatives have been prepared over the years that are active against both Gram-positive and particularly Gram-negative microbes; these are called "broad-spectrum" penicillins.

The many infectious diseases treated with penicillins include pneumonia, meningitis, tetanus, anthrax, gas gangrene, and syphilis. It is also used in combination with other antibiotics.

Generic penicillins have names ending in "cillin."

Depending on the penicillin derivative, of which there are more than 10, they can be taken by mouth or by intramuscular or intravenous injection.

Whereas penicillins are very safe drugs, their use poses a risk of causing an allergic reaction. Various sources report that anywhere from 1 to 10 percent of all individuals are penicillin allergic, although 2 percent may be closer to the mark.

Warning!

If you are allergic to penicillin, you should wear a bracelet or have another form of identification that alerts health-care workers of your condition. All doctors, dentists, pharmacists, and nurses with whom you interact should be notified of your allergy, and this should be entered on the medical records they maintain for you.

Signs of allergic response may vary in severity from a slight rash to a rare but life-threatening inability to breathe (caused by a constriction of airway passages) and a sudden drop in blood pressure. In such cases, emergency treatment involves an injection of epinephrine, in addition to mechanical support of breathing.

Individuals allergic to one penicillin are likely to be allergic to all other penicillins. If a severe penicillin-allergic reaction is experienced, no penicillin-, cephalosporin-, or carbapenem-like drugs should be taken.

Did You Know That ...?

As is true with all other allergic reactions to drugs, there is no relationship between the drug dose and the severity of the allergic reaction. For an allergic reaction to occur, at least one prior exposure to the drug is required.

Quinolones

Quinolones, such as ciprofloxacin, are active by mouth or injection against a wide range of Gram-positive and Gram-negative bacteria.

These drugs are primarily used for the treatment of infections caused by Gram-negative bacteria involving the urinary tract, prostate gland, respiratory tract, skin, and bones. They are also used to treat gonorrhea, anthrax, and respiratory infections caused by *Pseudomonas aeruginosa* in individuals with cystic fibrosis.

Generic quinolones usually have names ending in "floxacin."

Side effects are mild and infrequent and include nausea, vomiting, and diarrhea, as well as dizziness and nervousness.

On rare occasions, quinolones cause rupture of the tendons. Most often this involves the Achilles tendon and occurs in children under 18. Drug use should be discontinued at the first sign of pain or inflammation of the tendon.

The absorption of quinolones into the blood is reduced by antacids containing aluminum or magnesium, and by iron and zinc salts, and milk and other dairy products. This interaction may result in a reduction in their antibacterial effectiveness.

Quinolones can increase blood levels and the intensity of the effects of theophylline and the blood thinner warfarin. To avoid the risk of adverse effects, the doses of these drugs may have to be reduced.

Sulfa Drugs

The sulfa drugs (a.k.a. sulfonamides) appeared in the mid-1930s and were the first medicines used for the treatment of bacterial infections. Once widely used, sulfa drugs have been largely replaced by safer and less-toxic antibiotics.

Orally active sulfas, in particular sulfisoxazole, are used to treat urinary tract infections. Topical sulfas are used to treat eye infections (sulfacetamide) and infections associated with burns (silver sulfadiazine).

Generic sulfa drugs usually begin with "sulfa."

Sulfa drugs cause many side effects, which have contributed to their loss of popularity. These include hypersensitivity disorders, including skin rash and excessive sensitivity to sun, and the Stevens-Johnson syndrome, a life-threatening skin disorder. Individuals with a history of sulfa allergies should avoid using these drugs.

Other problems include red blood cell destruction (a.k.a. hemolytic anemia) and the deposition of bilirubin in the brains of newborns, causing brain damage (a.k.a. kernicterus).

Sulfamethoxazole in combination with the antibacterial drug trimethoprim (TMP-SMZ) is used around the world. Uses include urinary tract infections; ear infections; gastrointestinal infections caused by Gram-negative bacteria; and Pneumocystitis carinii infections, a pneumonia often seen in AIDS patients.

The most common side effects with TMP-SMZ are nausea, vomiting, and skin rash. Less commonly seen are the side effects caused by sulfa drugs when used alone.

Tetracyclines

The tetracyclines, such as doxycycline, are active against a very wide range of microbes including Gram-positive and Gram-negative microbes, *Rickettsia*, *Spirochetes*, *Chlamydia*, *Mycoplasma*, and *Heliobacter pylori*. Their widespread use in the past has led to the development of bacterial resistance, and they are now relegated to being backup drugs for many conditions. All tetracyclines are active orally but can also be given by injection.

Tetracyclines continue to be the first-choice medicines for the treatment of the following:

- *Richettsial disorders*, including Rocky Mountain spotted fever and typhus fever
- *Chlamydia infections* such as *trachoma* and selected sexually transmitted diseases
- *Cholera* and *brucellosis*
- *Mycoplasma pneumoniae*-caused pneumonia, the most common pneumonia in people ages 5 to 35
- Lyme disease and ehrlichioses, tick-borne diseases
- *Heliobacter pylori*, a stomach-dwelling bacterium that is a major cause of peptic ulcer disease
- Severe acne

Generic names of tetracyclines end in "cycline."

Gastrointestinal disturbances are the most common side effect, and these include indigestion, nausea, and diarrhea, which can be potentially dangerous.

Tetracyclines readily bind to calcium in newly formed teeth, including those of the fetus. This can lead to yellow-brown discoloration of teeth. If given to children, there is the risk of permanent tooth discoloration. Tetracyclines are not recommended for children under the age of 8.

Warning!

Tetracyclines should never be taken if they are outdated, have changed color or taste, look different, or if they have been stored in a setting that is too warm or too damp. Such medication should be discarded. Under such circumstances, tetracyclines can decompose into chemicals that may cause serious adverse effects, including kidney damage.

Tetracyclines can impair liver function, particularly when high doses are given intravenously to pregnant women. These drugs may worsen kidney function, particularly in individuals with a history of kidney disease.

These drugs increase sensitivity to the sun, with a greater risk of severe sunburn. Individuals, particularly those with fair skin, taking tetracyclines should limit their exposure to sun, use sunscreen, and wear protective clothing.

Tetracyclines bind to metals such as calcium, magnesium, aluminum, and iron, which interfere with their absorption into the bloodstream. Antibiotic levels in the blood are reduced, reducing their antibacterial effectiveness. Calcium supplements, most antacids, and iron supplements should be taken one hour before or two hours after tetracyclines.

Milk and other calcium-rich dairy products interfere with tetracycline absorption and lower their blood levels. Food interferes with the absorption of all tetracyclines, except doxycycline and minocycline. Other tetracyclines should be taken one hour before or two hours after meals and with a full glass of water.

Urinary Tract Antiseptics

After being taken by mouth, urinary antiseptics concentrate in the urine. Their concentrations in the blood are not sufficiently high to treat systemic infections.

Nitrofurantoin is used to treat active urinary tract infections and on a continuous basis to prevent the recurrence of such infections. Methenamine is only used to prevent infections. Neither drug is useful for the treatment of kidney infections.

The Least You Need to Know

♦ Antibacterial drug classes include the aminoglycosides (e.g., gentamicin), carbapenems (imipenem), cephalosporins (cefotaxime), erythromycins (a.k.a. macrolides such as erythromycin), penicillins (ampicillin), quinolones (ciprofloxacin), sulfa drugs (sulfamethoxazole), and tetracyclines (doxycycline).

♦ Some antibiotics treat infections caused by a limited number of microbes ("narrow-spectrum" antibiotics, such as the aminoglycosides), whereas others are effective against a wide range of different microbes ("broad-spectrum" antibiotics, such as tetracyclines and some cephalosporins and penicillins).

♦ The development of microbial resistance to antibiotics is the greatest challenge in the successful treatment of infectious diseases.

Drugs Used to Treat Bacterial Infections

Generic Name	Trade Name	How Taken: Oral (O) Topical (T) Injection (I)	Generic Available
Aminoglycosides ("micin" or "mycin" endings)			
Amikacin	Amikin	I	Yes
Gentamicin	Garamycin	I/T	Yes
Kanamycin	Kantrex	I/O	Yes
Netilmicin	Netromycin	I	No
Tobramycin	Nebcin	I/T	Yes
Carbapenems ("penem" endings)			
Ertapenem	Invanz	I	No
Imipenem + cilastatin	Primaxin	I	No
Meropenem	Merrem	I	No
Cephalosporins (start with "cef" or "ceph")			
First Generation			
Cefadroxil	Duricef, Ultracef	O	Yes
Cefazolin	Ancef	I	Yes
Cephalexin	Keflex	O	Yes
Cephradine	Velosef	I/O	Yes

continues

Drugs Used to Treat Bacterial Infections   (continued)

Generic Name	Trade Name	How Taken: Oral (O) Topical (T) Injection (I)	Generic Available
Cephalosporins (start with "cef" or "ceph")			
Second Generation			
Cefaclor	Ceclor	O	Yes
Cefamandole	Mandol	I	No
Cefmetazole	Zefazone	I	No
Cefonicid	Monocid	I	No
Cefotetan	Cefotan	I	No
Cefoxitin	Mefoxin	I	No
Cefprozil	Cefzil	O	No
Cefuroxime	Kufurox, Zinacef	I/O	Yes
Laracarbef	Lorabid	O	No
Third Generation			
Cefixime	Suprax	O	No
Cefdinir	Cefdinir	O	No
Cefditoren	Spectracef	O	No
Cefoperazone	Cefobid	I	No
Cefotaxime	Claforan	I	No
Cefpodoxime	Vantin	O	No
Ceftazidime	Fortaz, Tazicef, Tazidime	I	No
Ceftibuten	Cedax	O	No
Ceftizoxime	Cefizox	I	No
Ceftriaxone	Rocephin	I	No
Fourth Generation			
Cefepime	Maxipine	I	No
Erythromycins (Macrolides) ("mycin" endings)			
Azithromycin	Zithromax	I/O	Yes
Clarithromycin	Biaxin	O	No
Dirithromycin	Dynabac	O	No
Erythromycin	E-Mycin, Ery-Tab, Erythrocin, Ilosone	I/O/T	Yes

Generic Name	Trade Name	How Taken: Oral (O) Topical (T) Injection (I)	Generic Available
Penicillins ("cillin" endings)			
Narrow-Spectrum			
Cloxacillin	Cloxapen	O	
Dicloxacillin	Dycill, Dynapen Pathocil	O	Yes
Nafcillin	Unipen	I/O	Yes
Oxacillin	Bactocil	I	Yes
Penicillin G	Bicillin, Wycillin	I	Yes
Penicillin V	Veetids	O	Yes
Broad-Spectrum			
Ampicillin	Principen	I/O	Yes
Amoxicillin	Amoxil, Trimox	O	Yes
Amoxicillin + clavulanate	Augmentin	O	Yes
Carbenicillin	Geocillin	O	No
Piperacillin	Pipracil	I	Yes
Piperacillin + tazobactam	Zosyn	I	No
Ticarcillin	Ticar	I	No
Ticarcillin + clavulanate	Timentin	I	No
Quinolones ("floxacin")			
Ciprofloxacin	Cipro	I/O	Yes
Gatifloxacin	Tequin	I/O	No
Levofloxacin	Levaquin	I/O/T	No
Lomefloxacin	Maxaquin	O	No
Moxifloxacin	Avelox	I/O	No
Norfloxacin	Noroxin	O/T	No
Ofloxacin	Floxin	I/O/T	No
Trovafloxacin + alatrofloxacin	Trovan	I/O	No

continues

Drugs Used to Treat Bacterial Infections   (continued)

Generic Name	Trade Name	How Taken: Oral (O) Topical (T) Injection (I)	Generic Available
Sulfa Drugs (Sulfonamides) (start with "sulfa")			
Mafenide	Sulfamylon	T	Yes
Sulfacetamide	Sodium sulamyd	T	Yes
Sulfamethizole	Thiosulfil	O	No
Sulfamethoxazole	Gantanol	O	Yes
Sulfasalazine	Azulfidine	O	Yes
Sulfisoxazole	Gantrisin	O/T	Yes
Trimethoprim + sulfisoxazole, [Co-Trimoxazole, TMP-SMZ]	Bactrim, Septra	I/O	Yes
Tetracyclines ("cycline" endings)			
Demeclocycline	Declomycin	O	Yes
Doxycycline	Vibramycin	I/O	Yes
Minocycline	Minocin	I/O	Yes
Oxytetracycline	Terramycin	I	Yes
Tetracycline	Sumycin	O	Yes
Urinary Tract Antiseptics			
Cinoxacin	Cinobac	O	Yes
Fosfomycin	Monurol	O	No
Methenamine	Mandelamine	O	Yes
Nalidixic acid	NegGram	O	No
Nitrofurantoin	Furadantin, Macrodantin	O	Yes
Miscellaneous Antibacterial Drugs			
Aztreonam	Azactam	I	No
Chloramphenicol	Chloromycetin	I/O/T	Yes
Clindamycin	Cleocin	I/O/T	Yes
Linezolid	Zyvox	I/O	No
Metronidazole	Flagyl	I/O	Yes
Mupirocin	Bactroban	T	No
Vancomycin	Vancocin	I/O	Yes

Bipolar Disorder

Bipolar disorder is characterized by recurrent fluctuations in mood, energy level, and behavioral symptoms. Also called manic-depressive disorder, sufferers experience alternating episodes of mania and depression. The disease has a strong genetic predisposition.

During the manic phase, the mood is extremely elevated (called euphoria). Ideas rapidly come and go, talk is apparently never-ending, and energy levels are high, with no need to sleep. The individual is larger than life, has extreme self-confidence, and may engage in risk-taking behavior. In severe cases, schizophrenic symptoms may be present, with delusions and hallucinations.

The manic phase is followed by a depressive phase, in which the patient has a sad mood, experiences sleep disturbances and decreased energy, among other things.

Bipolar disorder has many variations. These differ based on the severity of the episode and how often the individual cycles between moods. Some individuals simultaneously experience mixed symptoms of mania and depression.

Drug Treatment of Bipolar Disorder: An Overview

Treatment of bipolar disorder has two primary objectives:

♦ Treatment of the immediate, or acute, condition. The immediate goal is to control the current mood, e.g., calm the patients so that they don't harm themselves or others.

♦ Maintenance therapy for preventing or reducing the severity of future manic-depressive episodes.

Lithium, divalproex, and lamotrigine have been shown effective for both acute treatment of bipolar disorder and to prevent mood swings. How they work is not clear. A number of antiseizure (such as carbamazepine) and antipsychotic drugs are used as backups. Combinations of drugs are often used, and psychotherapy is used with drugs.

Lithium

Lithium is the drug of choice for both acute and maintenance therapy. Feelings of extreme mood elevation and increased activity lessen within five to seven days after oral lithium. Maximum benefits do not occur for several weeks.

Until lithium takes hold, severely agitated patients may be given a benzodiazepine anti-anxiety drug. Severe behavioral symptoms are treated with antipsychotic drugs.

Lithium cautions:

- Toxic effects. Increasing blood levels of lithium are linked to toxicity. Early signs include nausea, vomiting, diarrhea, hand tremors, tired feeling, mental dullness, and excessive urination. Higher levels cause gross tremors, lack of coordination, and seizures.

> **Maximizing Your Medicine**
>
> Lithium doses are individualized and adjusted to maintain ideal blood levels. If levels are too high, toxicity results. Too low, lithium won't provide maximum benefits. Blood levels of lithium should be checked periodically until the most effective dose is determined.

- Long-term lithium use can depress thyroid function and can cause enlargement of the thyroid gland (goiter).

- Do not use if pregnant or nursing.

- Use with caution. Can cause toxicity in high doses if you have kidney or severe heart disease. Water pills (diuretics) increase the risk of lithium toxicity.

Divalproex

Divalproex (valproate) is used alone or in combination with lithium for acute and maintenance bipolar therapy. It may be better than lithium for individuals who rapidly cycle between mania and depression and those having mixed symptoms of both mania and depression.

Divalproex is also used to treat epilepsy and migraine.

Divalproex cautions:

- **Common side effects.** Loss of appetite, nausea, indigestion, mild diarrhea. With long-term treatment, weight gain may occur. Unlike lithium, divalproex does not cause severe toxicity when high doses are taken.

- **Do not take.** History of liver disease.

◆ **Use with caution.** If pregnant, because of potential birth defects. Risk may be reduced by taking folic acid. Pregnant women should discuss drug risks versus benefits of the drug with their doctors.

Lamotrigine

Originally used as an antiseizure drug, lamotrigine is used for bipolar disorder, in particular for patients showing strong depression.

Lamotrigine cautions:

◆ **Common side effects.** Headache, nausea, dizziness, drowsiness.

◆ **Caution.** May cause a potentially life-threatening skin rash. If a rash appears, it may not be possible to predict which are not serious and which are life-threatening. Lamotrigine should be discontinued at the first sign of a rash, unless it is certain that the rash is not caused by the drug.

The Least You Need to Know

◆ Drug treatment of bipolar disorder is intended to control the acute condition and prevent wide mood swings of mania and depression.

◆ Lithium, divalproex, and lamotrigine have been shown to effectively control and prevent these mood disorders.

Drugs Used for Bipolar Disorder

Generic Name	Trade Name	Generic Available
Lithium carbonate	Eskalith, Lithobid	Yes
Carbamazepine	Tegretol	Yes
Divalproex (valproate)	Depakote	No
Lamotrigine	Lamictal	No

Bladder Incontinence

Bladder incontinence, also called urinary incontinence, is the inability to control urination. Some of the leading causes of bladder incontinence are diseases, injuries, pregnancy and childbirth, menopause, as a complication of prostate surgery, and drugs. Incontinence mostly affects elderly individuals, and is more common in women than men.

To better understand this condition, let's briefly consider how the urinary tract works. Urine is produced by the kidneys and stored in the bladder. It is eliminated from the body through the urethra, a tube running from the bottom of the bladder. The process of urination is controlled by muscles called sphincters. When the sphincters contract, urine does not flow. When they relax, urine passes.

Types of Incontinence

There are several types of incontinence, two of the most common being stress incontinence and urge incontinence. Mixed incontinence is a combination of both.

- ◆ Stress incontinence is most common in women under 60 and in men who have had prostate surgery. Here, the sphincter does not completely contract, and small amounts of urine may be lost during exercise, coughing, laughing, or sneezing. Pelvic muscle exercises and prescription creams containing estrogen applied to the vagina or oral estrogens are often helpful for use by women after menopause. Specific drug treatments are not available to treat stress incontinence.

- ◆ Urge incontinence (also known as bladder overactivity) is most common in older individuals or those with Parkinson's disease or stroke patients. There is a sudden and intense urge to urinate and urination occurs frequently, including at nighttime. It is caused by an unexpected and unintended contraction of the bladder. Atropine-like drugs relax the bladder, preventing its contraction, and are effective in treating urge incontinence.

Atropine-Like Drugs

Drugs with atropine-like effects, such as oxybutynin, are the most effective drugs available for the management of urge incontinence. Oxybutynin is available as an immediate-release (IR) tablet and syrup, which is taken three times a day; an extended-release (XL) tablet taken once daily; and a transdermal or skin patch (TDS), applied twice weekly.

Extended-release oxybutynin is more effective than immediate-release in reducing incontinence episodes and it has fewer side effects.

Oxybutynin appears to be more effective than tolterodine for urge incontinence, with extended-release tolterodine working better than the immediate-release product. The most common side effect with these drugs is dry mouth, which may be so severe that the user can't speak or swallow. Other effects include blurred vision, constipation, indigestion, headache, and drowsiness.

> **Maximizing Your Medicine**
>
> Extended-release tablets (XL) continuously release the medication at a controlled rate over a 24-hour period. They should be swallowed whole and not chewed, crushed, or divided. The medication is contained in a tablet-like shell that is not absorbed by the body and is eliminated in the stool.

The Least You Need to Know

- Some of the leading causes of bladder incontinence are diseases, injuries, pregnancy and childbirth, menopause, as a complication of prostate surgery, and drugs.

- Urge incontinence, most common in the elderly, is effectively treated with atropine-like drugs, such as oxybutynin.

- Stress incontinence is most common in women under 60 and in men who have had prostate surgery.

Drugs Used for Urinary Incontinence

Generic Name	Trade Name	Generic Available
Oxybutynin	Ditropan	IR: Yes XL, TDS: No
Solifenancin	VESI care	No
Tolterodine	Detrol	No
Trospium	Sanctura	No

Blood-Clotting Conditions

Blood clotting prevents us from bleeding too much after an injury. However, when clots form abnormally within blood vessels, they may impede the flow of blood and cause potentially life-threatening consequences in the brain (stroke), in the heart (heart attack), in the lungs (thrombosis), and elsewhere in the body.

Did You Know That ...?

When you think about "thrombo," think blood clot. A thrombus is a blood clot present in a blood vessel. Thrombosis refers to the abnormal formation of such a clot. Thrombolytic drugs break down or dissolve such clots.

An embolus is a blood clot that forms in one location, then breaks away and blocks a blood vessel at another site, such as the lungs. The movement of that embolus in the blood is called embolism.

Let's take a quick look at the three stages by which the body acts to prevent blood loss:

1. A broken blood vessel constricts, reducing the loss of blood.

2. Platelets in the blood stick to each other and to proteins in the walls of injured blood vessels to form a platelet plug. For small wounds, this may be adequate to stem blood loss.

3. For larger wounds, the plug must be reinforced and strengthened. Fibers of a blood protein called fibrin are produced, then trap platelets, blood cells, and plasma to form a clot. Coagulation is the formation of a clot. Thrombin is needed for fibrin formation.

Blood-Clotting Medicines: An Overview

Two primary kinds of drugs are used for the treatment of abnormal blood-clotting conditions in the legs and lungs, and each works in a different way:

◆ Blood thinners or anticoagulants (such as warfarin and heparin) interfere with the coagulation of blood by preventing the formation of fibrin.

◆ Clot-dissolvers or fibrolytic drugs (such as alteplase [tPA] and streptokinase) promote the breakdown of fibrin, which causes the dissolution of the clot.

Blood Thinners (Anticoagulants)

Blood thinners, also called *anticoagulants*, are taken by mouth (warfarin) or by injection (heparin). Although they are both used to treat the same condition, they work in dramatically different ways.

def•i•ni•tion

Anticoagulants are commonly referred to as blood thinners, though this name is a bit deceiving. Anticoagulants don't actually thin the blood, nor do they dissolve clots that have been already formed. They do prevent clots from forming or becoming larger and, therefore, presenting a greater risk.

Oral Anticoagulants: Warfarin

Warfarin (Coumadin) is used on a chronic basis to prevent abnormal clot formation, in particular, in veins where blood flow tends to be slow. This may happen during prolonged periods of bed rest or extended plane flights. When they occur in the deep veins in the legs, the condition is called deep vein thrombosis (DVT). After such clots form, they may break away, and travel to and lodge themselves in such sites as the lungs (this is called a pulmonary embolism) where they block blood flow. This may lead to death of lung tissue and can be fatal.

Warfarin is also used on an ongoing basis to prevent clot formation in patients with artificial heart valves or abnormal heart rhythms (atrial fibrillation) when there is a high risk of stroke. Because warfarin's peak effects are not seen for days, it cannot be used to treat emergency problems; in these cases, heparin-like drugs are used.

Warfarin works by blocking the effects of vitamin K, a vitamin essential for the manufacture of clotting factors. Its effects may not be seen for up to several days after the drug has been started, and its effects continue for several days after the drug has been discontinued.

Maximizing Your Medicine

How much warfarin is required to balance clotting and excessive bleeding? If the dose is too low, the tendency for clot formation will continue. Too much drug, by contrast, increases the risk of bleeding, which can be life-threatening. Two measures are used to evaluate the degree of anticoagulation: the prothrombin test (PT) and the now-preferred international normalized ratio (INR). An INR of 2 to 3 is the usual target doctors seek to achieve.

Missed Doses

If a dose is missed, it should be taken as soon as possible, and the regular dosing schedule resumed. If the missed dose is not realized until the following day, forget the missed dose and don't double the next dose. Doubling the dose may increase the risk of bleeding. Just return to the regular dosing schedule.

Overdoses

Bleeding is the major problem caused by excessive doses of warfarin. Patients using anticoagulants should know the signs of overdoses and, if they appear, contact their doctor immediately.

These signs include bleeding from the gums when brushing teeth, sudden nosebleeds, skin bruising or purplish blotching of the skin, unusually heavy bleeding from cuts or wounds or during menstrual bleeding.

Signs of internal bleeding include abdominal or stomach pain or swelling; backaches; blood in the urine; bloody or tarry stools; coughing up or vomiting blood; constipation; severe and long-lasting headaches; joint pain, swelling, or stiffness.

Bleeding caused by excessive doses of warfarin can be stopped with vitamin K_1 (phytonadione), which can be taken by mouth or injection.

 Warning!

Make sure your doctor, dentist, and pharmacist know that you are taking warfarin. This drug should not be used for several days prior to elective surgical procedures. Carry or wear identification indicating that you are using warfarin. Consult your doctor or pharmacist before starting or stopping any other medicine.

Common Side Effects

Do not use warfarin if pregnant. It has been shown to cause bleeding in the fetus, resulting in deformities and even death.

In addition, warfarin should not be used by people with a vitamin K deficiency, liver disease, alcoholism, deficiency of platelets (thrombocytopenia), or uncontrollable bleeding. Warfarin should not be used during or immediately after surgery of the brain, spinal cord, or eye, or by patients having lumbar puncture (spinal tap) or regional anesthesia.

Use warfarin with great caution if you have gastrointestinal ulcers or severe high blood pressure.

Drug-Drug and Drug-Food Interactions

A large number of medicines—both prescription and OTC—may increase or decrease the effects of blood thinners. Check with your doctor or pharmacist before taking any new drugs or discontinuing old ones. These include prescription and OTC drugs and dietary supplements.

Drugs that may increase the effects of warfarin and increase the risk of bleeding include the following:

Acetaminophen

Alcohol

Antibiotics (oral)

Aspirin

Cimetidine

Clofibrate

Disulfiram

Heparin

Phenylbutazone

Sulfa drugs

Drugs that may decrease the effects of warfarin and increase the risk of clotting include the following:

Barbiturates

Cholestyramine

Ginseng

Green tea

Griseofulvin

Rifampin

St. John's wort

Vitamin K

Foods that may decrease the effects of warfarin and increase clotting risks include green, leafy vegetables that are rich in vitamin K.

Injectable Anticoagulants: Heparin-Like

Heparin and warfarin are different in several important ways. Heparin cannot be absorbed into the blood when taken by mouth, nor does it cross the placenta. So, unlike warfarin, heparin can be used during pregnancy. It is administered by intravenous injection or under the skin (subcutaneously). Unlike warfarin, heparin is a very rapid-acting blood thinner that can be used in emergency situations. It produces effects within minutes after it is injected intravenously and continues working for several hours.

Heparin is used as a blood-thinner to treat blood clots in the lungs, when a stroke is developing, for heart attack, and when blood clots are present in deep veins in the legs. It is also used to prevent clot formation during open-heart surgery and kidney dialysis.

Heparin works by inactivating thrombin and other clotting factors that are required for the formation of fibrin.

The major risk associated with heparin is bleeding. If bleeding does occur, as the result of an overdose, intravenous protamine sulfate can be used as an immediate-acting antidote. Signs of bleeding and cautions associated with its use are the same as for warfarin.

In addition, heparin may reduce the levels of platelets in the blood (a.k.a. thrombocy-topenia), which increases the risk of bleeding. Drugs that interfere with the function of platelets, in particular aspirin, can further increase this risk.

Heparin is obtained commercially from the lungs of cattle or the intestines of pigs. Individuals who have experienced unusual reactions or allergic responses to pork or beef may be at greater risk for being allergic to heparin. Common signs of allergy include chills, fever, and hives.

New Heparin-Like Drugs

In recent years, heparin has been broken into smaller units, which are referred to as low-molecular-weight heparins (a.k.a. LMWHs). These drugs can be used for the same conditions as heparin and have several advantages: they work for a longer period of time, give more reliable effects after a dose, and are less likely to reduce blood platelets.

In addition to preventing clot formation in deep leg veins, LMWHs are also used to prevent clots in patients having hip and knee replacement surgery.

Patients receiving LMWHs and undergoing spinal anesthesia or spinal tap are at increased risk of developing long-term or even permanent paralysis. This risk is increased when such individuals are also taking drugs that affect clotting, such as aspirin and related nonsteroidal anti-inflammatory drugs (NSAIDs).

Thrombin Inhibitors

Thrombin is needed for the formation of fibrin fibers, which serve as the backbone for clots. Thrombin inhibitors, a very new class of drugs, directly and immediately prevent thrombin from working—hence no fibrin fibers and no clot.

Did You Know That ...?

Leeches attach themselves to their victims and feed on their blood. When the leech is sucking their blood, it doesn't clot. The saliva of leeches contains hirudin, which has been found to be a potent thrombin inhibitor. Physicians have used leeches for medicinal purposes since the Middle Ages. Modern surgeons have used medicinal leeches to prevent clot formation in the fine blood vessels of reattached fingers. Lepirudin is a high-tech version of hirudin.

Drugs such as desirudin are used to prevent deep-vein clot formation in patients undergoing hip replacement therapy. The full potential of these drugs has yet to be determined.

Clot Dissolvers

After an injured blood vessel has healed, the body has no further need of the clot and disposes it. Plasmin is an enzyme present in the blood that breaks down fibrin fibers.

Unlike anticoagulants, which prevent the formation of clots, clot dissolvers are enzymes that cause dissolution of clots that have been formed. These drugs, called fibrinolytic or thrombolytic drugs, include alteplace (tPA) and streptokinase.

Clot dissolvers are injected intravenously and are used to break down clots in the heart, lungs, legs, and elsewhere in the body. Their use carries the potential risk of serious bleeding, and their benefits for these conditions have not been clearly proven. Hence, they are generally used only when anticoagulants have not been effective or when gangrene is present in the limb.

To reduce the risk of bleeding throughout the body, clot-dissolving drugs are generally applied directly to the clot. As discussed in the section on heart attacks, they are more often used to dissolve clots blocking blood flow in the arteries in the heart.

The Least You Need to Know

- ◆ Blood thinners (anticoagulants) are used to prevent the development of clots in the body and risk of these clots traveling to the lungs and brain.

- ◆ The dose of warfarin, the most widely used oral anticoagulant, must be carefully adjusted to fit the needs of each patient to prevent clotting while reducing the risk of bleeding.

- ◆ Persons taking warfarin must be careful to avoid activities that can cause bleeding.

- ◆ Persons taking warfarin and heparin must be careful to prevent drug-drug and drug-food interactions.

- ◆ Unlike warfarin, heparin-related drugs can be used during pregnancy and when it is necessary to rapidly produce an anticoagulant effect.

- ◆ Clot dissolvers (a.k.a. fibrinolytic drugs) are used intravenously to dissolve clots in the legs and lungs when blood thinners are ineffective or gangrene is present in the leg.

Drugs Used to Treat Coagulation Conditions

Generic Name	Trade Name	Generic Available
Oral Anticoagulants		
Warfarin	Coumadin	Yes
Injectable Anticoagulants		
Heparin	Liquaemin	Yes
Low-Molecular-Weight Heparins (LMWHs) (Generic Name Ending: "parin")		
Dalteparin	Fragmin	No
Enoxaparin	Lovenox	No
Tinzaparin	Innohep	No
Thrombin Inhibitors (Generic Name Ending: "irudin")		
Desirudin	Iprivask	No
Lepirudin	Refludan	No
Clot Dissolvers (Fibrinolytic Drugs)		
Alteplase [tPA]	Activase	No
Reteplase	Retavase	No
Streptokinase	Streptase	No
Urokinase	Abbokinase	No

Cancer

Cancer is a general term referring to a class of diseases in which normal cells change into abnormal ones. Such a change can occur in any of the body's cells or tissues. After this transformation has occurred, cancer cells don't look like or act like normal cells.

Major advances have been made in our understanding of cancer cells. This knowledge has led to the development of some exciting new drugs, a few of which can cure certain types of cancer. Many more drugs, given after surgery or radiation therapy, reduce the size of the cancer, slow its growth or spread, and even prolong life.

Cancer and Anticancer Drugs: An Overview

In our discussion, we talk about …

- The general nature of cancer.

- The most common kinds of cancer, in particular those for which drugs play a major role in their treatment.

- The challenges associated with the use of many anticancer drugs.

- The general properties of the major classes of anticancer drugs, with comments about specific drugs in each of these classes.

Three basic approaches are used to treat cancer: surgery, radiation, and drugs. Often two or more approaches are used in combination. Surgery and radiation are preferred for localized solid tumors. Likewise, drugs may be used for solid tumors as well as blood cancers and cancers that may have spread to multiple sites. Drugs also serve to kill tumor cells that have eluded the surgeon's blade or radiologist's beam.

Three categories of medicine are used to treat cancer:

- Cytotoxic drugs—those that kill cancer cells, often called chemotherapy

- Hormones and hormone antagonists

- Biological response modifiers that work by pumping up our natural immune defense system against cancer cells

We talk about all three kinds of drugs later in this chapter.

Cancer: The Big Picture

Second only to heart disease, cancer is a leading cause of death in the United States. In 2005, some 570,000 individuals died from all types of cancer, and about 1,373,000 new cases were identified.

Cancer is an umbrella term that refers to more than 100 conditions that share a number of common traits, among which include the following:

◆ The degree to which normal cells multiply is subject to genetic controls. Cancer cells do not respond to such control. They continue to grow aggressively and invade the space occupied by other cells interfering with their normal function.

◆ Cancer cells, unlike normal cells, can spread locally or break away from their primary sites to travel in blood or lymph to other parts of the body. Here they set up residence and grow new *neoplasms*, a process that is termed metastasis.

There is no single cause of cancer. Over the years, a number of cancer promoters, called carcinogens, have been identified. These include viruses, diet, chemical and physical agents, drugs (including anticancer drugs), and hormones.

def•i•ni•tion

A **neoplasm,** also called a tumor, is a collection of newly formed cells. A benign neoplasm is generally harmless, responds to genetic controls, and does not travel. A malignant neoplasm (cancer, carcinoma, or sarcoma) is harmful, grows aggressively, does not respond to genetic controls, and travels to other parts of the body where it grows into a new malignant tumor.

Common Cancers

In men, the most common new cases of cancer originate in the prostate, lung, blood and lymph, colon and rectum, urinary bladder, and skin. In women, cancers most commonly start in the breast, lung, colon and rectum, blood and lymph, and uterus.

In this section, we talk about cancers affecting the blood and lymphoid tissue, breast, colon and rectum, lung, prostate, skin, and uterus and ovaries. We also point out commonly used drugs used to treat each of these cancers.

How effective are drugs? When used alone, drugs can cure a limited number of cancers. These include cancers affecting white blood cells (called leukemias) and lymphoid tissues, as well as testicular cancer. In many more instances, drugs can produce cures or significant delays in tumor recurrence after the cancer has been eliminated by surgery or radiation. These include cancers of the breast, colon and rectum, ovaries, and bone.

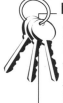

Did You Know That ...?

In cancer-language, a "cured" patient is entirely free of the cancer and has a normal life expectancy, the same as an individual without cancer. No cancer recurrence within five years is considered to be a cure; however, later relapses sometimes occur. A "complete response" is said to occur when the cancer is completely gone for at least one month after treatment. Many of these patients may relapse.

Blood Cancers

White blood cells, or leukocytes, serve as major defenders against attack by disease-causing bacteria and viruses. They are rapidly carried in the blood to the site of infection to search and destroy the troublesome invaders.

Leukemias are cancers of white blood cells. There are two general types of leukemias: lymphocytic leukemias and myelocytic leukemias. The names refer to the type of white cells affected. In the absence of treatment, acute leukemias may progress rapidly and cause death within months. On the other hand, chronic leukemias develop slowly over a 10- to 20-year period. Acute lymphocytic leukemia is the most common cancer in children, whereas acute myelocytic leukemia the most common leukemia in adults.

Most leukemias travel to surrounding organs, robbing them of their nutrients and causing their destruction. Some invade bone, causing intense pain and an increased tendency to fracture. Infection, anemia (decrease in red blood cells), and bleeding tendencies are common problems associated with leukemia.

Drug treatment of acute lymphocytic leukemia is complex and involves three phases:

- **Phase 1.** Attempt to bring the condition under immediate control. Drug combinations such as vincristine + prednisone + asparaginase + daunorubicin are used for one month.

- **Phase 2.** A more intensive phase of chemotherapy, over a one-to six-month period or longer. Use of drug combinations such as mercaptopurine, prednisone, vincristine, and methotrexate.

- **Phase 3.** Maintenance therapy for several years, using Phase 2 drugs given in cycles separated by drug-free periods.

Acute myelocytic leukemia is often treated with cytarabine and daunorubicin or idarubicin.

Lymph Tissue Cancers

Lymphomas are cancers that affect lymphoid tissue, which include lymphocytes and lymph nodes. Lymphocytes, a type of white blood cell, are major participants in the immune system. They protect the body against microbes, foreign tissues, and cancers by detecting and then destroying them.

Large numbers of abnormal lymphocytes are formed in lymphomas, reducing the effectiveness of the immune system. This makes the afflicted individual more susceptible to infections.

There are two primary groups of lymphomas: Hodgkin's and non-Hodgkin's lymphoma, with the latter eight times more common. There are many different types of non-Hodgkin's lymphoma, each with different prospects for recovery.

The most common symptom of Hodgkin's disease is a painless enlargement of lymph nodes. Other frequent symptoms include fever, night sweats, fatigue, and weight loss. Individuals with non-Hodgkin's lymphoma also have enlarged lymph nodes, as well as jaundice, abdominal cramps, diarrhea, and other gastrointestinal tract problems.

Both lymphomas are treated with cytotoxic anticancer drugs and radiation therapy. Far more favorable results are obtained when these lymphomas are detected and treated during their early stages.

A common combination of anticancer drugs for Hodgkin's disease is doxorubicin + bleomycin + vinblastine + dacarbazine. Another cocktail combines mechlorethamine + vincristine + procarbazine + prednisone.

Non-Hodgkin's lymphoma is often treated with single drugs, frequently chlorambucil or fludarabine. One common mixture (CVP) combines cyclophosphamide + vincristine + prednisone. The CHOP combination contains cyclophosphamide + doxorubicin + vincristine + prednisone.

Breast Cancer

Women rank breast cancer to be the most dreaded of all diseases. In 2005, some 211,000 new cases were diagnosed in women in the United States and, after lung cancer, breast cancer was the leading cause of cancer-related deaths.

Signs of breast cancer include: one or more lumps in the breast; dimpling or thickening or pulling of breast skin; ulceration of breast skin; an abnormal discharge from the nipple; a rash near the nipple area; a change in the position of the nipple; a lump in the underarm or above the collarbone. Breast cancer is generally painless.

There are different types of breast cancer, based on where the cancer started and how far it has spread:

- **Ductal cancers** are the most common form of cancer. They are cancers that have started in milk-carrying ducts, and can be further subdivided into two categories:

  Ductal cancer in situ refers to a cancer that has not spread to surrounding tissue.

  Invasive ductal cancer refers to cancer that has spread outside the milk ducts and sometimes throughout the body. This is the most common form of breast cancer.

- **Lobular cancers** are those starting in the milk-producing glands.

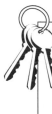

Did You Know That ...?

Breast cancer is classified, or staged, according to the size of the tumor and whether or not it has spread. The scale ranges from stage 0, indicating a very small tumor with no lymph node involvement and no spreading, to 4, a large tumor with multiple lymph node involvement and distant metastasis. Staging provides a basis for making treatment decisions and determining the patient's prognosis.

Treatment options for breast cancer include surgery, radiation, and such drugs as aromatase inhibitors (anastrozole, letrozole), anti-estrogens (tamoxifen, fulvestrant), anti-tumor antibiotics (doxorubicin), and plant products (docetaxel, paclitaxel).

Colorectal Cancer

Colorectal cancer caused more than 56,000 deaths in the United States in 2005, the second-leading cause of cancer deaths. Identified risk factors include a family history of this condition; cancer elsewhere in the body; polyps (i.e., a protruding tissue growth) in the rectum and colon (lower end of the large intestines); a high-fat, low-fiber diet; and a history of ulcerative colitis or Crohn's disease.

The tumor is very slow growing. When symptoms do appear, the cancer has generally spread to surrounding tissues and is far advanced. Early symptoms include either diarrhea or constipation and blood in the stool. Abdominal pain, loss of appetite, anemia, and weight loss are seen in the advanced stages.

Early detection and surgery are highly effective in producing a cure. In advanced cases, after the cancer has spread to lymph nodes or other parts of the abdominal cavity, drugs such as fluorouracil play a secondary role. Drugs are of limited value at this stage and are used to reduce the risk of further spread to the liver.

Lung Cancer

Lung cancer is the leading cause of cancer death in the United States, claiming more than 163,000 victims in 2005, or 3 out of every 10 deaths from cancer. Cigarette smoke and the carcinogens it contains are the most important causes of lung cancer. Some 80 to 90 percent of all cases are linked to smoking.

Did You Know That ...?

Lung cancer has claimed the lives of many celebrities, most only in their 50s. A very incomplete list includes musicians Leonard Bernstein, Jimmy Dorsey, Duke Ellington, George Harrison; actors Yul Brynner, Gary Cooper, Betty Grable; baseball players Joe DiMaggio and Roger Maris; TV newspersons Chet Huntley, Peter Jennings, Edward R. Murrow; and film producer Walt Disney.

Chronic cough is the most common sign of lung cancer, along with coughing up blood and breathing difficulties. Other signs include loss of appetite, weight loss, fatigue, and weakness. Lung cancer often spreads to other sites, including the lymph nodes, brain, bones, and liver.

Of all the common cancers, the prospects are among the bleakest for individuals with lung cancer. This is particularly the case when the cancer has spread and the individual continues to smoke.

Surgery is the preferred treatment while the cancer remains localized. When surgery is not an option, radiation therapy is used to slow tumor growth after it has spread.

Anticancer drugs, often used in conjunction with radiation, provide some benefit and may prolong life somewhat. Drug combinations include paclitaxel and carboplatin or cisplatin + vinorelbine + cisplatin.

Prostate Cancer

Prostate cancer is most common cause of cancer in men, with 232,000 newly diagnosed cases in 2005, and the second-leading cause of cancer deaths. It is usually such a very slow-growing tumor that far more men die *with* prostate cancer than *because of* it.

As the tumor grows in size, it compresses the urine tube (a.k.a. urethra), which interferes with the flow of urine. This is similar to what occurs in benign (noncancerous) prostate enlargement. Bones are often the site of tumor spread.

Depending on how extensive the cancer is and how far it has spread, a wide range of options is available. All have limitations. These options range from no treatment and watchful waiting, to surgery or radiation therapy, to treatment with hormones.

Prostate cancers require the male hormone (a.k.a. androgen) testosterone to grow and spread. Hormone blockers are used to treat this condition and act in one of two ways:

- ◆ Leuprolide and goserelin produce a "chemical castration" by preventing the testes from making testosterone.

- ◆ Flutamide and related testosterone receptor blockers ("tamides") prevent the male hormone from having its growth-enhancing effects on the cancerous prostate gland. Tamide drugs are used in combination with leuprolide.

Skin Cancers and Melanoma

Skin cancer is the most common cancer type in the United States, with some 1 million new cases diagnosed each year. Estimates suggest that by the age of 65, 40 to 50 percent of us will have at least one skin cancer. The risk of developing skin cancer is related to where we live, which in turn determines our exposure to harmful ultraviolet (UV) light.

def•i•ni•tion

The skin is the body's largest organ and weighs about 6 lbs. It has two primary layers: the outer layer or epidermis, and the inner dermis. The epidermis consists of flat, scale-like **squamous cells;** under which are round **basal cells;** and the deepest epidermal layer, the **melanocytes,** which give skin its color.

Skin cancers fall into two general categories: nonmelanoma and melanoma. *Squamous cell* and *basal cell* cancers, the most common nonmelanoma cancers, are slow growing and easily treated in early stages. Melanoma affects the *melanocytes*, the deepest epidermal skin layers, and can spread to other tissues and organs of the body. This is the most common of the 3 skin cancers. About 59,000 new cases of melanoma are diagnosed each year, and some 7,700 deaths occur annually from the disease.

At this time, cytotoxic drugs and biologicals play a relatively minor role in the treatment of skin cancers. They are far more often destroyed or removed by freezing, surgery, laser therapy, or radiation therapy.

Fluorouracil (5-FU), applied to the skin, is used for the treatment of precancerous skin lesions and selected types of basal cell cancers.

Clinical studies are underway evaluating the effectiveness of biological response modifiers against melanomas and nonmelanoma skin cancers. Such biological response modifiers include interferon (aldesleukin), interleukin-2, and imiquimod. They act by turning on the body's immune defense mechanisms to combat cancer cells.

Uterine and Ovarian Cancers

Cancers can attack any part of the female reproductive system. We are going to talk about two of the most common organs—the uterus and ovaries. There are two forms of uterine cancers:

♦ Endometrial cancer affects the endometrium, the lining of the uterus.

♦ Cervical cancer affects the cervix or the lower portion of the uterus, which opens into the vagina.

These cancers are first treated by their surgical removal. The woman may then receive radiation therapy or drugs. In advanced cases, when surgery is no longer possible, drugs may be given to prevent further growth or spread of the tumor beyond the walls of the uterus or to provide relief of symptoms.

Endometrial Cancer

Endometrial cancer is the most common cancer affecting the female reproductive system. In 2005, there were almost 41,000 newly diagnosed cases, and 7,300 deaths, most of which occurred in postmenopausal women ages 50 to 70.

Early signs of endometrial cancer are generally painless. Prior to menopause, irregular, heavier, or longer-lasting periods may occur. Abnormal vaginal bleeding may occur after menopause.

A progesterone-like drug (a female hormone), such as medroxyprogesterone, is given after surgical removal of the uterus (a.k.a. hysterectomy). If the cancer is detected early, surgery can provide significant benefit, curing up to 90 percent of women.

When progestin therapy ceases to be effective, or after the cancer has spread, more powerful (and potentially toxic drugs) are used. These include cisplatin, carboplatin, cyclophosphamide, doxorubicin, and paclitaxel.

Cervical Cancer

Cervical cancer is among the most common cancers of the female reproductive system, with more than 10,000 new cases in 2005. A major risk factor is infection by human papilloma viruses (HPVs), sexually transmitted viruses that cause genital warts.

Warning!

Gardasil, a newly developed vaccine, was found to be 100 percent effective in preventing cervical cancer two years after women were inoculated. In very promising clinical studies reported in 2005, this experimental vaccine blocked infection caused by two common human papilloma viruses (HPV), which together cause 70 percent of all cases of cervical cancer. Its long-term protective effects remain to be determined.

Early stages of cervical cancer usually have no symptoms. When symptoms are present, they include spotting or bleeding between periods, bleeding after intercourse, or heavier than normal bleeding. As the tumor spreads, heavy bleeding is common. Other symptoms include foul-smelling vaginal discharge, pain in the pelvis or lower back, and swelling of the legs. As the cancer spreads within the pelvis and beyond, prospects for recovery become reduced.

Did You Know That ...?

The Pap test (a.k.a. Pap smear) is simple, quick, and painless. It detects cervical cancer, even in early stages, more than 80 percent of the time. This test has led to early diagnosis and treatment and has reduced the death rate from this cancer by over 70 percent.

Drugs, such as cisplatin, fluorouracil, and ifosfamide, are reserved for cases of cervical cancer that cannot be adequately controlled with surgery and radiation therapy. Drug benefits are limited and short-lasting.

Ovarian Cancer

This is the second most common cancer affecting the female reproductive system, with 22,000 new cases reported each year.

The symptoms of ovarian cancer usually first appear after the tumor has spread beyond the ovaries and the pelvic region. The first signs are general and include indigestion, frequent urination, and constipation. The abdomen enlarges and fluid accumulates as the disease progresses. The ovary swells.

Treatment consists of surgery followed by such cytotoxic drugs as paclitaxel and cisplatin or carboplatin. In more advanced cases, bleomycin and etoposide are used.

Challenges in Cancer Chemotherapy

Drug treatment of cancer is tough! There are a number of major challenges associated with chemo, some of which severely limit or even prevent successful treatment. Because these problems apply to many of the most commonly used drugs, we talk about them now.

Cell Differences

The use of antibiotics to successfully treat microbial infections is based on very fundamental differences that exist between the cells of the microbe and the patient. Antibiotics zero in on and take advantage of these differences.

Cancer cells come from normal cells, so it is not surprising that there are few differences between them. Cytotoxic anticancer drugs damage both cancer cells and normal cells, causing toxic effects in the patient.

One Hundred Percent Kill

Successful cure of cancer requires the death of all—not most, but 100 percent—of the cancer cells. The high dose of the chemo drug needed to kill all cancer cells is very often a dose that also causes major harm to the patient. Thus, the highest dose that can be given is often limited by "dose-limiting toxicity."

Early Detection

The most successful treatment occurs after early detection before the cancer has spread, and while the cancer cells are most sensitive to chemo. With the notable exception of the Pap smear used to detect cervical cancer, few other diagnostic tests are so reliable at early stages.

Chemo Resistance

A major cause of treatment failure is the development of cancer cells that are resistant to chemo. In most instances, two or more drugs are used to treat cancers. Drug combinations: (1) reduce the development of drug resistance; (2) maximize the likelihood that 100 percent of the tumor cells will be killed; and (3) make it possible to reduce the dose of individual drugs in the combination, thus reducing toxicity to normal cells.

Adverse Effects of Cancer Chemotherapy

Chemo is most effective against cells that are rapidly dividing. Because of this, we find that the toxic effects of these drugs occur mainly in rapidly dividing normal cells. These include blood cells, cells of the digestive system, hair follicles, and sperm-producing cells.

Bone Marrow Suppression

Blood cells are produced in the marrow of bones, a site very susceptible to being depressed by chemo. White cell suppression raises the risk of developing severe and even life-threatening infections. Decreased blood platelets increase bleeding tendencies. Reduced red blood cells may lead to anemia.

Digestive System

Chemo often causes inflammation and ulcer formation of the mouth and lower portions of the digestive system. Severe diarrhea is not uncommon.

The profound and protracted nausea and vomiting very often experienced may serve as the tipping point for many cancer sufferers and result in their refusing to continue chemotherapy. Among the most effective drugs used to treat nausea and vomiting caused by chemotherapy include the following:

- Ondansetron (Zofran), often used in combination with the steroid dexamethasone (Decadron)

- Metoclopramide (Reglan)

- Prochlorperazine (Compazine)

- Marijuana (cannabis)-like drugs such as dronabinol (Marinol) and, in Canada, nabilone (Cesamet)

Hair Loss

Losses may occur about a week after the start of chemo, with greatest losses experienced within one to two months. Hair growth generally resumes within a few months after chemo has been discontinued.

Reproductive System Toxicity

Chemotherapy may produce irreversible sterility in males. When used by women during pregnancy, it may cause fetal deaths or fetal malformations. Because of the high risk of causing injury to the fetus, these drugs should not be used by pregnant women.

Other Effects

Some drugs are very irritating and may cause injury to surrounding tissues if they leak from veins after intravenous injection. Moreover, years after the use of some anticancer drugs and hormones, new cancers have appeared that may have been caused by the previous cancer chemotherapy.

Types of Anticancer Drugs

Medicines used for the treatment of cancer, which number about 100 and counting, fall into 4 general categories:

- Cytotoxic agents (i.e., drugs that kill cancer cells in different ways). These include the alkylating agents, antimetabolites, antitumor antibiotics, and plant drugs.

- Hormones and hormone antagonists. Some tumors require the presence of hormones to grow. Many of these drugs block the effects of hormones at its tissue receptors or prevent the manufacture of hormones by the body.

◆ Biological response modifiers. These drugs increase the body's immune system to detect and destroy the cancer.

◆ Miscellaneous drugs (i.e., those that don't conveniently fall into one of the other categories).

For most other conditions we have talked about in this book, we can talk about the general common effects of drugs in a given category or class. In essence, if you've seen one, you've seen them all—at least, to a greater or lesser extent. There are many differences between and among anticancer drugs, even among members of the same class.

Alkylating Agents

Adverse effects include bone marrow depression, which limits the highest doses that can be safely taken; nausea and vomiting; and hair loss.

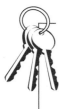

Did You Know That ...?

These drugs were discovered while the toxicity of mustard gases, used as chemical warfare agents during World War I, were being studied. Early attention was focused on their blistering effects on the skin, eyes, and breathing tubes. Later, it was noted they suppressed lymphoid tissue and bone marrow, and led to the use of nitrogen mustard derivatives as the first anticancer drugs in the 1940s.

These drugs interfere with male and female sex function. They should not be used by pregnant women and may cause sterility in men.

Commonly used alkylating agents include the following:

◆ **Carboplatin (Paraplatin).** Primarily used for ovarian and lung cancers. Adverse effects similar to but less severe than cisplatin.

◆ **Carmustine (BCNU).** Used for Hodgkin's disease, non-Hodgkin's lymphoma, brain cancer, multiple myeloma (an uncommon cancer that develops from abnormal plasma cells).

◆ **Cisplatin (Platinol-AQ).** Used intravenously in drug combinations for testicular and ovarian cancers, for which it is most effective. Also used for cancers of the bladder, head and neck, cervix, endometrium, lung, and colon and rectum. Nausea and vomiting can be very severe. Other adverse effects include kidney damage, hearing loss and ringing in the ears, and bone marrow suppression.

◆ **Cyclophosphamide (Cytoxan).** The most widely used alkylating agent. It is effective for the treatment of Hodgkin's disease; non-Hodgkin's lymphoma; acute and chronic lymphocytic leukemia; multiple myeloma; and solid tumors of the breast, ovary, lung, and cervix.

◆ **Ifosfamide (Ifex).** Used for cancer of the testes.

◆ **Mechlorethamine (Mustargen).** Used for Hodgkin's disease and non-Hodgkin's lymphoma.

◆ **Melphalan (Alkeran).** Used for multiple myeloma and tumors of the ovary and breast.

Antimetabolites

Adverse effects include bone marrow depression, which may limit the highest dose given; damage to cells of the gastrointestinal tract; and severe diarrhea.

Commonly used antimetabolites include the following:

◆ **Cytarabine (Cytosar-U).** Used for acute lymphocytic leukemia, acute myelocytic leukemia.

◆ **Fludarabine (Fludara).** Used for chronic lymphocytic leukemia.

◆ **Fluorouracil (Adrucil).** Widely used, often in combination with other drugs or radiation therapy, for solid tumors of breast, head, neck, lung, stomach. Applied topically (Efudex) for precancerous skin lesions.

◆ **Mercaptopurine (Purinethol).** Used for acute lymphocytic leukemia.

◆ **Methotrexate (Trexall).** Used for acute lymphocytic leukemia in children. In combination with other drugs for non-Hodgkin's lymphoma and solid tumors of the breast, head and neck, ovary, and bladder. Methotrexate (Rheumatrex) is also used for noncancerous conditions such as rheumatoid arthritis and psoriasis.

Plant Drugs

Plants have served as the source of a number of anticancer drugs. From the periwinkle plant of Madagascar come vinblastine and vincristine. The yew tree is the natural source of paclitaxel and its laboratory-modification docetaxel. The mandrake (may-apple) plant was used as medicines by American Indians and the early colonists. Derivatives of chemicals from this plant include etoposide and teniposide. Topotecan is an altered form of chemicals from a Chinese tree.

Common plant-based drugs include the following:

◆ **Etoposide (VePesid).** Used for testicular cancer and small cell cancer of the lung.

◆ **Teniposide (Vumon).** Used for acute lymphocytic leukemia in children. Doses of these drugs are limited by bone marrow depression. Nausea, vomiting, and diarrhea may occur, as does reversible hair loss.

◆ **Paclitaxel (Taxol) and docetaxel (Taxotere).** Used for metastatic cancers of the breast, ovaries, lung, head and neck, esophagus, and bladder. Doses are limited by bone marrow depression. Severe allergic reactions may occur, which can be decreased by giving the steroid dexamethasone and an antihistamine. Hair loss may occur suddenly but is reversible.

◆ **Topotecan (Hycamtin).** Used for small cell lung cancer and ovarian cancer no longer responding to other cytotoxic drugs. Bone marrow suppression, with increased susceptibility to infection, is the dose-limiting toxicity.

◆ **Vinblastine (Velban).** Used in combination for cancers of the testes and breast and Hodgkin's and non-Hodgkin's lymphoma. Doses are limited by bone marrow depression.

◆ **Vincristine (Oncovin).** Used in combination for cancers of the bladder and breast, Hodgkin's and non-Hodgkin's lymphoma, and acute lymphocytic leukemia. Doses are limited by nerve toxicity causing tingling, slowed reflexes, sensory impairments, weakness, constipation, and urinary difficulties.

Antitumor Antibiotics

Antibiotics are derived from compounds manufactured by microbes, and they are most often used to treat bacterial and fungal infections. A few have been found to work against cancers.

The "rubicin" antibiotics have adverse effects on the heart, including causing abnormal heart function and rhythm. Because of these toxic effects, all have limits on the total amount of a drug that can be given during a lifetime. They also may cause bone marrow depression, severe nausea and vomiting, and hair loss.

Commonly used antitumor antibiotics include the following:

- **Bleomycin (Blenoxane).** Used in combinations for Hodgkin's disease and cancers of the ovaries and testes. Minimal bone marrow suppression but may cause toxicity involving the skin and lungs.

- **Daunorubicin (Cerubidine).** Used for acute myelocytic leukemia.

- **Doxorubicin (Adriamycin).** Used for lymphomas, cancers of the breast, lung, soft tissue (sarcomas), and bone.

Hormones and Hormone Antagonists

Cytotoxic drugs kill cancer cells but are also toxic to healthy cells. Hormone anticancer drugs are much more selective in their effects and cause far fewer adverse effects to the patient.

Some tumors, such as those located in the breast, uterus, and prostate gland, depend on the presence of hormones to grow. Drugs are directed against the effects of female or male hormones, which can inhibit the growth of such tumors. They antagonize such hormones from working or interfere with the body's manufacture of such hormones.

Steroids are used to treat cancers involving white blood cells and lymphoid tissues.

Drugs Affecting Female Hormones

Several groups of medicines, primarily used to treat breast cancer, reduce the effects of estrogen, the female hormone. Two such groups of drugs are anti-estrogens and aromatase inhibitors.

Anti-estrogens (a.k.a. selective estrogen receptor modulators or SEMS), block the effects of estrogen on its receptor on the breast. Commonly used anti-estrogens include tamoxifen, toremiphene, and fulvestrant:

- **Tamoxifen (Nolvadex).** This is the most widely used and best-studied drug for the treatment of breast cancer. It is given by mouth after radiation therapy or surgical removal of the tumor or used alone for the treatment of metastatic breast cancer. It is most effective when taken for five years rather than shorter time periods. Tamoxifen only works in women who have estrogen-promoting breast tumors.

  Tamoxifen is also used to prevent breast cancer in women who are at high risk of developing this condition.

Common side effects include hot flashes, swelling (due to water retention), nausea and vomiting, and menstrual irregularities.

Warning!

The use of tamoxifen for periods over two years has been associated with an increased risk of endometrial cancer. This risk is greater in older, postmenopausal women. It also increases the risk of clotting disorders. The benefits of tamoxifen for treating cancer are far greater than these risks. But prior to using it to treat breast cancer, its risks should be carefully considered.

- **Raloxifene (Evista).** Recent studies have shown that raloxifene is as effective as tamoxifen in preventing breast cancer in high-risk women after menopause. Both drugs reduce this risk by one-half. But compared with tamoxifen, raloxifene produces these benefits while significantly reducing the dangers of getting uterine cancer or clotting disorders. Raloxifene is commonly used to prevent and treat osteoporosis in women after menopause.

- **Toremiphene (Fareston).** A tamoxifen-related drug also used to treat breast cancer.

- **Fulvestrant (Faslodex).** Given by injection once monthly for the treatment of advanced metastatic breast cancer. Common side effects include nausea, weakness, pain, hot flashes, and headache.

Aromatase inhibitors prevent the manufacture of estrogen. Anastrozole (Arimidex) and related drugs are considered by many to be a major advance in the treatment of early and advanced breast cancer in postmenopausal women.

Anastrozole is more effective than tamoxifen while causing fewer significant side effects. When compared with tamoxifen, anastrozole causes far less menstrual disorders, hot flashes, clotting disorders, and a lower risk of endometrial cancer. By contrast, bone pains are more common.

Other promising new drugs for the treatment of estrogen-dependent breast cancer include letrozole (Femara) and exemestane (Aromasin).

Did You Know That ...?

In 1941, Charles Huggins (1901–1997) showed that cancer cells don't grow on their own, as was believed, but depend on chemical signals, such as hormones, to grow and survive. Removal of these chemicals, by castration or by giving estrogens to decrease androgen production, caused prostate tumors to shrink. In 1950, he found that removal of ovaries, the source of female hormones, caused breast tumors to shrink.

Drugs Affecting Male Hormones

Prostate tumors require androgens, the male hormones, for growth. Medicines used to treat prostate cancer work by preventing testosterone production by the testes or by blocking the androgen receptor.

Production of androgens by the testes is under the control of a hormonal influence coming from the hypothalamus in the brain. This chemical is a gonadotropin-releasing hormone, commonly referred to as GnRH.

Leuprolide (Lupron), goserelin (Zoladex), and related "relin" drugs are GnRH-like chemicals manufactured in the laboratory used for advanced prostate cancer. When leuprolide is given by injection for several weeks, testosterone levels decline to levels seen after surgical removal of the testes.

Hot flashes, impotence, and loss of sex drive are common side effects. Bone pain may also be experienced.

Flutamide (Eulexin) and related "lutamide" drugs block the effects of androgens in prostate tumor cells needed for their growth. These oral drugs are generally given after surgical removal of the testes or leuprolide-induced "chemical castration."

Common side effects with "lutamide" drugs include enlargement of the breasts, hot flashes, nausea, and vomiting.

Progesterone-Like Drugs

Derivatives of progesterone (a.k.a. progestins), a female hormone, are used to treat cancers:

- **Medroxyprogesterone (Depo-Provera).** Used for advanced cancers of the endometrium and kidney

- **Megestrol (Megace).** Given for advanced cancers of the endometrium and breast

Common progestin side effects include swelling (due to water retention) and weight gain. Progestins have been shown to cause fetal abnormalities and must not be given during pregnancy.

Progestins are widely used as hormonal contraceptives, either alone or in combination with estrogens.

Steroids

Prednisone (Meticorten) and related steroids are used for acute and chronic lympho-cytic leukemias and cancers affecting lymphoid tissues, such as Hodgkin's disease and non-Hodgkin's lymphoma. They are of particular value when treating acute leukemia in children and lymphomas in children and adults.

When used at low doses or for rather brief periods of time, steroids are relatively safe drugs. Their long-term use may cause a very wide array of adverse effects including those involving bone and muscle, mood and behavior, and increased susceptibility to infection, fluid retention, and ulcers.

Biological Response Modifiers

Among the newest approaches to the treatment of cancer involves the use of drugs that increase the patient's natural immune defenses against tumors. The full potential of these drugs for the treatment of cancer has yet to be determined. They are all pro-teins and must be given by injection.

Interleukin and Interferon

Aldesleukin (interleukin-2, IL-2, Proleukin) is primarily used for advanced kidney cancer and malignant melanoma. When given at high doses, which are most effective against tumors, side effects often include a drop in blood pressure, retention of fluids, and kidney abnormalities.

Interferon is used for hairy cell leukemia and chronic myelogenous leukemia.

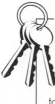

Did You Know That ...?

Monoclonal antibodies (MAbs) are used to determine minute amounts of hormones, infectious substances, and toxins in the blood as well as hidden cancer cells. They are also used detect the presence of abnormal proteins after a heart attack, to detect the virus that causes AIDS, to prevent tissue rejection after organ transplantation, and to serve as the basis for home pregnancy tests. All MAbs end in "umab," "ximab," or "momab."

Monoclonal Antibodies

After injection, monoclonal antibodies attach to specific chemicals on cancer cells. Several of these are being used for the treatment of cancers. Allergic reactions may occur after repeated injections.

The monoclonal antibodies used for cancers include ...

- **Alemtuzumab (Campath).** Used for lymphoma.

- **Bevacizumab (Avastin).** Used for metastatic colorectal cancer.

- **Cetuximab (Erbitux).** Used for metastatic colorectal cancer.

- **Rituximab (Rituxan).** Used for lymphomas.

- **Trastuzumab (Herceptin).** Used for breast cancer.

Miscellaneous Drugs

A wide range of miscellaneous drugs that don't fit neatly into any of the preceding categories work in different ways to combat cancer. Such drugs include the following:

- **Asparaginase (Elspar).** Used in drug combinations for acute lymphocytic leukemia. Adverse effects include allergic reactions, which can be very severe; blood clotting abnormalities; severe nausea and vomiting; and behavioral disturbances.

- **Dacarbazine (DTIC-Dome).** Used intravenously for malignant melanoma and in combination for Hodgkin's disease. Doses may be limited by bone marrow suppression. Nausea and vomiting may be severe.

- **Hydroxyurea (Hydrea).** Used orally for chronic myelocytic leukemia. Bone marrow suppression is the major dose-limiting effect. It is also used for sickle cell disease.

- **Procarbazine (Matulane).** Used orally in combination for Hodgkin's disease and for brain tumors. Doses may be limited by bone marrow suppression or nausea and vomiting.

Did You Know That ...?

Thalidomide first appeared on the market as a sleep-inducing drug in Europe in 1957. It was promoted as being extremely safe, even when taken in overdose and during pregnancy. Four years later, it was withdrawn after being shown to be responsible for causing 10,000 babies to be born with deformed limbs. It has recently reappeared and shows promise for treating multiple myeloma.

The Least You Need to Know

◆ Cancer is a collective term used to refer to some 100 conditions in which tumor cells continue growing without restraint, travel to other parts of the body, and establish new tumors.

◆ Cancer chemotherapy, when used alone, can cure several cancer types but is more often used after tumor elimination by surgery or radiation therapy.

◆ Cytotoxic drugs, the most widely used anticancer category, are effective but highly toxic to bone marrow and other normal cells, and resistance develops to their anticancer effects.

◆ Hormone-dependent tumors, located on the breast, uterus, and prostate, are treated with agents that block the manufacture, release, or effects of these hormones.

◆ Biological response modifiers, including monoclonal antibodies, act by increasing the immune defenses of the body against tumor cells.

Drugs Used for Treatment of Cancer

Generic Name	Trade Name	How Taken: Injection (I), Oral (O), Topical (T)	Generic Available
Alkylating Agents			
Busulfan	Busulfex, Myleran	I/O	Yes
Carboplatin	Paraplatin	I	Yes
Carmustine (BCNU)	BiCNU	I	No
Chlorambucil	Leukeran	O	No
Cisplatin (CDDP)	Platinol-AQ	I	Yes
Cyclophosphamide	Cytoxan, Neosar	I/O	No
Ifosfamide	Ifex	I	No
Lomustine (CCNU)	CeeNU	O	No
Mechlorethamine (HN2, Nitrogen Mustard)	Mustargen	I	No
Melphalan (L-PAM)	Alkeran	I/O	No

continues

Drugs Used for Treatment of Cancer (continued)

Generic Name	Trade Name	How Taken: Injection (I), Oral (O), Topical (T)	Generic Available
Oxaliplatin	Eloxatin	I	No
Streptozocin	Zanosar	I	No
Temozolomide	Temodar	O	No
Thiotepa	Thioplex	I	No
Antimetabolites			
Azacitidine	Vidaza	I	No
Capecitabine	Xeloda	O	No
Cladribine (CdA)	Leustatin	I	No
Cytarabine	Cytosar-U	I	Yes
Fludarabine	Fludara	I	No
Fluorouracil (5-FU)	Adrucil	I	Yes
	Carac	T	Yes
	Efudex	T	Yes
	Fluoroplex	T	Yes
Floxuridine	FUDR	I	No
Gemcitabine	Gemzar	I	No
Mercaptopurine (6-MP)	Purinethol	O	No
Methotrexate (Amethopterin, 6-MP)	Trexall	O	No
Permetrexed	Alimta	I	No
Pentostatin	Nipent	I	Yes
Thioguanine (TG)	Tabloid	O	No
Plant Drugs			
Docetaxel	Taxotere	I	No
Etoposide	Etopophos, Toposar, VePesid	I/O	Yes
Paclitaxel	Onxol, Taxol	I	No

Generic Name	Trade Name	How Taken: Injection (I), Oral (O), Topical (T)	Generic Available
Teniposide	Vumon	I	No
Vinblastine (VLB)	Velban	I	Yes
Vincristine (VCR)	Oncovin, Vincasar	I	Yes
Vinorelbine	Navelbine	I	No
Antitumor Antibiotics ("mycin", "rubicin")			
Bleomycin	Blenoxane	I	Yes
Dactinomycin (Actinomycin D)	Cosmegen	I	No
Daunorubicin	Cerubidine	I	Yes
Doxorubicin	Adriamycin, Doxil	I	Yes
Epirubicin	Ellence	I	No
Idarubicin	Idamycin	I	Yes
Mitomycin (MTC)	Mutamycin	I	No
Mitoxantrone	Novantrone	I	No
Plicamycin	Mithracin	I	No
Valrubicin	Valstar	I	No
Hormones and Hormone Antagonists			
Female Hormone (Estrogen) Antagonists			
Fulvestrant	Faslodex	I	No
Raloxifene	Evista	O	No
Tamoxifen	Nolvadex	O	No
Toremifene	Fareston	O	No
Aromatase Inhibitors			
Anastrozole	Arimidex	O	No
Exemestane	Aromasin	O	No
Letrozole	Femara	O	No
GnRH "relin" Drugs			
Goserelin	Zoladex	I	No
Histrelin	Vantas	I	No
Leuprolide	Eligard, Lupron, Viadur	I	No

continues

Drugs Used for Treatment of Cancer   (continued)

Generic Name	Trade Name	How Taken: Injection (I), Oral (O), Topical (T)	Generic Available
Triptorelin	Trelstar	I	No
Male Hormone (Androgen) Antagonists ("tamide")			
Bicalutamide	Casodex	O	No
Flutamide	Eulexin	O	No
Nilutamide	Nilandron	O	No
Estrogen and Progestins			
Estramustine	Emcyt	O	No
Medroxyprogesterone	Depo-Provera	I	No
Megestrol	Megace	O	Yes
Steroids			
Prednisone	Deltasone, Meticorten	O	Yes
Biological Response Modifiers			
Aldesleukin (IL-2, Interleukin-2)	Proleukin	I	No
Interferon alfa	Roferon-A	I	No
Bexarotene	Targretin	O/T	No
Bortezomid	Velcade	I	No
Denileukin	Ontak	I	No
Gefitinib	Iressa	O	No
Imatinib	Gleevec	O	No
Imiquimod	Aldara	T	No
Levamisole	Ergamisol	O	No
Thalidomide	Thalomid	O	No
Tretinoin	Vesanoid	O	No
Monoclonal Antibodies ("ximab," "umab," "momab")			
Alemtuzumab	Campath	I	No
Bevacizumab	Avastin	I	No
Cetuximab	Erbitux	I	No
Ibritumomab	Zevalin	I	No
Rituximab	Rituxan	I	No
Trastuzumab	Herceptin	I	No

Generic Name	Trade Name	How Taken: Injection (I), Oral (O), Topical (T)	Generic Available
Miscellaneous Drugs			
Altretamine	Hexalen	O	No
Arsenic trioxide	Trisenox	O	No
Asparaginase	Elspar	I	No
Dacarbazine (DTIC)	DTIC-Dome	I	Yes
Hydroxyurea	Hydrea	O	Yes
Mitotane (o,p'-DDD)	Lysodren	O	No
Pegaspargase	Oncaspar	I	No
Procarbazine	Matulane	O	No

Cholesterol, High

In atherosclerosis, fats penetrate artery walls and interfere with blood flow. The fatty deposits increase the danger of heart attack and stroke. Statins and related drugs are used to reduce elevated blood levels of fats, including cholesterol, thereby lowering the risk of these potentially fatal conditions. Let's get started by first talking briefly about the role cholesterol plays in normal body function.

Cholesterol's Role in Normal Body Function

Cholesterol is one of several kinds of fats, or lipids, in the body. It serves a number of important body functions, including being an integral component of cell membranes. It is also needed for the manufacture of certain hormones, such as the male and female sex hormones, and for bile acids, which are needed for the breakdown and absorption of dietary fats. There are two basic sources of body cholesterol: our diet and, far more important, cholesterol that is manufactured by our liver.

For a key to understanding how drugs reduce elevated levels of cholesterol, we need to talk about how it is carried around the body. Cholesterol can't dissolve in the blood and must be carried in the blood in other substances called lipoproteins. Three groups of lipoproteins are involved in the process:

♦ **VLDL (very low-density lipoproteins).** Important for the transport of triglycerides (other forms of fats). High triglyceride levels in the blood are thought to be involved in the development of atherosclerosis and are the second most important target of drug therapy. Target triglyceride levels are less than 150 mg/dL.

♦ **LDL (low-density lipoproteins).** Carries cholesterol to tissues. High levels of LDL ("bad" cholesterol) increase the risk of atherosclerosis. Low LDL levels decrease this risk. LDLs are the primary target of drug therapy. Target LDL levels are less than 100 mg/dL for most patients.

♦ **HDL (high-density lipoproteins).** Carries cholesterol away from tissues and back to the liver. By increasing the removal of cholesterol from tissues, HDL ("good" cholesterol) protects against the development of atherosclerosis. Low HDL levels increase this danger. Target HDL level: more than 40 mg/dL.

Cholesterol-Lowering Drugs: An Overview

Before using drugs to lower high cholesterol levels, individuals should attempt to reduce their risk factors for cardiovascular disorders. They should give up smoking, if they are smokers; lose weight, if overweight; increase physical activity, if sedentary; and cut back on high-fat, high-cholesterol foods.

Genetic factors may promote the development of atherosclerosis at an early age, which in the absence of effective treatment, leads to heart attacks in a high proportion of such individuals.

If lifestyle change approaches don't work, drugs should be tried. For a drug to be useful, it should lower LDL (bad cholesterol)—the most important single goal—as well as lower total cholesterol and triglycerides or increase HDL (good cholesterol). Target blood levels depend on the number of personal risk factors. The more risk factors, the more aggressive the targets.

LDL cholesterol levels return to their elevated levels if drugs are discontinued. Therefore, drug therapy must be continued for a lifetime.

There are four classes of drugs. Each works in a different way and has different side effects:

♦ Statins

♦ Binding resins

♦ Niacin

♦ Fibrates

Did You Know That ...?

Statins are among the most widely used of any class of medicines. In 2002, the two largest-selling drugs in the United States were Lipitor and Zocor, statins with combined sales of $10.3 billion.

Statins

Lovastatin and related statins are the most widely used class of drugs for reducing elevated cholesterol levels. Their great popularity can be attributed to their effectiveness and relatively few side effects.

Statins work in several complex ways to produce their beneficial effects. They significantly reduce both total cholesterol and LDL (bad) cholesterol and slightly increase HDL (good) cholesterol. These effects are evident after only a few weeks and are greatest within four to six weeks.

Clinical studies have shown that a wide range of individuals benefit from statins. These include healthy people, those with a history of heart disease, and those who have both elevated and normal cholesterol levels.

Benefits include fewer incidents of heart attack and stroke. Some doctors propose that statins be routinely used to prevent stroke and heart attacks in all individuals at risk. Moreover, several pharmaceutical manufacturers have formally attempted, but without success at present, to have their prescription-only statin drugs moved to an OTC status.

There are differences among the six statins with respect to their relative effectiveness, incidence of side effects, and drug interactions.

Maximizing Your Medicine

Statins are expensive and must be taken for a lifetime. How to save? Speak to your pharmacist about the costs of these different statins. Costs vary considerably. Ask your doctor if lovastatin is appropriate for you. It's available as a generic at half the cost of the brand. Also talk to your doctor and pharmacist about splitting the statin tablet you're using, essentially cutting your cost in half.

Statins need only be taken once daily. Lovastatin should be taken with meals, whereas the other statins can be taken without regard to meals. Taking statins in the evening is more effective than in the morning. These drugs work by reducing cholesterol manufacture by the liver, and most of this manufacturing takes place in the evening.

Warning!

If you have liver disease or are pregnant, do not take statins. Their use during the second and third trimester of pregnancy may cause injury and death to the developing fetus.

Side effects are generally uncommon and mild and include intestinal upset, rashes, and headache.

Liver toxicity and muscle injury are rare but very serious when they do occur. Individuals with liver disease and those who consume excessive amounts of alcohol are at greater risk for liver toxicity. Muscle aches, pains, and tenderness can progress to inflammation and breakdown of muscle. This has been associated with kidney failure.

Binding Resins

Unlike other drugs that reduce cholesterol, binding resins are not absorbed into the blood from the intestines. They are simply eliminated in the feces. Although not as effective as the statins, they are viewed as very safe alternatives.

In the intestines, these resins avidly bind to bile acids, preventing them from entering the blood. This promotes the elimination of bile acids in the feces. To replace the lost bile acids, the liver makes more using cholesterol, in particular LDL. As a consequence, blood levels of LDL (bad cholesterol) are reduced. LDL reduction is greatly increased when the resins are used with statins.

Common side effects include constipation, which is prevented by taking these granular resins with a full glass of water, and bloating and indigestion.

Resins can bind to and interfere with the absorption of other drugs. It is best to take them two hours before or after other medications. In particular, resins may reduce the effectiveness of warfarin, digoxin, levothyroxine, and tetracycline, as well as fat-soluble vitamins (A, D, E, K).

Niacin

Niacin (a.k.a. nicotinic acid) decreases LDL (bad cholesterol) and triglycerides and produces an impressive increase in HDL (good cholesterol).

Niacin is a B-complex vitamin found in yeast, liver, and lean meat.

Although niacin is highly effective, its usefulness is limited by side effects. The most common is an intense flushing of the face, with itching and feelings of warmth and tingling. The degree of flushing is often lessened if the dose is gradually increased and after repeated drug use. These effects, in particular flushing, are reduced when long-acting niacin is used.

Individuals with active liver disease or peptic ulcer should not take niacin. People with diabetes and gout should use niacin with caution.

Maximizing Your Medicine

Facial flushing can be reduced by taking an adult aspirin tablet (325 mg) 30 minutes before taking niacin. Avoid hot showers, hot drinks, and alcoholic beverages when taking niacin as these worsen the flushing.

Fibrates

Fibrates, also called fibric acids, lower triglycerides and increase HDL (good cholesterol). They have little effect on LDL (bad cholesterol). The primary use of fibrates is to reduce blood levels of triglycerides, thought to promote the development of atherosclerosis.

Fibrates should not be used by individuals with severe liver disease and severe kidney disease.

Fibrates may increase the risk of gallstones. Muscle toxicity may occur more often when fibrates are used in combination with statins.

Common side effects include rashes and indigestion.

Fibrates may increase the blood-thinning effects of warfarin, increasing the risk of bleeding.

The Least You Need to Know

- Elevated levels of cholesterol, in particular LDL (bad cholesterol), are associated with an increased risk of atherosclerosis.

- Atherosclerosis can increase the risk of stroke, heart attack, and other coronary artery diseases.

- Statins, the most effective and widely used drugs to reduce cholesterol levels, work by decreasing levels of LDL (bad cholesterol).

- Statins are well-tolerated medicines, whose major serious adverse effects are liver toxicity and severe muscle injury, which is associated with kidney failure.

- Binding resins are very safe drugs that lower LDL levels by working in the gastrointestinal tract.

- Niacin (nicotinic acid) is a highly effective drug whose usefulness is primarily limited by extreme flushing of the face and other potential side effects.

Drugs Used to Reduce Elevated Cholesterol

Generic Name	Trade Name	Generic Available
Statins (Generic Names End in "statin")		
Atorvastatin	Lipitor	No
Fluvastatin	Lescol	No
Lovastatin	Mevacor	Yes
Pravastatin	Pravachol	Yes
Rosuvastatin	Crestor	No
Simvastatin	Zocor	Yes
Binding Resins		
Cholestyramine	Questran	Yes
Colestipol	Colestid	No
Colesevelam	WelChol	No
Niacin (Nicotinic Acid)		
[Regular release]	Niacor	Yes
[Extended-release]	Niaspan, Slo-Niacin	Yes
Fibrates (Fibric Acids)		
Fenofibrate	Tricor	No
Gemfibrozil	Lopid	Yes
Other		
Ezetimide	Zetia	No

Contraception

Contraception is the prevention of pregnancy. Many contraceptive approaches are available, with varying degrees of effectiveness. Here we look at hormonal contraceptives, in particular those taken by mouth.

Hormonal Contraceptives: An Overview

Hormonal contraceptives are relatively safe, highly effective, and very widely used to prevent pregnancy. All contain the female hormones estrogen and progestin or progestin-only ingredients. They may be taken by mouth (oral contraceptives), injected, applied as skin patches, or inserted as a ring or IUD (intrauterine devise) into the uterus or vagina.

OTC Alternatives

Only one approved OTC chemical on the market kills sperm. Nonoxynol-9 is added to foams, gels, and suppositories. It doesn't protect against sexually transmitted diseases or HIV/AIDS.

In addition to being over 95 percent effective when used properly, their effects are reversible. After use is discontinued or they are removed, women have the potential to become pregnant.

Hormonal contraceptives work in one or more of the following ways:

◆ They prevent ovulation.

◆ They increase the thickness of mucus in the cervix, which interferes with the movement of sperm toward the egg.

◆ They prevent the fertilized egg from attaching to the wall of the uterus (a process called implantation), which is essential for its development.

Oral Contraceptives

Oral contraceptives (commonly referred to as "the pill") either contain both estrogen and progestin or progestin only ("mini-pill"). The several dozen products available differ with respect to their hormonal ingredients, the strength of these ingredients, and how they are taken.

All combination estrogen plus progestin products are equally effective in preventing pregnancy. Progestin-only products are slightly less effective than combination products.

Combination products are usually available in packages of 28 tablets, which simplifies the dosing schedule. Of these 28 tablets, 21 contain active hormones. The remaining 7 tablets contain an inactive ingredient or an iron supplement. Menstrual bleeding occurs three or four days after the last tablet containing the active hormone is taken.

Warning!

Although very highly effective in preventing pregnancy, oral and other hormonal contraceptives do not protect against sexually-transmitted diseases or HIV/AIDS.

Progestin-only products should be taken at the same time every day of the month throughout the year.

Dealing With Missed Doses

To avoid unintended pregnancy, the drugs must be taken without fail. What should be done if doses of combination products are missed?

- If only one dose is missed, take it as soon as possible or take two tablets the next day.

- If two consecutive doses are missed, take two tablets a day for the next two days, and on day three, resume taking the normal dose. Use an additional form of contraception (e.g., condom, diaphragm) for at least seven days after doses are missed.

- If three consecutive doses are missed, wait seven days and then start a new cycle of tablets. Use an additional form of contraception during the first two weeks of the new cycle.

Because progestin-only contraceptives are slightly less effective than combination products, a more conservative approach must be taken to dealing with missed doses:

- If only one dose is missed, take it as soon as possible or take two tablets the next day.

- If two or more consecutive tablets are missed, use a different method of contraception until a period occurs or pregnancy has been ruled out. These drugs should never be used during pregnancy or if there is a possibility of pregnancy.

Maximizing Your Medicine

To prevent pregnancy, oral contraceptives must be taken precisely as directed—day in, day out—regardless of whether sexual intercourse is on the "to do" list for that day. When days are missed, the odds for unwanted pregnancy increase. When women stop taking the combination products, more than half regain their fertility within three cycles after the last dose and about 90 percent within one year.

Other Benefits

In addition to preventing pregnancy, these drugs provide other benefits. They are able to relieve such menstrual problems as painful menstruation (dysmenorrhea) and irregular menstruation. Oral contraceptives are used to reduce the pain and bleeding seen in endometriosis.

They also reduce the risk of cancers of the ovaries and uterus (endometrium), as well as noncancerous fibrocystic breast disease and pelvic inflammatory disease.

 Warning!

Oral contraceptives should not be used by pregnant women or those with the following conditions:

- Breast cancer
- Blood clots in the veins
- Stroke or coronary artery disease
- Diabetes with damage to the kidneys, nerves, or retina
- Severe headaches
- Severely elevated blood pressure
- Liver disease
- Surgery requiring extended periods of immobilization or surgery of the legs
- Smokers of more than 20 cigarettes a day who are over age 35
- Nursing mothers less than six weeks after delivery

Oral contraceptives have many side effects, most of which are mild. These include nausea, breast fullness, water retention, weight gain, headache. With progestin-only products, unpredictable bleeding, spotting, or failure to menstruate is more common.

The nature of many of these side effects, and how often they occur, depends on the level of estrogen or progestin in a product. If any of these side effects are particularly troublesome, contact your doctor or pharmacist about changing your prescription for a more-favorable estrogen-progestin balance.

Potentially severe adverse effects include increased risk of blood clotting disorders, stroke, high blood pressure, and heart attacks. For nonsmokers, this risk is very small. It increases greatly for women who smoke more than 20 cigarettes a day and who are over 35.

Women should decide whether they want to continue to smoke or to take oral contraceptives. Doing both is an unhealthy option.

Drug Interactions

Prior to using oral contraceptives, a woman should consult her doctor or pharmacist with respect to any possible interactions with other drugs she is taking.

Using other drugs with oral contraceptives may reduce contraceptive effectiveness. These include certain antibiotics and selected medicines used for the treatment of seizures, HIV, and diabetes. Typical signs of reduced effectiveness include irregular bleeding and spotting. Increasing oral contraceptive dosage or using additional forms of contraception may be required.

Similarly, using oral contraceptives may decrease the effectiveness of other drugs. These include warfarin, a blood thinner, insulin, and other antidiabetic drugs taken by mouth. The dose of these drugs may need to be increased.

Oral contraceptives may increase the adverse effects and potential toxicity of other drugs. These include the tricyclic antidepressants and theophylline. Their dose may need to be reduced.

Non-Oral Hormonal Contraceptives

Some women might prefer not to take hormonal contraceptives every day. A variety of products deliver hormones over extended times ranging from one week up to five years after a single dose or application. Their side effects are similar to those seen with oral contraceptives. Here are the most popular alternatives:

- ◆ **Patch.** Ortho Evra is a patch containing estrogen and progestin that is applied to the upper body, upper outer arm, abdomen, or buttocks. A new patch is applied once weekly for a total of three weeks. During the fourth week, no patch is worn and menstruation occurs.

◆ **Ring.** NuvaRing is inserted into the vagina for three weeks, during which time it releases a hormonal combination. During the fourth week, when it is removed, the woman has a period.

◆ **Long-acting injections.** A single injection of progestin-only Depo-Provera into the muscle provides relatively safe and effective contraceptive protection for three months or more. This contraceptive approach has been used by millions of women worldwide since the 1960s. Menstrual irregularities are the most common side effects seen with this product.

Lunelle is an estrogen plus progestin combination injected at monthly intervals.

◆ **IUD.** These T-shaped devises slowly release progestin. They are relatively safe, very effective, and rather economical approaches to contraception. Progestasert and Mirena are inserted into the uterus and are left in place for 12 months and 5 years, respectively.

The major potential problem with IUDs is pelvic inflammatory disease resulting from sexually transmitted diseases. IUDs are most safely used by monogamous women whose partners are also monogamous.

The Least You Need to Know

◆ Hormonal contraceptives all contain estrogen plus progestin or progestin only.

◆ Minor side effects are common and are caused by too much or too little estrogen or progestin.

◆ Hormonal contraceptives may be taken by mouth (oral contraceptives), injected, applied as skin patches, or inserted as a ring or IUD (intrauterine devise) into the uterus or vagina.

◆ Because of other medical conditions or drugs being taken, some women should not use hormonal contraceptives or should use them with great caution.

Hormonal Contraceptive Products

Combination oral contraceptives	Alesse, Demulen, Estrostep, Loestrin, Lo/Ovral, Necon, Norinyl, Ortho-Novum, Ortho-Tricyclen, Ovcon, Seasonale, Tri-Levlen, Triphasil
Progestin-only oral contraceptives	Errin, Nor-QD, Ortho Micronor
Estrogen + progestin patch	Ortho Evra
Estrogen + progestin ring	NuvaRing
Long-acting injections	Depo-Provera, Lunelle
Progestin-containing IUDs	Progestasert, Mirena

Depression

Depression is a common psychiatric disorder in which there is extreme sadness over extended periods of time ranging from six months to two years, if untreated. Pleasure and satisfaction are no longer derived from family, work, or hobbies. The nature of the symptoms may vary but often include feelings of apathy, negativism, pessimism, and a lack of motivation. Loss of appetite and sleep disturbances are common. Suicide may be considered.

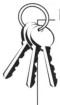

Did You Know That ...?

The old spiritual tells us that "I'm sometimes up and I'm sometimes down." Fluctuations in mood are a very normal part of living. We all experience degrees of sadness after personal, social, or monetary stresses, failures, and losses. These are relatively short-lived and do not interfere with work, life, or relationships. We spring back and return to normal even in the absence of medical treatment. This is not clinical depression.

Depression is among the most common psychiatric conditions. Over a lifetime, 15 percent of us will have a major depressive illness. Twice as many women experience depression as men.

Drug Treatment of Depression: An Overview

Without medical treatment, depression usually continues for about six months before mood returns to normal. Treatment approaches include psychoanalysis, electroconvulsive therapy (ECT), and, most often, drugs. Psychotherapy, in combination with drugs, provide additional benefits.

There are four primary groups of prescription antidepressant medications: tricyclics, selective serotonin-reuptake inhibitors (SSRIs), monoamine oxidase inhibitors (MAOIs), and a group of other, unrelated drugs.

Many theories have been proposed attempting to describe the causes of depression. Many theories revolve about abnormalities in serotonin and norepinephrine, two neurotransmitters in the brain. Different classes of antidepressants work in different ways, but they all seem to increase the amount of serotonin or norepinephrine available to act at their target sites in the brain.

OTC Alternatives

St. John's wort is a very popular dietary supplement. In clinical trials conducted to date, it appears to be effective for mild to moderate depression. Side effects are far less common than with tricyclics and about the same as SSRIs. St. John's wort reduces the blood levels and clinical effectiveness of other drugs. Batch-to-batch variation may exist in the content of hypericin, its active ingredient.

In general, 65 to 70 percent of persons receiving any antidepressant will have their depression lifted. However, we cannot predict whether the drug will be effective for a specific person. If one antidepressant fails to work, often another one will.

All antidepressants must be taken for several weeks before they begin to work, and they are usually taken for 12 months after the symptoms of depression have passed.

Distinct differences exist among the different drug classes with respect to their side effects and precautions.

 Warning! _____

Many drugs begin to provide real benefit after only a few doses. Not so with antidepressants. All of them must be taken for several weeks before the mood begins to improve. People suffering from depression commonly think about death and possibly suicide. Users of these drugs should be advised of this normal time delay. They must be encouraged to continue taking their medication and to not give up hope.

Tricyclic Antidepressants

For many years, tricyclics, such as imipramine (Tofranil) and amitriptyline (Elavil), were the most widely used antidepressants. Although tricyclics are as effective as other drugs, the extent of their usage has declined. Newer drugs have fewer side effects and are safer when taken in excess.

Side effects include dry mouth, blurred vision, constipation, difficulty in urinating, sedation, dizziness, increased heart rate, impairment of memory, weight gain, and impairment of sexual function. Side effects may be more pronounced in the elderly.

Tricyclic cautions:

- **Overdoses.** These drugs are potentially dangerous, even deadly, when taken in excessive doses. They interfere with normal heart rhythms. This is an obvious problem for persons bent on taking their own lives.

- **Drug withdrawal.** Don't stop using drugs abruptly. Dizziness, nausea, diarrhea, sleep difficulties, and nervousness may result.

- **Drug interactions.** Tricyclics should not be used together with MAOIs, depressant drugs (e.g., morphine-like opioids, sedating antihistamines, Valium-like benzodiazepines), and other drugs with atropine-like properties.

Selective Serotonin-Reuptake Inhibitors (SSRIs)

Prozac-like drugs are the most widely used class of antidepressants. They are as effective as tricyclics, but do not cause as many side effects and are far safer when taken in excessive doses.

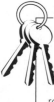

Did You Know That ...?

Many SSRIs are used for other medical conditions such as anxiety disorders, obsessive-compulsive disorders, panic reactions, and premenstrual dysphoric disorder (PMDD).

Side effects are generally mild and include nausea, vomiting, diarrhea, insomnia, weight gain, and interference with sexual function in both men and women.

SSRI caution:

- **Drug withdrawal.** Don't stop using SSRIs abruptly. Flu-like symptoms may result including dizziness, headache, nausea, and nervousness. Dosage should be gradually reduced over a two-to three-week period.

Monoamine Oxidase Inhibitors (MAOIs)

Nardil and Parnate are effective, but they are reserved for patients who don't benefit from other types of antidepressants. Their usage is limited because of side effects, restrictions in diet, and potentially dangerous drug interactions.

When assuming an erect position, users may experience dizziness and lightheadedness that results from a sudden drop in blood pressure (orthostatic hypotension). If these effects occur, sit or lie down.

Other side effects include nervousness, weight gain, impairment of sexual function, dry mouth, and constipation.

MAOI cautions:

◆ **Drug interactions.** MAOIs may interact with many other drugs including tricyclic and SSRI antidepressants, decongestants often found in cold preparations, drugs for high blood pressure, and meperidine (Demerol).

◆ **Food interactions.** MAOIs should not be taken with tyramine-rich foods and drinks, including (but not limited to) figs, avocados, fermented or smoked meats and fishes, most cheeses, yeast, Chianti wine, and some beers. Headache, increase in heart rate, nausea, vomiting, a sharp rise in blood pressure, and stroke may occur. This potentially fatal reaction is called a hypertensive crisis.

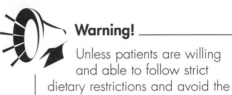

Warning!

Unless patients are willing and able to follow strict dietary restrictions and avoid the use of tyramine-rich foods and drinks, they should not take MAOIs.

Other Antidepressants

A number of miscellaneous antidepressant drugs are available that cannot be neatly placed in one of the previously listed categories. Each has distinctive side effects. It's not possible to generalize about their characteristics.

The Least You Need to Know

◆ Depression is a common psychiatric condition that 15 percent of us will experience during a lifetime.

◆ Most antidepressants provide benefit to 65 to 70 percent of treated individuals, although it is not possible to predict which patients will respond to given drugs.

◆ Antidepressants must be given for several weeks before mood improves and are generally taken for 12 months after symptoms are relieved.

◆ In addition to their effectiveness in a given patient, drug selection is based on side effects and other precautions.

- Prozac-like SSRIs are the most widely used antidepressants because of their generally mild side effects and relative safety when taken in overdose.

- Tricyclics cause an extensive array of side effects and are quite dangerous when taken in excessive doses.

Drugs Used for Depression

Generic Name	Trade Name	Generic Available
Tricyclics		
Amitriptyline	Elavil	Yes
Clomipramine	Anafranil	Yes
Desipramine	Norpramin	Yes
Doxepin	Sinequan	Yes
Imipramine	Tofranil	Yes
Nortriptyline	Aventyl, Pamelor	Yes
Protriptyline	Vivactil	Yes
Trimipramine	Surmontil	No
Selective Serotonin-Reuptake Inhibitors (SSRIs)		
Citalopram	Celexa	No
Duloxetine	Cymbalta	No
Escitalopram	Lexapro	No
Fluoxetine	Prozac, Sarafem	Yes
Fluvoxamine	Luvox	Yes
Paroxetine	Paxil	Yes
Sertraline	Zoloft	Yes
Monoamine Oxidase Inhibitors (MAOIs)		
Phenelzine	Nardil	No
Tranylcypromine	Parnate	No

Generic Name	Trade Name	Generic Available
Other Drugs		
Amoxapine	Asendin	Yes
Bupropion	Wellbutrin	Yes
Mirtazepine	Remeron	No
Nefazodone	Serzone	No
Trazodone	Desyrel	Yes
Venlafaxine	Effexor	No

Diabetes Mellitus

Diabetes mellitus afflicts more than 18 million Americans, yet only 2 out of 3 of those with the condition know they have it. To reduce, or preferably prevent, the long-term complications of diabetes and increase life expectancy, it's critically important that diabetics be treated and effectively managed.

Did You Know That ...?

There are two different conditions called diabetes, both associated with thirst and a voluminous urine output: Diabetes insipidus ("water" diabetes) is a rare disease related to a hormone from the pituitary gland. By contrast, diabetes mellitus ("sugar" diabetes) is a common disease involving insulin, a hormone from the pancreas. In this section, we focus on diabetes mellitus, which we simply refer to as diabetes.

Diabetes is a condition in which there is a problem with insulin, a hormone made by and released from the pancreas. Insulin's major function is to facilitate the movement of sugar from the blood into cells, where it is metabolized to supply the energy needs of the body.

One of two basic problems may exist in diabetes. Either there is too little insulin or cells are insulin resistant and don't adequately respond to its effects. In either case, *sugar* remains in the blood and is unable to enter many cells, where it is used for energy. In addition, sugar can't be saved for use at a later time.

def•i•ni•tion

When we talk about **sugar**, we specifically mean glucose. "Glycemia" means sugar in the blood. Normal blood sugar levels range from 70 to 110 mg/dL (1 dL = 100 ml, a little more than 3 oz). Excessive sugar levels in the blood (more than 110 mg/dL) are called hyperglycemia, which may be associated with diabetes. Low blood sugar levels are referred to as hypoglycemia.

The most conspicuous sign of diabetes is an increase in blood sugar, a condition called hyperglycemia. Blood sugar can be easily self-monitored using simple, affordable testing devices and a drop of blood.

Other common signs of diabetes, many resulting from excessive blood sugar levels, include sugar in the urine (glycosuria); excretion of large amounts of water (polyuria); and excessive hunger (polyphagia).

The uncontrolled diabetic cannot metabolize sugar for energy and must use fats instead. When large amounts of fat are broken down they form substances called ketones, which makes the blood more acidic. This condition, ketoacidosis, may cause unconsciousness (diabetic coma) and death if not promptly treated. Diabetic coma has been often mistaken for severe alcohol intoxication.

Types of Diabetes

There are two major types of diabetes: type 1 and type 2. They differ in their prevalence, cause, when and how rapidly they appear, and how they are treated.

Type 1 diabetes was formerly called insulin-dependent diabetes mellitus (IDDM) or juvenile-onset diabetes. Far more common is type 2, which was previously known as non-insulin-dependent diabetes mellitus (NIDDM) or adult-onset diabetes.

Type 1 Diabetes

Only about 10 percent of all diabetics have type 1 diabetes, a condition in which most of the insulin-producing cells of the pancreas are destroyed. This results from an autoimmune condition in which the body's immune system destroys its own cells. The cell destruction may be triggered by a viral infection. Because the body can no longer make its own insulin, outside sources of insulin are required for survival.

Although type 1 may occur at any age, it almost always makes its appearance, and typically without warning, during the childhood or adolescent years. Type 1 is a severe condition and difficult to fully control. Here the diabetic is subject to rapidly developing, life-threatening ketoacidosis. Continued good health into adulthood depends on managing diet and adhering to the dosing schedule for insulin.

Type 2 Diabetes

Most diabetics, about 90 percent, have type 2 diabetes, also known as insulin-resistant diabetes. With this condition, insulin secretion may or may not be impaired; regardless, tissues fail to respond properly to available insulin (i.e., insulin resistant), and sugar does not move into cells and is not adequately consumed for energy. The risk of ketoacidosis is low because some insulin production generally presists. There is a strong genetic disposition to developing type 2, and most people with the condition are obese. An increased risk is seen in African-Americans and Hispanics.

Historically, type 2 first occurred after the age of 30. There is now growing concern that an increasing proportion of teenagers, who are obese, are developing this condition.

Type 2 diabetes typically develops slowly over many years.

Short-Term and Long-Term Complications

Each diabetic patient has unique medication and dosage requirements that have been individualized by their doctors. The diabetic should understand that the right dose of medication must be taken at the right time.

Too low a dose of insulin will not control the condition, potentially resulting in keto-acidosis in the type 1 patient. By contrast, an excessive dose of insulin causes an exaggerated drop in blood sugar leading to drowsiness, fatigue, confusion, and fainting. If deprived of adequate sugar supplies for an extended period of time, brain damage can result.

Taking insulin or oral antidiabetic drugs reduce the acute risks of diabetes. The long-term complications, however, continue to progress in both type 1 and type 2 diabetes and are responsible for more than 90 percent of deaths in diabetics. These chronic complications include degenerative changes to small blood vessels, kidneys (with kidney failure), eyes (a major cause of adult blindness), and nerves. Reduced blood flow to the extremities causes slow wound healing, infections, ulceration, and in advanced cases, gangrene. The diabetic runs a greater risk of developing atherosclerosis (a.k.a. hardening of the arteries) and coronary artery disease (e.g., angina and heart attack).

> **Maximizing Your Medicine**
>
> Several very important, large-scale studies have shown that when blood sugar levels are carefully and closely maintained at normal levels, these long-term complications can be substantially reduced.

Diabetic Treatment Overview

Successful treatment of diabetes involves keeping blood sugar within normal limits. Diet, exercise, and drugs are used to achieve this objective.

Antidiabetic drugs fall into two general categories: insulin taken by injection and drugs taken by mouth that reduce blood sugar levels, called oral hypoglycemics. Which drugs are used for which patients?

◆ All type 1 diabetics require insulin to control their blood sugar. Some type 2 diabetics may also require insulin.

◆ Oral hypoglycemics are often effective for treating type 2, but never type 1, diabetes.

◆ Adequate control of blood sugar in type 2 diabetics may require the use of a combination of oral drugs or an oral drug plus insulin.

Insulin

Insulin is a hormone that is made in and released by the pancreas. Pharmaceutical insulin was formerly obtained from either the pancreas of beef or pigs. Today, human insulin can be produced in the laboratory using cutting-edge techniques of molecular biology. Human insulin is most commonly used, although porcine (pig) insulin is still available.

If insulin is taken by mouth, it is rapidly broken down and inactivated, so it must be injected or inhaled.

Maximizing Your Medicine

There is a need for non-injectable insulins. Oral insulin preparations have not been promising thus far. Successful use of an insulin nasal spray has been complicated by the difficulty of ensuring that accurate doses are delivered to the blood.

Exubera, a dry powder that is inhaled into the lungs, is the first new way to take insulin since it was discovered in the 1920s. This rapid-acting inhaled insulin was approved by the FDA in 2006 for types 1 and 2 diabetes. It is not expected to replace long-acting insulin injections for type 1 diabetics. It is not intended to be used by diabetics with asthma or poorly controlled lung disease or by smokers.

Types of Insulin

Pharmaceutical insulin preparations are categorized primarily with respect to time considerations: their onset of action, time of peak effects, and duration of action.

Insulin Preparations Based on Approximate Time

Insulin Type	Onset	Peak	Duration
Rapid acting	15–30 min	1–2 hrs.	4–6 hrs.
Intermediate acting	2–4 hrs.	4–12 hrs.	12–18 hrs.
Long acting	4–8 hrs.	10–16 hrs.	18–24 hrs.

Regular insulin rapidly reduces blood sugar after injection, but its effects are relatively short-lived and several injections are needed each day. Zinc or the protein protamine added to insulin make products that reduce blood sugar for extended periods of time. This product is a cloudy suspension that must be carefully and completely mixed before use.

Subtle changes in the complex chemistry of insulin produce such "designer" insulin products as insulin lispro, which acts more rapidly than regular insulin. Insulin glargine, by contrast, acts to reduce blood sugar for 24 hours after a single injection.

Different dosing schedules are used to administer insulin. Patients need to work closely with their doctors to determine which insulin preparation and schedule of insulin administration best meets their diabetic needs, their willingness to have multiple daily injections, and their lifestyle.

Warning!

If the insulin is cloudy, make sure that it is completely mixed before use. Mix by slowly rolling the bottle between your hands or gently tipping over the bottle several times. Never shake the bottle vigorously.

Some schedules are preferred because they are simple to follow or require only a single injection a day. More complex schedules combine rapid and intermediate-acting preparations and require several injections a day. They provide greater control of blood sugar, the key to reducing long-term complications. Many of these insulin combinations are pre-mixed and commercially available.

How Insulin Is Taken

Insulin is normally injected under the skin into the underlying layer of fat. These injections are usually made into the upper arms, thighs, and abdomen.

In addition to injections given by typical syringe and needle, insulin may be given by …

- ◆ **Jet injectors.** No needle is needed; instead, insulin is shot directly through the skin. These devices are expensive and not easy to use.

- **Pen injectors.** Pen-like devices that are equipped with a disposable needle and prefilled cartridge. Suitable for more convenient and less publicly visible injections.

- **Insulin pumps.** Available as an external portable pump, it is smaller than a deck of playing cards and can be attached to a belt. The pump can be programmed to deliver a fixed dose of insulin or extra amounts to fit special circumstances. Insulin is injected subcutaneously into the abdomen. Surgically implantable insulin pumps are being developed.

In emergency situations, regular (natural) insulin can be given by intravenous (IV) injection. Only regular insulin can be safely given via IV.

To simplify calculation of dosage and reduce the risk of errors, only two concentrations of insulin are available in the United States: 100 units/ml (U-100), which is used routinely; and 500 units/ml (U-500), for use in emergencies and by diabetics with high insulin dosage requirements. U-40 is available in some other countries.

Maximizing Your Medicine

Storage considerations: unopened insulin should be refrigerated (but never frozen) prior to use. The expiration date appearing on an insulin vial specifically refers to an unopened, refrigerated product. Check the manufacturer's recommendations for product stability at room temperature (59–86°) after it has been opened. In general, it's good for 28 days, without loss of potency.

Adverse Effects

Insulin's most common adverse effect is an excessive drop in blood sugar. Hypoglycemia results when too much insulin is given relative to the body's actual needs. This situation can arise as the result of missed meals, too much alcohol, illness, or greater than normal exercise.

Early signs of low blood sugar include feelings of hunger and weakness, sweating, nausea, and nervousness. In more advanced stages, the patient will experience mental confusion, incoherent speech, double vision, and loss of consciousness. If untreated, permanent brain damage and death may occur.

Warning!

Diabetics should know and be alert to the early signs of low blood sugar. They are advised to carry lump sugar or hard candy or take a sugar-containing liquid at its first signs. Moreover, they should carry cards or medic alert tags that identify themselves as diabetics.

Prior to the availability of human insulin, repeated injections of insulin from animal sources caused abnormalities in the fatty tissue at the sites of injection—either a loss or a buildup of fat. Localized allergic reactions can also occur, these caused by contaminants in animal insulin products. These problems are quite rare when human insulin is used.

Oral Hypoglycemic Drugs

Oral hypoglycemic drugs lower blood sugar after being taken by mouth and are the primary medicines used for type 2 diabetes. These drugs should only be used when high blood sugar levels cannot be controlled by dietary modifications or increases in physical activity in sedentary individuals.

There are five classes of oral antidiabetic drugs, and they produce their effects by working in different ways:

- **Sulfonylureas and glinides.** Increase the release of insulin from the pancreas. These drugs can only work if the cells in the pancreas are able to produce insulin.

- **Biguanides.** Increase tissue sensitivity to insulin and decrease the body's manufacture of additional sugar.

- **Glitazones.** Increase the sensitivity of tissues to available insulin by decreasing insulin resistance.

- **Glucosidase inhibitors.** Slow the speed at which dietary carbohydrates are broken down into smaller sugar units. This slows their normally rapid absorption into the blood after meals, leading to a rise of blood sugar.

Sulfonylureas

Seven glyburide-like sulfonylureas are marketed in the United States. These drugs mainly differ based on how long they work (i.e., their duration of action). Newer versions of these drugs work at lower doses; when given in comparable doses, however, they all lower blood sugar to the same extent. Sulfonylureas can be used in combination with insulin and other oral antidiabetic drugs.

The most common adverse effect is an over-response, where blood sugar is excessively reduced (i.e., hypoglycemia). These drugs also stimulate appetite, which may cause weight gain. This complicates the problems of most type 2 diabetics, most of whom are already obese.

A greater than anticipated drop in blood sugar can occur when sulfonylureas are taken with some other drugs. These include alcohol, aspirin and related nonsteroidal anti-inflammatory drugs (NSAIDs), and sulfa drugs.

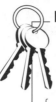

Did You Know That ...?

Based on the chance observation that a sulfa drug, used to treat typhoid fever, caused a drop in blood sugar, the sulfonylureas were developed. These were the first oral hypoglycemic drugs available.

Glinides

Glinides also work by stimulating the release of insulin from the pancreas. They start working faster than the sulfonylureas and continue to work for a shorter period of time. They must be given 30 minutes before meals and are intended to reduce the rise in blood sugar that normally occurs after meals.

Their most common side effect is hypoglycemia, but this occurs far less often than with sulfonylureas. Weight gain may also occur.

Biguanides

Metformin is the only biguanide marketed in the United States. It is an effective drug and is even more effective when used with a sulfonylurea. It is the only oral drug found to reduce the risk of diabetes-related deaths and those caused by heart attacks.

Hypoglycemia and weight gain are not a problem with metformin. Upset stomach, loss of appetite, and diarrhea are problems, and they occur commonly. Weight loss often occurs, which on average is greater than 5 lbs.

Metformin should only be used in individuals with effective kidney and liver function. It should be avoided in heart failure patients who require medications. Toxic metformin levels can build up, and dire consequences can result in individuals with diseases of these organs.

Glitazones

Glitazones slowly reduce blood glucose levels. Their greatest effects are not seen until they have been taken for three to four months.

They also cause a decrease in fats (a.k.a. triglycerides) and increase levels of "good" (HDL) cholesterol. These changes are positive for diabetic patients prone to heart disease. Unfortunately, "bad" (LDL) cholesterol levels may also be increased.

Glitazones tend to cause weight gain and fluid retention. The latter can lead to or worsen heart failure. They should not be given to diabetics with a history of heart failure.

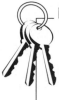

Did You Know That …?

When the first glitazone, troglitazone, appeared on the market in 1995, the medical community greeted it with great enthusiasm. It worked in a novel way and was highly effective. Less than five years later, it was withdrawn from the market after causing liver toxicity and 28 deaths resulting from liver failure. Happily, these problems have not been seen with the currently available glitazones.

Glucosidase Inhibitors

Glucosidase inhibitors are used to reduce blood sugar levels after meals and are taken at the start of each meal.

The usefulness of these drugs is limited by their frequently causing intestinal gas, bloating, abdominal discomfort, and diarrhea.

The Least You Need to Know

- An increase in blood sugar (a.k.a. hyperglycemia) is the most important sign in diabetes and is responsible for its symptoms.

- Type 1 diabetes must be treated with injected insulin, whereas type 2 can be managed with lifestyle change, oral hypoglycemic drugs, and/or insulin.

- The risk of the long-term complications of diabetes, including degenerative changes to small blood vessels, the kidneys, eyes, and nerves, can be reduced by keeping blood sugar at normal levels.

◆ Insulin preparations primarily differ with respect to how rapidly they reduce blood sugar, when they produce their peak effects, and how long they continue to work.

◆ An excessive decrease in blood sugar (a.k.a. hypoglycemia) is the most common adverse effect associated with the use of insulin.

◆ Oral hypoglycemic drugs primarily act by increasing the amount of insulin released by the pancreas or by making tissues more sensitive to available insulin.

◆ The most common adverse effects caused by many hypoglycemic drugs include hypoglycemia and weight gain.

Drugs Used for Diabetes Mellitus

Generic Name	Trade Name	Generic Available
Insulin		
Rapid Acting		
Aspart insulin	NovoLog	No
Glulisine insulin	Apidra	No
Lispro insulin	Humalog	No
Regular insulin	Humulin R	No
	Novolin R	No
Intermediate Acting		
Lente insulin	Humulin L, Lente Iletin	No
NPH (Isophane) insulin suspension	Humulin N, Novolin N, NPH Iletin	No
Long Acting		
Glargine insulin	Lantus	No
Ultralente insulin	Humulin U	No
Oral Hypoglycemic Drugs		
Biguanides		
Metformin	Glucophage	Yes

continues

Drugs Used for Diabetes Mellitus   (continued)

Generic Name	Trade Name	Generic Available
Glinides		
Nateglinide	Starlix	No
Repaglinide	Prandin	No
Glitazones		
Pioglitazone	Actos	No
Rosiglitazone	Avandia	No
Glucosidase Inhibitors		
Acarbose	Precose	No
Miglitol	Glyset	No
Sulfonylureas		
Acetohexamide	Dymelor	Yes
Chlorpropamide	Diabinase	Yes
Glimeparide	Amaryl	No
Glipizide	Glucotrol	Yes
Glyburide	DiaBeta, Glynase, Micronase	Yes
Tolazamide	Tolinase	Yes
Tolbutamide	Orinase	Yes

Diarrhea

Diarrhea is an increase in the number, amount, or wateriness of bowel movements.

The causes of diarrhea are many and varied; they include infections caused by bacteria, viruses, and parasites; as well as certain foods; inflammation, tumors, malabsorption, stress; and many drugs or chemicals.

Treatment: An Overview

In most instances, diarrhea is simple, mild to moderate in severity, and temporary, lasting for less than two days. Treatment is likewise simple—eliminate the offensive agent if possible, replace the lost fluids, sugar, and salts (i.e., electrolytes, such as sodium, potassium, magnesium, chloride), and if needed, take an OTC product to stem the flow. At times, it is preferable not to give anti-diarrheal drugs. The body may be attempting to rid the body of toxins or bacteria.

In more severe cases, a doctor should be consulted. There is good reason for concern if the diarrhea persists for more than 48 hours or if, at any time, temperature exceeds 101°F, there is abdominal pain, severe chills, or bloody stools. Young children, elderly individuals, and those with severe health problems (such as diabetes or heart disease) are at greater risk of becoming severely dehydrated. If uncorrected, fatalities may occur.

Did You Know That ...?

The body judiciously safeguards its important resources, among the most important of which are body fluids. Every day some 9 quarts of fluids enter our digestive tract, but only 4 oz. are eliminated in the stools. Some 98.5 percent of the total fluids are captured and returned to the blood after their absorption in the intestines.

An attempt should be made to identify and specifically treat the cause of the diarrhea, such as by using antibacterial medicines.

Prescription drugs used to treat diarrhea are all opioids.

OTC Alternatives

Adsorbents bind not only toxins and microbes that may be causing diarrhea, but also drugs and nutrients. Such adsorbents include bismuth subsalicylate (BSS; Pepto-Bismol; Kaopectate) and polycarbophil (FiberCon). OTC products often contain several drugs. BSS also relieves intestinal inflammation. BSS and loperamide (Imodium) are quite effective.

Opioids

The antidiarrheal effects of opium have long been recognized. Opium tincture (a.k.a. laudanum), paregoric (camphorated tincture of opium), and codeine are effective antidiarrheal medications. They have been replaced by related drugs (opioids) that are safer and not subject to abuse.

Warning!

If the cause of diarrhea is bacteria that has penetrated the walls of the intestines or if the patient has a fever, neither loperamide nor diphenoxylate should be used.

In addition to quieting the intestines, opioids work in multiple and complex ways to control diarrhea. By slowing the passage of materials down the intestines, more time and opportunity is available for fluids and electrolytes to return to the bloodstream and not be lost in the stools. Opioids are so effective that constipation may result from their use.

Two of the most commonly used opioids are loperamide and diphenoxylate.

Loperamide

The same loperamide (Imodium) is available both as a prescription and an OTC product. When obtained as an OTC product, lower doses are recommended.

Unlike opium and diphenoxylate, which get into the brain and cause behavioral side effects, loperamide only works in the intestines. It is used for the control of diarrheal condition, including *traveler's diarrhea.*

Side effects, although uncommon, may include dizziness and constipation.

def•i•ni•tion

Traveler's diarrhea is a common souvenir of trips to Latin America, southern Europe, Africa, and Asia. In addition to avoiding high-risk foods and drinks, some travelers take BSS for prevention. Active treatment includes BSS, loperamide (faster than BSS), and such antibacterials as a quinolone antibiotic or trimethoprim-sulfamethoxazole.

Diphenoxylate

Diphenoxylate is a prescription-only drug to which a small amount of atropine has been added to discourage intentional overdose for purposes of abuse.

Unlike loperamide, both diphenoxylate and atropine enter the brain, which accounts for behavioral side effects. These include dizziness, drowsiness, and confusion. Atropine-like effects may include flushing, dry skin, fever, increases in heart rate, and retention of urine.

When used with MAO inhibitor antidepressants, diphenoxylate may dangerously increase blood pressure. It may also increase the depressant effects of barbiturates, tranquilizers, and alcohol.

The Least You Need to Know

- ◆ Whereas mild to moderate cases of diarrhea can be treated with OTC drugs, a doctor should be consulted for severe cases, as you might need prescription medication.

- ◆ The most widely used and effective drugs to control diarrhea are opioids, such as loperamide.

- ◆ Traveler's diarrhea is treated with both antidiarrheal drugs and with antibacterial medication.

Drugs Used for Treatment of Diarrhea

Generic Name	Trade Name	Generic Available
Opioids		
Diphenoxin + atropine	Motofen	No
Diphenoxylate + atropine	Lomotil	Yes
Loperamide	Imodium	Yes
Paregoric (Camphorated opium tincture)	—	Yes

continues

Drugs Used for Treatment of Diarrhea (continued)

Generic Name	Trade Name	Generic Available
Antibacterials		
Ciprofloxacin	Cipro	Yes
Norfloxacin	Noroxin	No
Trimethoprim + sulfamethoxazole (Co-Trimethoxazole)	Bactrim DS, Septra DS	Yes

Eczema (Dermatitis)

Eczema, also called dermatitis, is a catchall name for skin disorders having a red and itching rash. Drugs applied to the skin are used to treat eczema.

Contact Dermatitis

Contact dermatitis results from direct exposure to certain cosmetics, jewelry, chemicals, and plants, such as poison ivy. More than half of all eczemas are of this type. If the cause is known, try to avoid it.

Atopic Dermatitis

Atopic dermatitis, also called chronic or hand dermatitis, is common in infants and young children and often, but not always, disappears by the teenage years. This condition is most often seen in folks with asthma or hay fever. Often the sufferer has an itchy rash and very dry skin, but its cause is not known. There is no permanent cure for this condition, and soaps and detergents, rough clothing, and temperature extremes worsen it.

Did You Know That ...?

Poison ivy, poison oak, and poison sumac all contain the plant oil urushiol. Exposure to this oil is responsible for the itching, red rash, and blisters. The itching and rash last for several weeks. Topical steroids relieve the symptoms, but the rash remains for the usual period.

Topical Steroids

Some 20 different prescription-only steroids are available for application to the skin. Most of these products are available in different concentrations and in different dosage forms (e.g., ointments, creams, gels).

Topical steroids should be applied in a thin film and gently rubbed into the skin. They relieve the redness, itching, and swelling that may be present, with improvement generally seen within a week.

OTC Alternatives

Several categories of OTC products may be useful for the treatment of eczema, including moisturizers. Some other products relieve pain and itching and protect injured skin. Topical hydrocortisone, in strengths of up to 1 percent, is the only steroid drug available OTC.

Some topical preparations are preferred for the treatment of different types of dermatitis:

- Ointments and creams provide greater moisturizing effects than solutions, lotions, or gels.

- Lotions are preferred for oozing rashes.

- Solutions, lotions, and gels are easier to apply to hairy areas.

Common adverse effects include skin irritation, thinning of the skin with stretch marks, and extension of scars.

Just because a drug is applied to the skin, it doesn't mean that it can't enter the bloodstream and cause adverse effects in other parts of the body. This can be the case with topical steroids. Don't use these drugs more often or for longer periods than your doctor has recommended.

Patients should not bandage or wrap the skin being treated unless their doctor advises them to do so. Wrapping the skin may increase the beneficial effects of steroids but may also increase their potential for causing adverse effects.

> **Warning!**
>
> If you have a skin reaction shortly after starting any medication, contact your doctor or pharmacist immediately. You may be having a drug-induced allergic reaction.

The Least You Need to Know

- Eczema, also called dermatitis, has many causes, only some of which can be identified.

- Topical steroids are highly effective in providing rapid relief of the redness, itching, and swelling seen in eczema.

- Topical steroids should not be used more often or for longer periods of time than prescribed.

Topical Steroids Used for Eczema

Generic Name	Trade Name(s)	Generic Available
Aclometasone	Aclovate	No
Amcinonide	Cyclocort	No
Betamethasone	Diprolene, Diprosone, Valisone	Yes
Clobetasol	Temovate	Yes
Desonide	DesOwen, Tridesilon	Yes
Desoximetasone	Topicort	Yes
Fluocinolone	Synalar	Yes
Fluocinonide	Lidex	Yes
Flurandrenolide	Cordran	Yes
Halcinonide	Halog	
Hydrocortisone	Cortaid, Cortizone, Hytone	Yes
Triamcinolone	Aristocort, Kenalog	Yes

Endometriosis

The endometrium is the tissue lining the uterus, which is shed during menstruation. For reasons we don't understand, with endometriosis, endometrial tissue can be found in abnormal locations, including the ovaries, fallopian tubes, intestines, vagina, bladder, and between the rectum and the vagina.

Female hormones, responsible for the monthly period, cause these misplaced endometrial tissues to menstruate. These shed tissues have nowhere to go and remain to form scar tissue and cause irritation and pain.

Symptoms and the location of the endometriosis differ considerably among women. Abdominal bloating is common. Pain usually occurs and can be extreme, particularly in the days immediately prior to and during menstruation. Sexual intercourse is very painful at this time. Interestingly, some women experience no pain.

Endometriosis occurs in 10 to 15 percent of women during their reproductive years and may be responsible for one third of all cases of infertility.

Drug Treatment of Endometriosis: An Overview

Endometriosis can be treated with surgery or drugs. Both approaches may relieve symptoms, but neither cures the disease.

OTC nonsteroidal anti-inflammatory drugs (NSAIDS) are used for pain relief. Other drugs change the hormonal environment to shrink displaced endometrial tissue, reducing pain and bleeding. These include the oral contraceptives, progestins, gonadotropin-like drugs, and Danazol. Preventing periods reduces pain but also the possibility of pregnancy.

OTC Alternatives

Nonsteroidal anti-inflammatory drugs (NSAIDs), such as ibuprofen (Motrin) and naproxen (Aleve), are used to relieve pain. Long-term use may cause adverse effects to the gastrointestinal tract and kidneys. NSAIDS are commonly used for pain relief in osteoarthritis.

Estrogen and Progestin Oral Contraceptives

Oral contraceptives have estrogen and progestin ingredients. They shrink nonuterine endometrial tissue and decrease menstrual flow. Several dozen oral contraceptives are available, with no major differences in benefit (see "Contraception" for more information on oral contraceptives).

Warning!

Oral contraceptives should not be used by pregnant women or those with the following conditions:

- ◆ Breast cancer
- ◆ Blood clots in the veins
- ◆ Stroke or coronary artery disease
- ◆ Diabetes with damage to the kidneys, nerves, or retina
- ◆ Severe headaches
- ◆ Severely elevated blood pressure
- ◆ Liver disease
- ◆ Surgery requiring extended periods of immobilization or surgery of the legs
- ◆ Smokers of more than 20 cigarettes a day who are over age 35
- ◆ Nursing mothers less than six weeks after delivery

Cautions

There are many side effects, most of which are mild. These include nausea, breast fullness, water retention, weight gain, and headache.

The nature of many of these side effects, and how often they occur, depends on the level of estrogen or progestin in the product. If any of these side effects are particularly troublesome, contact your doctor or pharmacist about changing your prescription to a product with a more favorable estrogen-progestin balance.

Potentially severe adverse effects include increased risk of blood clotting disorders, stroke, high blood pressure, and heart attacks. For nonsmokers, this risk is very small. It increases greatly for women who smoke more than 20 cigarettes a day and who are over 35.

Women should decide whether they want to continue to smoke or to take oral contraceptives. Doing both is an unhealthy option.

Drug Interactions

Prior to using oral contraceptives, a woman should consult her doctor or pharmacist with respect to any possible interactions with other drugs she is taking.

Use of oral contraceptives may decrease the effectiveness of other drugs, including warfarin (a blood thinner), insulin, and other antidiabetic drugs taken by mouth. The dose of these drugs may need to be increased.

Use of oral contraceptives may increase the adverse effects and potential toxicity of other drugs. These include the tricyclic antidepressants and theophylline. Their dose may need to be reduced.

Progestins

Progestins are female hormones used for contraceptive purposes and treatment of endometriosis. The most widely used progestin is medroxprogesterone, taken orally (Provera) or by an injection into the muscle (Depo-Provera) every three months. Relief of pain occurs in 80 to 90 percent of treated women.

Common side effects include irregular periods, water retention, weight gain, and mood swings. Women may experience a delay in becoming pregnant after injection therapy has ended. Progestins cause fewer side effects and are less expensive than the gonadotropin-like drugs.

Gonadotropin-Like Drugs

Naturally-produced estrogen stimulates growth of endometrial tissues. Gonadotropin-releasing hormone (GnRH) prevents estrogen release.

Three laboratory-manufactured GnRH-like drugs are available:

◆ Leuprolide is injected into the muscles once every three months.

◆ Goserelin is injected under the skin once monthly.

◆ Nafarelin is taken daily as a nasal spray.

After being used for a 6-month period, 85 to 100 percent of women are pain-free. However, after five years of use, only one half remain pain-free.

Common side effects include hot flashes, dryness of the vagina, insomnia, and bone loss after three months of treatment. Estrogen and other treatments are being tested to prevent bone loss without interfering with the GnRH benefits.

Danazol

Oral danazol shrinks the size of endometrial tissue, both outside and within the uterus. Effects on the uterine endothelial tissues interfere with pregnancy. Some 80 to 90 percent of women will have reduction of symptoms within two months of therapy.

Danazol's benefits are offset by side effects. It has male hormone-like effects, which cause acne, deepening of the voice, and facial hair. It also interferes with liver function, causes water retention, and produces adverse effects to the female fetus.

The Least You Need to Know

◆ OTC nonsteroidal anti-inflammatory drugs (e.g., ibuprofen, naproxen) are used to relieve pain associated with endometriosis.

◆ Drugs used for the treatment of endometriosis shrink the size of endometrial tissues outside the uterus and may also reduce menstrual flow.

◆ Female hormones, gonadotropin-like drugs, and danazol do not cure endometriosis but relieve pain in a high proportion of women.

Drug Treatment of Endometriosis

Generic Name	Trade Name	Generic Available
Oral Contraceptives		
Estrogen + Progestin	Alesse, Demulen, Estrostep, Loestrin, Lo/Ovral, Necon, Norinyl, Ortho-Novum, Ortho-Tricyclen, Ovcon, Ovral, Ovrette, Seasonale, Tri-Levlen, Triphasil	Yes
Progestin	Errin, Nor-QD, Ortho Micronor	No

continues

Drug Treatment of Endometriosis   (continued)

Generic Name	Trade Name	Generic Available
Gonadotropin-Like Drugs (GnRH)		
Goserelin	Zoladex	No
Leuprolide	Lupron	Yes
Nafarelin	Synarel	No
Other		
Danazol	Danocrine	Yes

Erectile Dysfunction

Prior to the appearance of some very suggestive and catchy direct-to-consumer ads on TV and in popular magazines in the late 1990s, there was little public discussion of erectile dysfunction.

Erectile dysfunction (ED or impotence) is the persistent inability to initiate or maintain an erection. More recently, this definition has been significantly extended to also include the inability to sustain an erection that is suitable for satisfactory sexual performance—very subjective criteria, to be sure. By no means an uncommon problem, ED affects some 30 million American men and leads to 500,000 doctor office visits each year.

To achieve an erection, there must be adequate blood flow into the penis and restrictions upon its prematurely flowing out. Nerve impulses are required for this to occur. Not surprisingly, ED may have many causes, and these include disorders of blood circulation to the penis, nerve injuries, stroke, low levels of the male hormone testosterone, various drugs, and chronic alcoholism. Among the most common causes is diabetes mellitus—ED affects 35 to 75 percent of all diabetics.

Doctors use many approaches to treat ED: surgery (penile implants); mechanical devices and supports; and drugs, some of which require injection into the penis. By far, the safest, most effective, and user-friendly ED treatment has been sildenafil (Viagra) and related drugs.

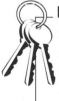

Did You Know That ...?

Using natural drugs to enhance sexual function is nothing new. The Song of Solomon refers to the root mandrake's aphrodisiacal properties. "Spanish fly," obtained from a shining golden-green colored beetle, was used by the ancient Greeks and Romans, a practice that continued until several decades ago. Use of yohimbine, from a West African tree bark, has peaked and waned over the past 100 years.

Viagra-Like Drugs

Viagra and related drugs are effective in the treatment of ED, arising from a variety of causes, in about 75 percent of men. These drugs act by increasing the blood flow to the penis. For Viagra to work, the man must be sexually aroused. No desire, no erection.

Two other commonly used Viagra-like drugs are equally effective in treating ED. The major difference between these drugs and Viagra is time—how quickly do they act (onset) and how long do they work (duration) after being taken by mouth.

Sildenafil (Viagra) must be taken at least one hour prior to anticipated sexual activity, and the desired effects continue for four to five hours. By contrast, the newer drugs tadalafil (Cialis) and vardenafil (Levitra) begin acting within only 15 to 30 minutes and continue for up to 36 hours. (Note the "afil" ending of the generic names.)

Contrary to expectations, there is no established evidence that, when used by men with normal erectile function, these drugs will further improve an erection or its duration. Moreover, when taken by women, they do not appear to improve the quality of sexual satisfaction or the ability of a woman to have an orgasm.

Viagra-like drugs must never be used in combination with nitrates, such as nitroglycerin, medicines used for the treatment of angina and heart attacks. When used in combination, these drugs can produce a life-threatening drop in blood pressure.

Warning! _____

Men with a recent history of heart failure, angina, stroke, abnormal heart rhythms, or high blood pressure are generally warned by their doctors to take reasonable precautions when engaged in sexual activity. To prevent an increased risk of heart attack under such circumstances, patients should consult their doctors before using Viagra-like drugs.

Common side effects include headache, facial flushing, and upset stomach.

Too much of a good thing can be dangerous. A number of cases of painful erections lasting for more than six hours (known as priapism) have been reported after using these drugs. In the event that the erection persists for more than four hours, medical assistance should be obtained immediately to prevent potential permanent damage to the penile tissue.

More than 20 million men worldwide have used Viagra. In very rare instances, men taking Viagra and related drugs have suddenly experienced loss of vision. This optic nerve disease is referred to as NAION. A direct linkage between Viagra and NAION has not been clearly established to date.

The Least You Need to Know

◆ Viagra-like drugs don't produce erections in the absence of sexual arousal.

◆ Regardless of the cause of ED, Viagra-like drugs are highly effective in producing erections and differ only with regard to how fast and how long they work.

◆ Viagra-like drugs should never be used in combination with such nitrates as nitroglycerin and should be used with great caution in patients with a recent history of heart disease.

Drugs Used for Erectile Dysfunction

Generic Name	Trade Name	How Taken	Generic Available
Viagra-Like drugs			
Sidenafil	Viagra	Oral	No
Tadalafil	Cialis	Oral	No
Vardenafil	Levitra	Oral	No
Other Drugs			
Alprostadil,	Caverject	Injection—penis	Yes
Prostaglandin E1	Muse	Pellet—urethra	No
Phentolamine + papaverine		Injection—penis	Yes

Fungal Infections

This section covers a number of common infections caused by fungi. These include superficial infections affecting the genital areas, feet, skin and nails, and mouth, as well as far more serious life-threatening infections that primarily attack the lungs. We consider their treatment with drugs that specifically work against fungi.

Fungal Infections: An Overview

Fungal infections, also called mycoses, are generally classified as being either superficial or systemic:

> ◆ Superficial fungal infections commonly affect the mucous membranes of the mouth and genital area as well as the skin, scalp, and nails.

> ◆ Systemic fungal infections are generally acquired by inhalation of or contact with fungal spores and commonly affect the lungs and skin. These conditions can develop in healthy individuals but are more common in people with impaired immune function, as seen in AIDS.

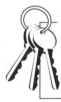

Did You Know That ...?

There are said to be 1.5 million species of fungi, which are classified as molds and yeasts.

In many cases, different antifungal drugs are used to treat the different types of infections.

Superficial Fungal Infections

Superficial fungal infections include …

> ◆ Candidiasis, which is a yeast infection commonly affecting the mucous membranes of the mouth and genital area.

> ◆ Ringworm (tinea) infections of the skin, scalp, and nails.

Topical and oral antifungal drugs are used to treat these conditions.

Candidiasis

The fungus Candida is normally present and causes no harm in the mucous membranes of the vagina, mouth, and digestive system. It is also in moist skin areas.

A variety of factors lead to Candida overgrowth. Antibiotics, for example, kill bacteria and disrupt the normal microbial balance. Candidiasis is seen in individuals who have a depressed immune system as the result of disease (e.g., AIDS) or drugs they are taking (e.g., steroids).

Vaginal candidiasis (also called vulvovaginal candidiasis or yeast infection) is associated with sexual intercourse, but is not a sexually transmitted disease. It occurs in three out of four women at least once during their lifetime. The most characteristic sign is a cottage-cheese-like discharge. Also common are intense itching, soreness, and a burning sensation when urinating.

A wide variety of nonprescription topical and prescription topical and oral products are available. They are able to clear vaginal candidiasis in one to three days. Vaginal candidiasis associated with uncontrolled diabetes mellitus or with a depressed immune system generally requires 10 to 14 days of treatment.

OTC Alternatives

Highly effective OTC vaginal creams, suppositories, and tablets are available to treat uncomplicated vaginal candidiasis. They are usually 85 to 90 percent effective after being used for only one to three days. These "azole" drugs include butoconazole (Femstat), clotrimazole (Gyne-Lotrimin, Mycelex), miconazole (Monistat), and ticonazole (Monostat).

White patches on the tongue and on the inside surfaces of the mouth are common signs of oral candidiasis (also called thrush). Although the patient may not experience any distressing symptoms, thrush is treated to prevent its spread. In severe cases, it may interfere with eating and drinking.

The first treatment approach for thrush typically involves a topical azole in the form of a lozenge or cream. Alternatively, nystatin suspension is swished around in the mouth several times daily. To be effective, these drugs need to be in contact with the affected areas for 20 to 30 minutes, which is sometimes difficult to accomplish.

If topical preparations prove ineffective or cannot be tolerated, systemic azole tablets are used for periods that range from 7 to 21 days.

Ringworm Infections

Fungal infections of the skin are classified according to their location on the body:

◆ **Athlete's foot** (tinea pedis), the most common fungal infection, usually responds well to topical antifungal creams, many of which can be purchased OTC and clear the infection within two to four weeks. Severe cases may require prescription oral azole therapy.

◆ **Jock itch** (tinea cruris), an infection involving the inner thighs and buttocks, is more common in men than women. Topical antifungal drugs should be used one to two weeks after the symptoms disappear. Itching and burning can be relieved by using topical steroids for several days.

◆ **Body ringworm** (tinea corporis) is treated like athlete's foot and jock itch.

◆ **Scalp ringworm** (tinea capitis) is more difficult to treat. Daily shampooing is recommended for removal of the scales and oral antifungal drugs (azoles, griseofulvin, terbinafine) may need to be used for several months.

◆ **Nail ringworm** (tinea unguium) is a common nail problem that far more often affects the toenails than the fingernails. Topical drugs are of little value and oral antifungal drugs must be taken daily for a minimum of three months for affected toenails and for a somewhat shorter period for fingernails. Terbinafine and itraconazole are the preferred drugs, and these are not always effective.

Systemic Fungal Infections

Systemic fungal infections, including blasto*mycosis*, coccidioido*mycosis*, and histo*plasmosis*, affect the lungs. These fungal infections, often severe, are commonly seen in individuals whose immune system is impaired. This can result from AIDS or other medical conditions or drugs taken to treat kidney failure, organ transplantation, or cancer.

def•i•ni•tion

Mycosis refers to any disease caused by a fungus. The prefixes denote the specific fungus, such as Histoplasma, Blastomyces, and Coccidioides.

Histoplasmosis

Inhaled spores containing the Histoplasma fungus are found in the soil and are associated with the droppings of birds and bats. Most individuals with this infection experience mild flu-like symptoms, which pass within several weeks. No treatment is needed.

In older individuals or those with an impaired immune response, histoplasmosis may slowly progress over a period of several years, first interfering with breathing and later spreading to other parts of the body. This expansion more commonly occurs in infants and those with impaired immune function. In the absence of treatment, in very severe cases, the disease may progress exceedingly fast and death occurs within one to two months.

Oral itraconazole or ketoconazole is used for six months to two years to treat histoplasmosis. In severe cases, particularly those with impaired immune function, intravenous amphotericin B is used.

Did You Know That ...?

Fungi reproduce by making tiny spores, each containing nuclei and a set of chromosomes. Spores are resistant to heat, drought, and other adverse conditions in the environment. When conditions once again become favorable, spores germinate and are carried in air currents to repeat the sexual cycle. These fungal conditions are usually contracted after inhaling the spores.

Blastomycosis

The lungs are the primary site for blastomycosis. Symptoms include fever, breathing difficulties, chest pain, and cough. The infection may spread to the skin, bones, the genital area in men and, more rarely, to the brain. In the absence of treatment, the disease slowly progresses, and is ultimately fatal. For reasons that are not clear, this disease is not more common in AIDS patients.

Blastomycosis responds well to treatment with oral itraconazole or ketoconazole given for periods of at least six months. Amphotericin B is used in more severe cases, where the disease has spread to the brain, or in patients with depressed immune function.

Coccidioidomycosis

Coccidioidomycosis, also called San Joaquin fever, can range in severity from a lung infection without symptoms to an illness with flu-like symptoms. In the most severe cases, the infection spreads from the lungs to the lymph nodes, liver, kidney, skin, and covering of the brain (the meninges). Untreated fungal meningitis is invariably fatal.

Infections limited to the lungs, without symptoms, are generally left untreated. When the infection spreads to other parts of the body, oral azoles or intravenous amphotericin B is used.

Spread of coccidioidomycosis to the meninges is reason for great concern. Fluconazole or itraconazole are used by mouth to treat meningitis. If they are not effective, amphotericin B is injected directly into the spinal fluid. Because fluconazole may only keep the fungal infection under control, and not produce a cure, lifetime drug therapy may be needed.

Antifungal Drugs: An Overview

Antifungal drugs are used for the treatment of …

- ◆ Both superficial and systemic fungal infections, such as the azoles.

- ◆ Primarily superficial infections, such as terbinafine, griseofulvin, and nystatin.

- ◆ Primarily systemic infections, such as amphotericin B.

Amphotericin B

Amphotericin B is the most important drug for the treatment of a wide variety of life-threatening systemic fungal infections. It is very valuable for fungal infections in cancer patients or those with impaired immune function. Treatment with amphotericin B may vary in length from six weeks to four months. When the infection has been brought under control, patients are usually switched to much safer azole drugs.

Because amphotericin B is not absorbed from the gastrointestinal tract, it must be given by injection, in particular, intravenously. Because insufficiently high drug concentrations enter the brain or spinal cord after intravenous injection, fungal meningitis is treated with injections directly into the spinal fluid.

Topical amphotericin B is used to treat skin ringworm.

The benefits that amphotericin B confers as a highly effective, life-saving antifungal drug more than outweigh its many serious side effects. These adverse effects occur when it is administered by intravenous infusion and afterward.

Intravenous infusion consistently causes fever, chills, vomiting, and headache. These effects can be reduced with antihistamines and acetaminophen or aspirin.

Kidney toxicity is the most common and severe adverse effect caused by this medicine. It occurs to a greater or lesser extent in all patients and is more severe when higher doses are given. Impaired liver function, a decrease in blood platelets, and anemia may also occur.

The risk of kidney toxicity increases when amphotericin B is given with other cyclosporine or aminoglycoside antibiotics, or other drugs that cause kidney toxicity.

Azoles

Ketoconazole and related azoles (all of which have generic names ending in "azole"), used topically, orally, and by injection, are effective against a wide range of fungal infections:

- Applied topically, many azoles are in prescription and nonprescription products to treat superficial candidiasis of the vagina and mouth. They are very effective against such ringworm infections as athlete's foot, jock itch, and ringworm of the body. Clotrimazole is particularly useful.

- Orally, azoles such as itraconazole can treat nail ringworm.

- Orally, and less often by injection, azoles such as itraconazole and ketoconazole can treat systemic infections.

- Orally and intravenously, the specific azole fluconazole enters the spinal fluid and is very effective for treating fungal meningitis.

In general, the side effects associated with the oral azoles are mild. These most often include nausea, vomiting, digestion, and diarrhea. Some azoles cause skin rash and liver disturbances.

Individuals taking ketoconazole and itraconazole should be aware that they interact with many other drugs. Ketoconazole reduces the ability of drug metabolizing enzymes in the liver from breaking down many other medicines, potentially increasing their toxicity.

Warning!

Individuals taking azoles, in particular ketoconazole and itraconazole, should be aware that these drugs interact with many other medicines used to treat many conditions. Before starting to take or discontinuing taking other drugs, including prescription, OTC, or herbals, consult your physician or pharmacist.

Anti-ulcer drugs that reduce stomach acid decrease the absorption of ketoconazole. Similar interactions occur with other azoles, although it is less a problem.

Griseofulvin

Griseofulvin is given orally to treat ringworm of the skin, hair, and nails. Infections of the skin may respond within four to eight weeks, whereas those of the toenails may require a year or more of drug therapy.

Take griseofulvin with a fatty meal to increase absorption.

Side effects are infrequent and include headache and indigestion. Allergic reactions, such as rashes and fever, may also occur.

Griseofulvin may decrease the effectiveness of the blood thinner warfarin.

Did You Know That ...?

An antibiotic is a substance produced by a mold or bacteria that prevents the growth of other living cells. Amphotericin B and nystatin, antibiotics produced by soil microbes, are effective against fungi but not bacteria.

Nystatin

Nystatin does not enter the bloodstream after being taken by mouth or when applied to the skin. It is used for the treatment of candidiasis of the intestines, mouth (thrush), and skin.

Nystatin may cause nausea, vomiting, and diarrhea when taken by mouth and irritation when applied to the skin.

Terbinafine

Oral terbinafine is perhaps the most effective drug for the treatment of toenail ringworm infections. Terbinafine must be taken daily for three months. It is applied topically for one to two weeks to treat ringworm infections of the skin.

Common side effects or oral terbinafine include headache, diarrhea, and indigestion. Skin rashes may also occur.

The Least You Need to Know

♦ Superficial fungal infections, including vaginal candidiasis (yeast infection) and thrush, are effectively treated with topical azole derivatives or nystatin.

◆ Ringworm infections of the skin, athlete's foot, and jock itch are effectively treated with azoles.

◆ Treatment of ringworm of the nails, particularly toenails, is difficult and prolonged, and uses such drugs as terbinafine, itraconazole, and griseofulvin.

◆ Amphotericin B, a life-saving drug in systemic fungal infections, causes potentially serious adverse effects to the kidneys as well as frequent side effects during its intravenous infusion.

◆ Oral itraconazole and ketoconazole are effective for the long-term treatment of systemic fungal infections, and fluconazole is used for fungal meningitis.

Drugs Used for Fungal Infections

Generic Name	Trade Name	How Taken: Topical (T), Injection (I), Oral (O)	Generic Available
Superficial Infections			
Azoles ("azole" ending)			
Clotrimazole	Lotrimin Mycelex	T	Yes
Econazole	Spectazole	T	Yes
Fluconazole	Diflucan	O	No
Itraconazole	Sporanox	O	No
Ketoconazole	Nizoral	T	No
Miconazole	Fungoid, Monistat-Derm	T	Yes
Oxiconazole	Oxistat	T	No
Sertaconazole	Ertaczo	T	No
Sulconazole	Exelderm	T	No
Others			
Amphotericin B	Fungizone	T	No
Butenafine	Mentax	T	No
Ciclopirox	Loprox	T	No
Griseofulvin	Fulvicin P/G, Grifulvin, Grisactin, Gris-PEG	O	Yes

continues

Drugs Used for Fungal Infections　(continued)

Generic Name	Trade Name	How Taken: Topical (T), Injection (I), Oral (O)	Generic Available
Haloprogin	Halotex	T	No
Naftifine	Naftin	T	No
Nystatin	Mycostatin, Nilstat	O/T	Yes
Terbinafine	Lamisil	O/T	No
Triacetin	Fungoid	T	No
Systemic Infections			
Azoles			
Fluconazole	Diflucan	I/O	No
Itraconazole	Sporanox	I/O	No
Ketoconazole	Nizoral	O	Yes
Voriconazole	Vfend	I/O	No
Others			
Amphotericin B	AmBisome, Amphocin, Fungizone	I	Yes
Caspofungin	Cancidas	I	No
Flucytosine	Ancobon	O	No

Glaucoma

Glaucoma affects three to four million people in the United States and is a leading cause of blindness. Risk increases in those over 40, in African Americans, and people with a family history of this condition. Other predisposing factors include diabetes, eye injury, infection, inflammation, tumor, long-term steroid use, and near- or far-sightedness.

Eye Fluids and Glaucoma

Fluid in the eye permits it to keep its shape. Normally, the amount of fluid being formed in the eye is equal to the outflow of fluid leaving the eye. This keeps constant pressure within the eye.

Fluid builds up if more is produced than can be drained, and when that happens, eye pressure increases. In time, this greater pressure compresses the retina and nerves, which can cause visual loss and eventual blindness. Pressure can increase slowly or rapidly.

In open-angle glaucoma, the rate of fluid drainage gradually slows, and pressure increases slowly, with few symptoms. Open-angle glaucoma accounts for some 90 percent of all cases. Drugs are highly effective in controlling pressure.

In many cases of narrow-angle (a.k.a. closed-angle) glaucoma, there is a sudden blockade of fluid outflow, and eye pressure rises rapidly. Blurred vision and severe eye pain are experienced. Permanent blindness may result unless there is effective treatment within several hours. Drugs rapidly reduce eye pressure prior to surgery, which increases fluid outflow.

Warning!

A number of OTC products, including those intended for the treatment of coughs and colds and for allergies, should not be used by people with glaucoma. Before buying such products, first consult your pharmacist or very carefully read the labels of OTC products regarding their precautions.

Drug Treatment of Glaucoma: An Overview

More than 15 antiglaucoma drugs are available. Based on how they work and their effects, they are placed into five classes:

- Beta-blockers
- Carbonic anhydrase inhibitors
- Epinephrine-like drugs
- Prostaglandin-like drugs
- Pilocarpine-like drugs

In general terms, some drugs reduce eye pressure by decreasing the formation of fluid—e.g., beta-blockers, carbonic anhydrase inhibitors. Others work by increasing fluid outflow from the eye—e.g., prostaglandins and epinephrine and pilocarpine-like drugs.

Antiglaucoma drugs, usually eye drops, reduce excessive pressure to prevent further loss of vision or to maintain pressure within safe limits. These drugs control pressure but do not correct the underlying problem and must be taken on a regular basis, for a lifetime. Beneficial changes in pressure are often seen within a week.

Most doctors follow a similar sequential procedure to treat open-angle glaucoma, but the choice of drugs may vary.

A single drug is first tried, most often a beta-blocker. If eye pressure does not fall enough or significant side effects occur, a drug from a different class is substituted. If results are still unsatisfactory, a second drug from another class is added. If the combination doesn't work, surgery is performed to increase fluid outflow.

Beta-Blockers

Beta-blockers are also used by mouth for the treatment of high blood pressure and a variety of heart conditions. Their use as eye drops are usually the first medicine doctors select for the treatment of open-angle glaucoma.

Name hint: Generic names for beta-blockers all end in "olol."

The most common side effect is temporary eye stinging. Beta-blockers can enter the blood from the eye and can slow the heart rate and cause heart blockage. They can also narrow the breathing tubes. Individuals with asthma or other severe breathing disorders are at greater risk.

Carbonic Anhydrase Inhibitors

Some carbonic anhydrase inhibitors, such as acetazolamide, are taken orally. Others, including brinzolamide and dorzolamide, are used as eye drops.

These medicines are backups if other drugs don't work, or they are used in combination with other drugs, such as beta-blockers (e.g., Cosopt). They produce a rapid reduction in eye pressure that is essential in narrow-angle glaucoma.

Name hint: Generic names for carbonic anhydrase inhibitors all end in "zolamide."

Common side effects with oral drugs include a sick and crumby feeling, loss of appetite, nausea, and diarrhea. Stinging sometimes occurs with eye drops.

Epinephrine-Like Drugs

Epinephrine-like drugs are used as eye drops alone or in combination with other drugs for open-angle glaucoma.

Common side effects include headache, brow ache, and blurred vision. If they enter the blood, they can cause increases in heart rate and blood pressure.

Prostaglandins-Like Drugs

Prostaglandin drops may be used as the first choice drugs, rather than the beta-blockers, for patients with asthma or certain heart conditions.

Name hint: Generic names for prostaglandin-like drugs usually end or have in their name "oprost."

Some of these drugs may color eyes brown or cause the eyelids and eyelashes to darken.

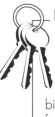

Did You Know That ...?

Prostaglandins play a role in many body functions, including blood clotting, causing contractions of the uterus during childbirth, and protecting the stomach from digesting itself like a piece of meat.

Pilocarpine-Like Drugs

Pilocarpine and related drugs (known as cholinergic drugs) act on muscles in the eye to increase fluid outflow and also constrict the pupils (miotics). Pilocarpine eye drops

(Isopto Carpine, Pilocar) must be used three to four times daily; gels are used only at bedtime.

Pilocarpine is also used for the emergency treatment of narrow-angle glaucoma.

Constriction of the pupils may interfere with near vision, such as reading. Eye pain and irritation, headache, and brow ache are also common.

If too much drug enters the blood, it may narrow the breathing tubes, slow the heart rate, increase sweating or salivation, or cause nausea and diarrhea.

The Least You Need to Know

 ♦ The rate of formation of fluid in the eye is normally the same rate as its drainage from the eye.

 ♦ Acute-angle glaucoma, caused by increased eye pressure, develops slowly, causing vision loss and potential blindness.

 ♦ Narrow-angle glaucoma, caused by blockade of fluid outflow, often requires immediate medical treatment.

 ♦ Beta-blockers and carbonic anhydrase inhibitors decrease excessive eye pressure by reducing fluid formation.

 ♦ Prostaglandins and epinephrine- and pilocarpine-like drugs decrease pressure by increasing fluid outflow.

 ♦ Effective treatment often requires taking two drugs from different classes for a lifetime.

Drugs Used for Glaucoma

Generic Name	Trade Name	Generic Available
Beta-Blockers		
Betaxolol	Betoptic	Yes
Carteolol	Ocupres	Yes
Levobetaxolol	Betaxon	Yes
Levobunolol	Betagan, AK-Beta	Yes

Generic Name	Trade Name	Generic Available
Metipranolol	OptiPranolol	Yes
Timolol	Timoptic, Betimol	Yes
Carbonic Anhydrase Inhibitors		
Acetazolamide	Diamox	Yes
Brinzolamide	Azopt	No
Dorzolamide	Trusopt	No
Epinephrine-Like Drugs		
Apraclonidine	Iopidine	No
Brimonidine	Alphagan	Yes
Dipivefrin	AKPro,Propine	Yes
Epinephrine	Epifrin, Epinal, Glaucon	Yes
Prostaglandin-Like Drugs		
Bimatoprost	Lumigan	No
Latanoprost	Xalatan	No
Travoprost	Travatan	No
Unoprostone	Rescula	No
Pilocarpine-Like Drugs		
Pilocarpine	Akarpine, Isopto Carpine, Pilocar	Yes

Gout

In gout, uric acid crystals deposit in the joints causing inflammation, swelling, and extreme pain. The large toe is most often affected, although it also occurs in ankles, heels, wrists, knees, elbows, and fingers. Gout is far more common in men than women, usually occurs in middle age, and often runs in families. Attacks can be precipitated by consuming large volumes of alcohol.

Uric Acids and Gout

Uric acid is produced by the body's own cells and is also introduced into the body through purine-rich foods. Cells are continuously building up and breaking down. In the process, purines are released into the blood and from it, uric acid forms. Purine-rich foods include all organ meats, such as sweetbreads, liver, beef kidneys; and shellfish, scallops, anchovies, herring, nuts, and dried legumes.

Uric acid is normally excreted in the urine. If the kidneys can't remove the high levels of uric acid in the blood, uric acid salts (a.k.a. urates) are deposited as sharp crystals in the joints. Inflammation with sharp pain and swelling results.

Some drugs relieve pain caused by an acute attack. Others prevent attacks by reducing uric acid levels in the blood.

Treatment of Acute Attacks

Colchicine, nonsteroidal anti-inflammatory drugs (NSAIDs), and steroids are used to relieve the pain and inflammation caused by an acute gout attack (called gouty arthritis).

Colchicine

Colchicine relieves pain within hours after being taken by mouth, and signs of inflammation disappear within several days. It is most effective if taken within 24 to 48 hours of the onset of symptoms. Small doses can be taken daily to prevent acute attacks.

The most common signs of too much colchicine are nausea, vomiting, diarrhea, and abdominal pain, and these may be seen in most patients. If any of these signs occur, drug use should be discontinued immediately. Colchicine should be used cautiously by patients with liver or kidney disease.

> **Maximizing Your Medicine**
>
> Oral colchicine dosing for an acute attack is interesting. Patients undergoing an acute attack are instructed to take 0.6 to 1.2 mg every 2 hours until pain is relieved, abdominal cramping or diarrhea occurs, or a maximum of 8 mg (approximately 13 tablets) are taken.

Indomethacin and Other NSAIDs

Among the NSAIDs, prescription indomethacin (Indocin) is most effective in providing symptomatic relief of pain and inflammation. After being taken orally, pain is generally relieved within hours and inflammation is relieved in three to five days.

Indomethacin may cause severe headaches and dizziness. The gastrointestinal distress and bleeding often seen when NSAIDs are used, is less likely to occur when these drugs are used for a short period of time.

Steroids

If colchicine and indomethacin or other NSAIDs don't relieve pain, prednisone or a related steroid can be used. These drugs are given orally or injected directly into the affected joint.

Prevention of Attacks

When blood uric acid levels are low, crystals are not deposited in joints, and the risk of attacks is reduced. Drugs lower uric acid levels by either increasing their excretion in the urine or by decreasing their formation.

Probenecid and Sulfinpyrazone

Probenecid and sulfinpyrazone increase the excretion of uric acids in the urine. They provide no benefit during an acute attack, and may precipitate attacks during their first few months of use.

These drugs are generally well-tolerated. Common side effects include nausea, vomiting, and abdominal pain, effects reduced when they are taken with food. To prevent uric acid stones forming in the urinary tract, take these drugs with several quarts of fluids daily.

Allopurinol

Allopurinol prevents uric acid formation from purine. It prevents new uric acid crystals from depositing in joints and causes existing deposits to become smaller. It is also used to reduce uric acid levels caused by some anti-cancer drugs.

Warning!

Although it may seem reasonable, never use aspirin to combat an acute gout attack. Aspirin interferes with the increased excretion of uric acid by probenecid and sulfinpyrazone.

Mild side effects include stomach upset, drowsiness, and headache. Periodic eye exams are important, because allopurinol may cause cataracts when used for more than three years. If a rash or fever develop, allopurinol should be immediately discontinued. They may signal a rare but potentially fatal allergic reaction.

The Least You Need to Know

◆ Gout results from uric acid crystals deposited in the joints.

◆ Colchicine, indomethacin, and steroids are used to treat acute attacks of gout.

◆ Probenecid, sulfinpyrazone, and allopurinol reduce blood uric acid levels and prevent attacks.

Drugs Used for the Treatment of Gout

Generic Name	Trade Name	Generic Available
Relief of Pain and Inflammation		
Nonsteroidal Anti-Inflammatory Drugs (NSAIDs)		
Celecoxib	Celebrex	No
Diclofenac	Cataflam, Voltaren	Yes
Diflunisal	Dolobid	Yes

Generic Name	Trade Name	Generic Available
Fenoprofen	Nalfon	Yes
Flurbiprofen	Ansaid	Yes
Ibuprofen	Advil, Motrin	Yes
Indomethacin	Indocin	Yes
Ketoprofen	Orudis, Oruvail	Yes
Meloxicam	Mobic	No
Nabumetone	Relafen	Yes
Naproxen	Aleve, Naprosyn	Yes
Oxaprozin	Daypro	Yes
Piroxicam	Feldene	Yes
Sulindac	Clinoril	Yes
Tolmetin	Tolectin	Yes
Other Drugs		
Colchicine		Yes
Prednisone	Meticorten, Deltasone	Yes
Prevention of Attacks		
Allopurinol	Zyloprim	Yes
Probenecid	Benemid	Yes
Sulfinpyrazone	Anturane, Novopyrazone (Canada)	Yes

Hair Loss

From the number of ads I have seen, it appears that the hair-replacement industry is thriving. Sudden and unexpected hair loss, in particular, from the head, can be very traumatic. Its causes are many and include severe illnesses with high fever, emotional stress, hormonal disorders, pregnancy, thyroid disorders, and certain drugs (e.g., cancer chemotherapy). Happily, this type of hair loss is temporary, and hair generally returns.

But by far, the most common cause of hair loss from the head, also known as baldness, is aging, and it is permanent. This "natural" occurrence (called pattern baldness) is seen in more than one half of all men and 20 to 30 percent of women.

Increased levels of the male hormone dihydrotestosterone (DHT) and a balding gene work together to thin our hair. "What about me?" you ask. Pull out the old family photos, they may provide some clues.

Pattern baldness can be treated with two drugs: the prescription-only drug, Propecia; and Rogaine, an OTC product. These drugs are different in all respects but one: they only work, when they do work, as long as they are used.

Propecia (Finasteride)

Finasteride interferes with the ability of the body to convert the male hormone testosterone to dihydrotestosterone. DHT is not only responsible for causing male-pattern baldness, but it also causes the prostate gland to enlarge to such an extent that it interferes with normal urination.

When used to treat baldness, finasteride is called Propecia. At five times the dose, this same drug is taken for prostate enlargement and is marketed as Proscar.

Propecia is only recommended for the treatment of pattern baldness in men. It is taken by mouth and must be used for three months or more before early

Warning!

Propecia is not recommended for hair loss in women. More important, it should never be taken or even handled by women who are pregnant or who might become pregnant. The drug has the potential to produce abnormalities of the male genital tract of the fetus.

signs of benefit are seen. Hair growth occurs in two thirds of the users and, in most men, additional loss of hair is stopped.

Propecia may interfere with sexual function in some men.

Rogaine (Minoxidil)

After being applied to the hair, Rogaine may work by increasing blood flow to the scalp. Under the best of conditions, users should not expect that all their lost hair will return. Minimal growth ("peach fuzz") is more common than bushy real hair. In other cases, the benefits can be measured by the stopping or slowing down of additional hair loss.

Rogaine is applied to the hair twice daily. The hair should not be allowed to get wet for at least four hours after it is applied.

Although it's good to have a positive feeling about the medicines you're taking, Rogaine users need not rush to make a hair-cutting appointment after its first application. Early favorable results do not occur for several months, with the best responses generally after only after 8 to 12 months. Although not inexpensive, Rogaine costs much less than Propecia. If drug use is discontinued, new hair will be lost within three to four months.

Did You Know That …?

Not all side effects are bad. Minoxidil (Loniten) was first brought to the market to lower high blood pressure. It worked. But early on it was seen to stimulate the growth of body hair in both men and women. The rest is history.

The Least You Need to Know

◆ Propecia, intended to be taken by mouth and only by men, is considerably more expensive than Rogaine, but is also more effective in increasing hair gain and preventing additional hair loss.

◆ Propecia should never be taken or handled by women who might become pregnant because of its dangers to her male fetus.

◆ Rogaine, applied to the scalp, promotes hair growth and stops hair loss in some men and women.

◆ Within months after discontinuing the use of Propecia and Rogaine, hair loss returns.

Drugs Used for Hair Loss

Generic Name	Trade Name	Generic Available
Finasteride	Propecia	No
Minoxidil	Rogaine	Yes

Heart Conditions

Conditions affecting the heart are the leading cause of death in the United States. The good news is that many medicines are available that can treat these conditions as well as reduce major disability and death.

The heart is a muscular pump that propels blood around the body. The blood carries nutrients and oxygen to cells and removes waste materials from cells for their elimination from the body. The amount of blood pumped by the heart each minute (cardiac output) is a measure of its effectiveness as a pump. Cardiac output depends on the amount of blood expelled from the heart each time it contracts and the number of times the heart contracts each minute.

In this section, we talk about common conditions affecting the heart. These include ...

◆ Heart failure, in which the heart is not an effective pump.

◆ Abnormal heart rhythms, in which the chambers of the heart fail to contract in synchrony, causing the heart to pump blood inefficiently.

◆ Coronary artery disease, including angina and heart attack, in which the blood supply to the heart muscle is reduced or blocked.

Many of these heart conditions are treated with the same kinds of drugs.

Heart Failure

In heart failure, the heart fails to meet the body's need for blood. As a consequence, cells are deprived of sufficient amounts of oxygen and nutrients that they require to function normally. Feelings of fatigue and even exhaustion and shortness of breath result. In addition, adequate amounts of blood are not returned to the heart, which leads to an accumulation of fluids in the lungs, tissues, and bloodstream. The heart tries to keep up by beating rapidly, but each contraction is weak.

Heart failure is primarily seen in seniors and is the leading cause of hospital admissions in individuals over 65. Lifetime drug treatment is required for this chronic disorder.

Heart failure has many causes. It may appear suddenly and without warning or progressively develop over many years. The most common causes are uncontrolled high blood pressure and coronary artery disease, more specifically, angina and heart attack.

Treatment Overview

Drug therapy of heart failure is intended to improve the quality of the patient's life, reduce symptoms of the condition and the need for hospitalization, slow the worsening of the disease, and increase life expectancy.

Specific treatment guidelines have been recommended for patients based on the severity of heart failure. Multiple drugs are commonly prescribed for heart failure. These typically include an ACE inhibitor, a water pill (a.k.a. diuretic), a beta-blocker, and digoxin. ARBs (angiotensin-receptor blockers) and spironolactone may also be used as backup drugs.

Maximizing Your Medicine

The American College of Cardiology (ACC) and the American Heart Association (AHA) recently issued guidelines for the evaluation and treatment of heart failure. In addition to classifying patients into four increasingly advanced stages (A–D) and recommending treatments, the guidelines also proposed measures designed to reduce risk factors and prevent (or slow) the progressive worsening of the condition.

ACE Inhibitors

ACE (short for angiotensin-converting enzyme) inhibitors are the most important drugs used for the treatment of heart failure. They improve the function of the cardiovascular system. The heart becomes a more effective pump, the rapid heartbeat is slowed, and elevated blood pressure is reduced.

Did You Know That ...?

Angiotensin is a hormone produced by the kidney that helps control blood pressure. Excessive angiotensin contributes to heart failure by increasing blood pressure and decreasing the loss of salt and water. ACE (angiotensin-converting enzyme) inhibitors interfere with the manufacture of angiotensin and ARBs (angiotensin-receptor blockers) interfere with angiotensin's effects.

Clinical studies have shown that ACE inhibitors and ARBs (discussed later in this chapter) reduce symptoms of the disease, slow the progressive nature of the condition, and improve the patient's quality of life. Most important, they reduce mortality rates by 20 to 30 percent.

Water Pills (Diuretics)

Buildup of excessive fluids in the bloodstream and congestion in the lungs is common in heart failure. Hence the descriptive name "congestive heart failure." Water pills reduce fluid accumulation by promoting water loss in the urine. Patients feel better very fast after beginning treatment. Unfortunately, diuretics don't slow the progression of the heart condition and don't prolong life.

There are many classes of water pills. Loop diuretics, such as furosemide, are highly effective in promoting the loss of fluids and salts and are most commonly used in heart failure.

Beta-Blockers

Low doses of selected beta-blockers improve heart function, reduce heart failure symptoms and hospitalizations, and increase life expectancy.

Beta-blockers are recommended treatment for all patients, regardless of the severity of their heart failure. Of the many beta-blockers, bisprolol, carvedilol, and metoprolol succinate CR/XL have been found to be most effective for heart failure.

Maximizing Your Medicine

Metoprolol tartrate (Lopressor) is an immediate-acting product that is available as an inexpensive generic. This product has not been shown to be as effective nor provide the same therapeutic benefits as metoprolol succinate XL (Toprol), an extended-release product.

Digoxin

Digoxin, obtained from the foxglove, or Digitalis plant, long enjoyed use as the first drug choice for the treatment of chronic heart failure. Its beneficial effects were thought to result from an increase in the amount of blood pumped out with each heartbeat. We now know that its effects on the heart are far more complex.

Although digoxin no longer enjoys its preeminent role in heart failure, it continues to be used for the treatment of this condition. It

Did You Know That ...?

In 1785, the English physician William Withering reported that the foxglove plant (Digitalis) was effective for the treatment of dropsy (fluid accumulation), an important symptom of congestive heart failure. Digoxin, the active ingredient in Digitalis lanata, is one of the most prescribed of all drugs.

reduces the symptoms of heart failure and improves the quality of patient life, but does not increase survival.

> **Warning!** _____
>
> Digoxin is a potentially dangerous drug and may, itself, cause abnormal heart rhythms. Blood levels only slightly higher than those that are medically effective increase the risk of toxicity. This risk is increased when blood levels of potassium are depressed. To reduce the risk of toxicity, digoxin must be carefully taken as prescribed.

ARBs

The role of ARBs (angiotensin-receptor blockers) for the treatment of heart failure has not been resolved. Clinical studies conducted to date have not shown them to have fewer side effects nor be more effective than the ACE inhibitors. Some question whether they are even as effective as ACE inhibitors, and they are more expensive.

ARBs are only recommended for use in patients who cannot take ACE inhibitors. Valsartan is one ARB approved for heart failure.

Spironolactone

Aldosterone is a hormone made by the adrenal cortex that plays a critical role in conserving the body's sodium. When sodium is retained, so is water. Excessive aldosterone levels can cause fluid retention, one of the primary problems associated with heart failure. This hormone also causes adverse effects to the heart.

Spironolactone blocks the effects of aldosterone. It reduces hospitalizations due to heart failure and the risk of death.

Maximizing Your Medicine

African-Americans have a higher risk of heart failure, with more than 700,000 suffering from this condition. The combination drug BiDil has been approved specifically for the treatment of heart failure in blacks, the first drug that has been approved for use in a specific racial group. BiDil consists of isosorbide dinitrate, used alone to treat chest pain (angina), and hydralazine, used to reduce high blood pressure.

Abnormal Heart Rhythms

The heart has four chambers: two on top, called atria; and two beneath, the ventricles. Every minute the heart beats 60 to 100 times. With each beat, blood flows from the atria into the ventricles. The blood-filled ventricles then contract, driving the blood to the lungs or throughout the body.

Specialized tissue in the heart serves as its pacemaker, generating electrical signals that travel through the heart into the ventricles and triggering each heartbeat.

Sometimes the atria or the ventricles begin to contract independent of one another and at different rates, which might be either too fast or too slow. When this occurs, the heart chambers do not fill or empty normally, and the heart becomes a less efficient, or even an inefficient, pump. When this happens, blood flow is compromised and an oxygen deficiency can result. Moreover, clots can form, become dislodged, and block blood flow to critical organs, such as the brain. A stroke can result.

Abnormal heart rhythms, often called *arrhythmias* or *dysrhythmias*, have many causes, the most common of which are heart diseases. More specifically, these include coronary artery diseases and heart attack, in which blood flow to the heart muscle is blocked; disorders of the heart valves; high blood pressure; heart failure; thyroid disease; birth defects; and old age.

Additionally, some drugs (e.g., cold preparations, allergy medication, stimulants) and foods (e.g., coffee and alcohol), as well as smoking and illicit drug use (e.g., cocaine and crack), can provoke abnormal rhythms. Stress can take its toll as well.

There are many different types of arrhythmias. Some are merely annoying to the patient and require no drug treatment. Others can cause immediate death. Drug treatment is intended to reduce the severity of the symptoms and incidence of death.

def•i•ni•tion

The terms **arrhythmias** and **dysrhythmias** are generally used interchangeably. The more commonly used is arrhythmia, which means the absence of a heart rhythm. Dysrhythmia is an abnormal rhythm, which is a much more accurate description of these conditions.

Common symptoms of arrhythmias include awareness of the heartbeat (palpitations), shortness of breath, dizziness, weakness, cold sweats, chest pain, and feeling faint. Arrhythmias are classified as to whether …

◆ The condition starts in the atria or in the ventricles. Atrial arrhythmias (e.g., atrial flutter, atrial fibrillation) are less dangerous than ventricular arrhythmias (e.g., ventricular fibrillation).

◆ The heart rate is increased (tachycardia) or decreased (bradycardia).

Treatment Overview

Arrhythmias may be managed using either nondrug approaches, such as implantable artificial pacemakers or defibrillators—which are often preferred—or with drugs. Anti-arrhythmic drugs are given to prevent or suppress the formation of abnormal rhythms.

Such drugs cause side effects and often potentially serious toxicity when used over extended periods of time, and their use by doctors is declining. Finding an ideal drug and a dose of that drug, one that effectively controls the arrhythmia while minimizing adverse effects, is often a great challenge.

No all-purpose drugs exist that are effective against all types of abnormal rhythms. Some drugs are given intravenously on an emergency basis for life-threatening arrhythmias, whereas others are used orally on a chronic basis to prevent symptoms.

Based on how they work, most of the some 15 drugs are placed in 1 of 4 primary classes or types (Type I–Type IV). We focus our attention on selected drugs from each type.

Type I: Sodium Channel Blockers

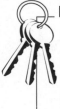

Did You Know That …?

Lidocaine is one of the most widely used local anesthetics. It is applied topically and injected to prevent pain in a limited area.

Disopyramide is used orally for ventricular arrhythmias. Side effects include blurred vision, dry mouth, constipation, and difficulty urinating.

Lidocaine is given intravenously to treat and prevent ventricular arrhythmias, most frequently during and immediately after heart attacks. Side effects may include drowsiness, confusion, and convulsions.

Type II: Beta-Blockers

Propranolol is taken orally to prevent and treat rapid and irregular heartbeats and reduce fatalities after heart attacks. Adverse effects may include excessive slowing of the heart rate and closure of breathing tubes in asthmatic patients.

Type III: Potassium Channel Blockers

Amiodarone is a highly effective and widely used drug whose potential benefits are limited by its toxic effects. It is given intravenously for the prevention and treatment of life-threatening ventricular arrhythmias not helped by safer drugs. It is used orally on a long-term basis to prevent atrial and ventricular arrhythmias.

Adverse effects are many and include lung damage as well as visual and skin problems, which may continue even after the drug is discontinued; thyroid abnormalities; and nerve and gastrointestinal disturbances. This drug can, itself, cause disturbances in heart function.

Type IV: Calcium Antagonists

Verapamil is used intravenously and orally to slow the rate at which the ventricles contract in cases where the atria are contracting in an uncoordinated manner. Of the many calcium antagonists available on the market, only verapamil and diltiazem have been found to be safe and effective for the treatment of a rapid abnormal heart rhythm.

Adverse effects with calcium antagonists are generally few but may include excessive slowing of the heart rate and heart failure.

 Warning!

Verapamil and diltiazem can increase blood levels of digoxin, which can increase the risk of digoxin toxicity. The dose of digoxin may need to be reduced.

Coronary Artery Disease

Cardiovascular diseases—those affecting the heart and blood vessels—cause 1 million deaths each year in the United States, more than any other condition. The most common of these cardiovascular diseases is coronary artery disease, which accounts for almost one half of these deaths. Some 13 million Americans have a history of angina, heart attack, or other types of coronary artery disease.

Let's take a quick look at who is affected by coronary artery disease and why. Overall, men die at higher rates than women. This is especially true for men ages 35 to 55. After 55, the rate for men decreases, whereas that for women increases. After 70, more women than men die. Blacks are at particularly high risk, especially men.

A number of factors increase the risk of developing coronary artery disease, some of which are beyond our control. These include genetic predisposition (heredity), male gender, and advanced age. On the other hand, having high cholesterol levels or high blood pressure, being obese, eating fat-rich foods, smoking, and being physically inactive are things we can change.

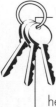

Did You Know That ...?

The heart muscle pulls more oxygen out of the blood than any other tissue. With strenuous exercise, blood flow to the heart may be 10 times greater than at rest. The coronary artery supplies the heart with blood and oxygen.

def•i•ni•tion

Coronary artery disease is also called **ischemic heart disease.** *Ischemia* means lack of oxygen to the heart muscle and a great reduction or absence of blood flow to it.

Coronary artery disease, also called *ischemic heart disease* or coronary insufficiency, results from decreased blood flow and diminished oxygen to the heart muscle. In most instances, coronary disease results from a progressive buildup of cholesterol and fatty plaques, called atheromas, within the walls of the artery. Clot formation may arise from disrupted atheroma. The clot may further obstruct blood flow or may break off and block another segment of the artery.

There are two primary consequences of coronary artery disease: angina (angina pectoris, chest pain) and heart attack. In angina, there is a partial and temporary interruption in the blood and oxygen supply. During a heart attack, blood flow is completely blocked.

Angina

Angina attacks are typically brought on when the oxygen demands of the heart are greatly increased because of exercise or stress. In other variations of angina, spasms of the coronary artery may occur which temporarily interrupt blood flow. These often occur when the patient is at rest or while asleep.

Individuals with angina—which number about 6.5 million in the United States—typically complain that during an attack they feel as though there is a great weight or pressure on their chests, although symptoms can mimic heartburn, muscle spasms, and other less critical conditions.

Primary drug treatment reduces the intensity of angina symptoms by decreasing the heart's demand for oxygen. Other drugs prevent the clumping of platelets, which is responsible for clot formation on the walls of the arteries. These anti-angina drugs include nitrates, calcium antagonists, beta-blockers, anticoagulants, antiplatelet drugs, and clot busters.

Nitrates

The finding that nitrates relieve angina symptoms dates back to 1867, and they have been used ever since. Nitroglycerin tablets are fast acting, highly effective, and very inexpensive.

Nitrate is the first choice for the treatment of angina, when attacks occur no more often than once every few days. Nitroglycerin is also taken to prevent symptoms when the patient is going to participate in activities likely to precipitate an attack.

Beta-Blockers

Propranolol and other beta-blockers are widely used to prevent angina symptoms. They reduce the oxygen demands of the heart muscle by reducing the amount of work the heart does. They do this by reducing the rate and the force with which the heart contracts.

Beta-blockers are the preferred drugs to treat stable angina. They are most effective in controlling the symptoms and reducing the risk of heart attack and death. They are not good for angina that results from spasms of the coronary arteries.

Calcium Antagonists

Calcium antagonists, also called calcium channel blockers or CCBs, effectively control both stable angina and angina resulting from spasms of the coronary artery. They are considered to be useful backup drugs for patients who cannot take beta-blockers.

Antiplatelet Drugs

When a blood vessel is injured, platelets contained in the blood rush to the scene. They clump together to help form a clot, thereby preventing the loss of blood. As discussed earlier, coronary artery disease may result from the formation of clots in the artery, which may obstruct blood flow. Antiplatelet drugs prevent the clumping of platelets and the resulting clot formation.

Aspirin and related antiplatelet drugs can be used for patients with either stable or spastic angina. Individuals who have previously had heart attacks are excellent candidates for these drugs. One aspirin tablet a day is recommended.

Clopidogrel or ticlopidine are alternatives for patients who cannot take aspirin. They are much more expensive and not necessarily more effective.

Heart Attack

A heart attack, also called a myocardial infarction or MI, occurs when the blood supply to the heart muscle is abruptly blocked and the heart loses its supply of oxygen. This is a medical emergency that requires immediate action! Half of all MI deaths occur within three to four hours after the first appearance of symptoms.

Individuals even vaguely suspecting that they are having a heart attack should call for emergency assistance and then chew an aspirin tablet. Breaking the aspirin into smaller pieces speeds the rate at which it is absorbed into the blood and begins to work.

There are two phases in the treatment of a heart attack. The first, or acute, phase in the treatment facility seeks to restore the oxygen supply to the heart so that it meets the demand. This is the time between the start of symptoms and discharge from the hospital, usually about six days. Thereafter, long-term drug therapy begins to prevent a recurrence and promote recovery.

In the treatment facility, a beta-blocker is given to slow the rate at which the heart is beating, reducing its oxygen needs. If a blood clot is responsible for blocking coronary blood flow, a clot buster (a.k.a. a thrombolytic drug), such as streptokinase or alteplase (tPA), is given. They are only effective for the first six hours after the beginning of symptoms.

Morphine, given intravenously, relieves pain, calms the anxious patient, and also reduces the amount of work done by the heart.

Did You Know That ...?

Typical symptoms of a heart attack are a crushing pain that travels down the arm (usually the left one) and up to the jaw. Other symptoms include sweating, nausea, weakness, and a feeling of impending death. One out of every five individuals experience no symptoms.

ACE inhibitors, when given during this critical acute phase, have been shown to decrease the risk of heart failure and reduce deaths. These benefits have been particularly impressive for patients who have high blood pressure or diabetes.

After hospital discharge, doctors prescribe a range of drugs to prevent the recurrence of a heart attack. These include ACE inhibitors for at least several weeks after the initial symptoms. On a chronic and often life-long basis, beta-blockers have been shown to decrease the risk of future heart attacks. Antiplatelet drugs and cholesterol-lowering statins are also used.

Drug Treatment of Heart Conditions

In this section, we talk in greater detail about the drugs used for the treatment of heart conditions. Because many of the same drugs keep reappearing and are used for a number of such conditions, it's convenient for us to consider them all in one place. We present them in alphabetical order and focus on their use for heart conditions.

ACE Inhibitors and ARBs

ACE (short for angiotensin-converting enzyme) inhibitors and ARBs (angiotensin-receptor blockers) are the most important group of drugs available to treat heart failure, particularly in patients with high blood pressure. They make the heart a more efficient pump by slowing the heartbeat and reducing elevated blood pressure. Their use lowers the risk of future hospitalizations, future heart attacks, or death caused by heart failure.

Name hint: the generic names of ACE inhibitors end in "pril." ARBs end in "sartan."

The most common side effect of ACE inhibitors is a dry, nonproductive cough, which is seen in 5 to 10 percent of users. This is more often seen in women than men and is the most common reason why people stop using these medications. Far less common, but far more serious, is the possibility of kidney damage. ACE inhibitors can also cause an allergic reaction, which is initially seen as a sudden swelling of the lips, face, and cheeks. If such symptoms appear, drug use should be stopped and the patient should seek immediate medical attention.

Warning!

Do not take ACE inhibitors or ARBs if pregnant. Their use during the second and third trimester of pregnancy may have harmful effects on the developing fetus.

With ARBs, dizziness is sometimes seen, but they don't produce a cough or an allergic reaction.

Antiplatelet Drugs

To form a clot, platelets must clump together. Aspirin and other antiplatelet medicines work by preventing this clumping. These drugs can prevent angina and heart attacks and treat heart attacks in progress.

At the first signs of a possible heart attack, chewing an aspirin tablet and then immediately getting to an emergency room can save one's life. The antiplatelet effects kick in within 60 minutes.

Maximizing Your Medicine

Aspirin is highly effective and even lifesaving when taken at the first signs of a heart attack or stroke. Regular use can reduce the risk of them occurring. The most effective dose has not been determined, but less is probably better and causes fewer side effects. One children's aspirin (81 mg) or ½ an adult's aspirin (160 mg), taken daily, is recommended. A generic brand is quite effective.

At the low doses of aspirin recommended to prevent heart attack and angina, side effects are few. They include an increased risk of bleeding and indigestion, abdominal pain, and diarrhea.

Clopidogrel (Plavix) is used to prevent platelet clumping in patients with a history of heart attack. It is only slightly more effective than aspirin.

At a monthly cost of $115 to $130, and with no apparent advantages over aspirin, Plavix is most appropriate for those who cannot take aspirin or who do not benefit from it. It causes similar side effects as aspirin and to the same extent, such as abdominal pain, indigestion, diarrhea, and rash.

 Warning! _____

Aspirin-allergic individuals must avoid any dose of aspirin and should consider taking another antiplatelet drug.

Antiplatelet drugs increase the risk of bleeding. Individuals should inform their doctors and dentists that they are taking such medicines before any elective surgery is scheduled. Aspirin should never be given within 24 hours of the clot buster tPA, because tPA increases the risk of bleeding.

Beta-Blockers

Beta-blockers are among the most widely used group of drugs for heart failure, abnormal rhythms, angina, and heart attack. They reduce the force of each heartbeat and decrease the rate at which the heart beats.

There are some 10 beta-blockers available, and of these 3 stand out for the treatment of heart failure: bisprolol, carvedilol, and metaprolol succinate CR/XL.

Name hint: generic names for beta-blockers all end in "lol" and most in "olol."

Because heart disease medications are typically taken for a lifetime, their cost becomes a major consideration. A month's supply of a beta-blocker may vary in cost from $10 to more than $250. Look for generic products. With the notable exception of the metoprolol talked about earlier, generics are just as effective as the trade-name medicines at only a fraction of the cost.

Common side effects include slowing of the heartbeat; reduction of good cholesterol (HDL) levels in the blood; breathing difficulties in individuals with asthma, bronchitis, emphysema, or a history of severe allergic reactions; sleep disturbances; and erectile dysfunction. Beta-blockers also may mask the signs of low blood sugar in diabetics and may worsen the mood of persons with depression.

> **Warning!**
> Beta-blockers should never be abruptly discontinued, because a rebound rapid and irregular heartbeat may occur. This is a particular risk for angina patients.

Calcium Antagonists

Calcium antagonists (also called calcium channel blockers or CCBs) are used to treat angina and abnormal heart rhythms and reduce elevated blood pressure. Many experts warn against their use in heart failure because they may mask the symptoms of this condition.

They have not been conclusively shown to reduce the death rate from heart attacks or stroke in individuals who have high blood pressure or angina. Some assume that they may do so.

In addition to treating stable angina, they are also effective for the management of angina resulting from spasms of the coronary artery. They are useful backup anti-angina drugs (but not first choices) for patients who cannot take beta-blockers.

Only two of these drugs—verapamil and diltiazem—are effective for the treatment of abnormal rhythms that are associated with a rapid heart rate.

Common side effects include dizziness, constipation, headache, swelling of the feet and ankles, and inflammation and overgrowth of the gums. Some calcium blockers can reduce heart rates to dangerously slow levels.

Eight calcium antagonists are on the market in the United States. All are FDA approved for high blood pressure and five are approved for angina. There is no reason to believe that the other three are not also effective. Products are either short acting and must be taken up to four times daily or are "sustained release" (SR) or "continuous release" (CR) and taken only once daily.

Brand-name products of these once-a-day drugs are no more effective than their generic equivalents but are far more expensive (e.g., $77 vs. $32 per month for treating angina). Similarly, for drugs used to treat abnormal heart rhythms, it's $66 vs. $22. Take-home lesson: ask your pharmacist to help you get an inexpensive, yet effective, generic equivalent of a calcium antagonist.

Clot Busters

Alteplase (tPA) is highly effective in dissolving blood clots and significantly reducing disability caused by heart attacks. It is also used for the emergency treatment of strokes caused by clots.

To be effective, tPA must be administered intravenously no later than six hours after the symptoms of a heart attack have begun. A strict set of criteria has been established to determine which patients are eligible to receive tPA. The decision to use this potentially dangerous drug, which can increase the risk of bleeding, is not taken lightly.

Loop Diuretics

There are many classes of diuretics (a.k.a. water pills), drugs that increase the loss of fluids and salts in the urine. Of these, the most powerful and effective are the loop diuretics, such as furosemide. These are preferred for the treatment of congestive heart failure.

Loop diuretics (so-called because of where they work in the kidney) can be given intravenously, when a rapid effect is needed, or by mouth.

Loop diuretics can cause a profound drop in blood pressure and an excessive loss of fluids and salts, in particular, sodium, chloride, and potassium. Low potassium levels increase the risk of toxicity from digoxin, a drug commonly used in heart failure.

Nitrates

Nitroglycerin is the first choice for the treatment of angina in patients not having symptoms more often than several times a week. It is also taken to prevent symptoms when activities are likely to precipitate an attack.

Nitroglycerin is taken under the tongue (sublingual), either as a tablet or a spray, or placed between the upper lip and the gum cheek (buccal). Relief of symptoms is almost immediate! These products begin to relieve chest pain within 1 to 3 minutes and continue to work for 30 to 60 minutes.

When symptoms occur more often than once a day, long-acting nitrates can be used to prevent such attacks. Such products include nitroglycerin oral tablets (intended to be swallowed) and patches or ointment applied to the skin. Tablets containing isosorbide dinitrate are also effective. These slower-acting drugs are not intended to be used to stop acute symptoms.

> ### Maximizing Your Medicine
>
> Nitroglycerin sublingual tablets should never be swallowed. If one tablet fails to relieve pain, one or two additional tablets can be taken at 5-minute intervals. If pain is not relieved within 15 minutes, medical assistance should be sought immediately.

When first used, nitroglycerin can produce a severe headache. This effect decreases (i.e., tolerance develops) after the drug is taken regularly for several weeks. Other early adverse effects include dizziness and a drop in blood pressure after rapidly arising (a.k.a. orthostatic hypotension). Tolerance also develops to these effects.

To prevent the development of tolerance to the long-acting nitrates, so that they continue to work effectively to prevent angina symptoms, patients should not use these products for at least 8 hours during every 24-hour period.

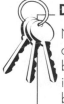

Did You Know That ...?

Nitroglycerin (a.k.a. TNT) is an explosive. During the first days of employment handling TNT, new workers often experience severe headaches, dizziness, and a drop in blood pressure. With regular exposure to nitroglycerin, these symptoms rapidly diminish but are quick to return after employee absence after a long weekend. This has been referred to as the "Monday disease."

Nitroglycerin and other nitrates can increase the blood pressure–reducing effects of other drugs. Such drugs not only include beta-blockers and calcium channel blockers used to treat angina, but also alcohol. A life-threatening drop in blood pressure can occur if nitrates are used within 24 hours of sidenafil (Viagra), widely used for erectile dysfunction.

Statins

Lovastatin and related statins are the most widely used drugs for reducing elevated cholesterol levels, a significant risk factor in coronary artery disease. Statins are effective and cause relatively few side effects.

They significantly reduce both total cholesterol and LDL (bad cholesterol) and slightly increase HDL (good cholesterol). These effects are evident after only a few weeks and are greatest within four to six weeks.

Clinical studies have shown that with their use there are fewer deaths from heart attack and stroke and decreases in the incidence of these conditions. Some advocates have proposed that statins be routinely used to prevent heart attacks in all individuals at risk.

There are differences among the six available statins with respect to their relative effectiveness, incidence of side effects, and drug interactions.

Maximizing Your Medicine

Statins are expensive and must be taken for a lifetime. Speak to your pharmacist about the relative costs of the different statins; they vary considerably. Ask your doctor whether lovastatin is appropriate for you. It's available as a generic equivalent at half the cost of the brand-name product. Also talk to your doctor and pharmacist about splitting the statin tablet you're using.

Statins need only be taken once daily. Lovastatin should be taken with meals, whereas the other statins can be taken without regard to meals. Taking statins in the evening is more effective than in the morning. These drugs work by reducing cholesterol manufacture by the liver, and most of this manufacturing takes place in the evening.

Side effects are generally uncommon and mild and include intestinal upset, rashes, and headache.

Liver toxicity and muscle injury are rare but very serious when they do occur. Individuals with liver disease and who consume excessive amounts of alcohol are at greater risk for liver toxicity. Muscle aches, pains, and tenderness can progress to inflammation and breakdown of muscle. This has been associated with kidney failure.

If you have liver disease or are pregnant, do not take statins. Their use during the second and third trimester of pregnancy may cause injury and death to the developing fetus.

The Least You Need to Know

- Treatment of heart failure with ACE inhibitors, water pills (diuretics), beta-blockers, and digoxin are intended to make the heart a more efficient pump, which reduces symptoms and increases life expectancy.

- Drug treatment of abnormal heart rhythms (a.k.a. arrhythmias or dysrhythmias) is far from satisfactory because of their undesirable effects and difficulty in adjusting dosage.

- Coronary artery disease, including angina and heart attack, is the most common cause of death in the United States.

- Drug treatment of angina reduces the oxygen needs of the heart or prevents the formation of clots in the walls of the coronary arteries, which block blood flow.

- Early drug treatments of heart attacks restore adequate blood flow to the heart by reducing its needs and by breaking down clots that block blood flow.

- Long-term drug treatment with beta-blockers, antiplatelets, and cholesterol-lowering statins is intended to prevent the recurrence of a heart attack.

Drugs Used for Heart Diseases

Generic Name	Trade Name(s)	How Taken: Topical (T), Injection (I), Oral (O), Sublingal (S)	Generic Available
ACE Inhibitors ("prils")			
Captopril	Capoten	O	Yes
Enalapril	Vasotec	I/O	Yes
Lisinopril	Prinivil Zestril	O	Yes
Quinapril	Accupril	O	No
Ramipril	Altace	O	No

continues

Drugs Used for Heart Diseases   (continued)

Generic Name	Trade Name(s)	How Taken: Topical (T), Injection (I), Oral (O), Sublingal (S)	Generic Available
Anti-Arrhythmic Drugs			
Type I			
Disopyramide	Norpace	O	Yes
Flecainide	Tambocor	O	Yes
Lidocaine	Xylocaine	I	Yes
Mexiletine	Mexitil	O	No
Moricizine	Ethmozine	O	No
Procainamide	Procanbid, Pronestyl	I/O	Yes
Propafenone	Rythmol	O	Yes
Quinidine	Quinaglute	I/O	Yes
Type II			
Acebutolol	Sectral	O	Yes
Esmolol	Brevibloc	I	No
Propranolol	Inderal	I/O	Yes
Type III			
Amiodarone	Cordarone	O/I	Yes
Bretylium	—	I	Yes
Ibutilide	Corvert	I	No
Sotalol	Betapace	O	Yes
ARBs ("sartans")			
Losartan	Cozaar	O	No
Valsartan	Diovan	O	No
Anti-Platelet Drugs			
Aspirin		O	Yes
Clopidogrel	Plavix	O	No
Ticlopidine	Ticlid	O	No

Drugs Used for Heart Diseases

Generic Name	Trade Name(s)	How Taken: Topical (T), Injection (I), Oral (O), Sublingal (S)	Generic Available
Beta-Blockers ("lol" or "olol")			
Acebutolol	Sectral	O	Yes
Atenolol	Tenormin	I/O	Yes
Bisprolol	Zebeta	O	No
Carvedilol	Coreg	O	No
Metoprolol	Lopressor, Toprol	I/O	Yes
Nadolol	Corgard	O	Yes
Propranolol	Inderal, Trandale	I/O	Yes
Calcium Antagonists			
Amlodipine	Amvaz, Norvasc	O	No
Diltiazem	Cardizem, Dilacor	I/O	Yes
Nifedipine	Adalat, Procardia	O	Yes
Verapamil	Calan, Isoptin, Verelan	I/O	Yes
Clot Busters (Thrombolytic Agents) ("plase")			
Alteplase	Activase	I	No
Reteplase	Retavase	I	No
Streptokinase	Streptase	I	No
Tenecteplase	TNKase	I	No
Loop Diuretics			
Bumetanide	Bumex	I/O	Yes
Ethacrynic acid	Edecrin	I/O	No

continues

Drugs Used for Heart Diseases   (continued)

Generic Name	Trade Name(s)	How Taken: Topical (T), Injection (I), Oral (O), Sublingal (S)	Generic Available
Furosemide	Lasix	I/O	Yes
Torsemide	Demadex	I/O	Yes
Nitrates			
Isosorbide dinitrate	Isordil, Sorbitrate	O/S	Yes
Isosorbide mononitrate	Imdur	O	Yes
Nitroglycerin	Nitro-Bid IV, NitroQuick, Nitrostat	I/O/S/T	Yes/No
Statins			
Atorvastatin	Lipitor	O	No
Fluvastatin	Lescol	O	No
Lovastatin	Mevacor	O	Yes
Pravastatin	Pravachol	O	Yes
Rosuvastatin	Crestor	O	No
Simvastatin	Zocor	O	Yes
Miscellaneous			
Adenosine	Adenocard	I	No
Digoxin	Lanoxin	I/O	Yes
Spironolactone	Aldactone	O	Yes

Heartburn and Peptic Ulcers

Digestive disorders are among the most common health problems experienced by Americans and are varied in nature. Sometimes referred to by the vague designations indigestion or dyspepsia, individuals may complain of abdominal pain, heartburn, gas, nausea, and diarrhea.

In this section, we talk about heartburn, acid reflux, and peptic ulcers. These conditions involve stomach acid, and their treatment involves many of the same drugs.

Before we start talking about these conditions, let's take a quick look at the digestive system, in particular, the stomach and esophagus.

Digestive System Overview

After being swallowed, food travels down the throat, through the esophagus, and into the stomach. To ensure that food only moves in one direction—from the esophagus to the stomach—a round muscle called the gastro-esophageal sphincter securely closes after food has entered the stomach.

Food is stored in the upper portion of the stomach. As it moves down through the stomach, food is mixed with acid and digestive juices that cause its breakdown into smaller pieces. Cells lining the stomach are coated with a mucus layer that normally protects them against the highly corrosive effects of the stomach's acid and juices. The broken-down food moves into the small intestine, where it is further broken down and absorbed into the blood.

Heartburn

If the gastro-esophageal sphincter fails to shut tightly closed, the acid and juices can move backward (reflux) into the esophagus. This often occurs during pregnancy. Because the esophagus lacks a protective coat of mucus, it is subject to tissue damage and erosion.

Patients complain of *heartburn* and indigestion, which may be common symptoms of acid reflux (gastro-esophageal reflux disease or GERD). Heartburn most commonly occurs after meals, especially large or fatty meals, or when the sufferer lies down at night.

def•i•ni•tion

Heartburn is a burning feeling behind the breastbone that travels from the stomach toward the neck. If the stomach contents move up to the mouth, they cause a sour or bitter taste. Heartburn may be mild and occasional or a symptom of the more serious and recurring condition called acid reflux (a.k.a. gastro-esophageal reflux disease or GERD). Here there is actual damage to the walls of the esophagus. Occasionally, burning reflux stomach contents are nearly or partially inhaled, causing extreme discomfort, coughing, and even life-threatening blockage of the upper airway.

Peptic Ulcer

Prolonged exposure of the stomach walls and upper portion of the small intestine to acid and digestive juices leads to their irritation and erosion. This condition, called peptic ulcer disease, is very common, and affects 10 percent of us at some point during our lifetime.

Ulcers may affect the stomach (gastric ulcers) or, far more commonly, the upper segment of the small intestine (duodenal ulcers). Common symptoms of duodenal ulcers include a burning, aching feeling, accompanied by steady pain. Rapid or slow bleeding can occur if blood vessels are eroded during ulceration. Milk, food, or antacids relieve duodenal ulcer pain for several hours. By contrast, food may relieve or bring on the pain of gastric ulcers.

There are three causes of peptic ulcers:

- An infection caused by the intestinal bacterium Helicobacter pylori, which is implicated in most cases

- Aspirin and other nonsteroidal anti-inflammatory drugs (NSAIDs)

- Stress-related factors

Treatment Overview

Tissue damage in peptic ulcer disease and acid reflux are both caused by acid. Some of the same drugs are used to treat both conditions. These include the acid-reducing drugs and antacids. Antibacterial and protective drugs are used to treat peptic ulcer disease.

Peptic Ulcer Disease

Past treatments of peptic ulcer disease were focused on the symptoms, which kept reappearing. With the discovery that the microbe Helicobacter pylori is implicated in most cases, treatment now seeks to eliminate the source of the disease and cure it. When the microbe is not eliminated, ulcers return virtually 100 percent of the time. After its effective elimination, recurrences may only occur in 1 percent of individuals.

When the microbe has been found to be present, antibacterial medicines are typically prescribed to eradicate the infection. Two or three such drugs are used simultaneously to prevent the development of drug-resistant strains. In addition, drugs are given that reduce acid secretion. These are either ranitidine (Zantac)-related histamine-2 blockers or omeprazole (Prilosec)-like proton pump inhibitors (PPIs).

Drug therapy lasts from 7 to 14 days, with longer periods of treatment leading to a higher rate of microbial eradication.

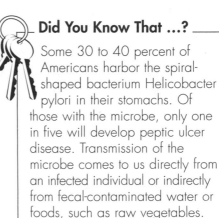

Did You Know That …?

Some 30 to 40 percent of Americans harbor the spiral-shaped bacterium Helicobacter pylori in their stomachs. Of those with the microbe, only one in five will develop peptic ulcer disease. Transmission of the microbe comes to us directly from an infected individual or indirectly from fecal-contaminated water or foods, such as raw vegetables.

Should an NSAID be responsible for the ulcer, it should be discontinued and an acid-reducing drug or a protective barrier drug (such as sucralfate, Carafate) be prescribed. Patients who must continue taking an NSAID may also take an acid-reducer or misoprostol (Cytotec), the latter reducing acid and increasing protective mechanisms in the stomach lining.

Maximizing Your Medicine

Antacids neutralize stomach acid and rapidly relieve the pain and burning sensations of ulcers, heartburn, and acid reflux. They don't coat or protect the stomach against acid or digestive juices. Examples of such OTC drugs, all available as generic products, include aluminum hydroxide (Amphojel), magnesium hydroxide (Riopan), calcium carbonate (Maalox, Mylanta, Tums), and sodium bicarbonate. Diarrhea or constipation is a common side effect.

Acid Reflux

The symptoms associated with mild and occasional cases of heartburn or acid reflux can be treated and immediately relieved with OTC antacids. This relief lasts between 30 minutes when antacids are taken on an empty stomach to three hours if taken after meals. Patients needing antacids frequently should consider acid-reducing drugs.

Drugs that reduce acid secretion are most effective for providing symptomatic relief of acid reflux and promoting its healing. These are the ranitidine-related histamine-2 blockers or omeprazole-like proton pump inhibitors (PPIs).

Within 12 months after discontinuing use of these medications, 70 to 90 percent of patients relapse. To maintain the benefits, patients must often remain on long-term therapy with these drugs.

We'll now talk about the drugs used for peptic ulcer disease and acid reflex in greater detail.

Histamine-2 Blockers

Histamine-2 blockers were the first drugs found to be effective in reducing the release of stomach acid. Treatment with these drugs promote healing of tissue damage caused by gastric and duodenal ulcers and acid reflux. Stress ulcers are also prevented by these drugs.

These drugs, including ranitidine and famotidine, have good safety records, and all are available OTC and by prescription. Most can be purchased as less expensive generic products.

Name tip: all generic names end in "tidine."

Cimetidine may cause confusion and reduced sexual desires. It interferes with the breakdown of such drugs as warfarin and phenytoin, and thereby increases their potential adverse effects. Few of these problems occur with other histamine-2 blockers.

Proton Pump Inhibitors

Proton pump inhibitors (PPIs) are the most effective drugs for inhibiting the secretion of stomach acid. PPIs provide greater benefit in peptic ulcers and acid reflux to more people and in a shorter period of time than the histamine-2 blockers. They are not recommended for the relief of occasional heartburn—antacids should be used instead.

Omeprazole and related PPIs are the preferred drug class for acid reduction in peptic ulcer disease and acid reflex. Drug therapy usually lasts for four to eight weeks. Some 60 to 70 percent of users get complete relief of symptoms of acid reflux, and 85 to 90 percent experience healing of their esophagus after eight weeks. To maintain these benefits, and prevent recurrence of ulcers, continuous treatment may be required in some patients.

Name tip: all generic names end in "prazole."

Very few side effects are reported with PPIs, and these occur infrequently. The most common include nausea, abdominal pain, constipation, diarrhea, and intestinal gas.

> **Maximizing Your Medicine**
>
> There are no noteworthy differences in the effectiveness or side effects among the five available PPIs. The generic brand of non-prescription omeprazole is as effective and costs much less than branded prescription or OTC products.

Sucralfate

Sucralfate is used for the acute and chronic treatment of peptic ulcers. It promotes healing by providing a coat that covers the ulcer and protects it against the corrosive effects of acid and digestive juices for up to six hours. It has no effect on acid or its release.

Sucralfate should be taken on an empty stomach one hour prior to meals. Constipation is the most common side effect.

> **Warning!**
>
> Sucralfate reduces the absorption of a number of drugs including phenytoin, digoxin, and ciprofloxacin and related fluoroquinolone antibiotics. To avoid this problem, take sucralfate two hours after these drugs.

Misoprostol

Aspirin and related NSAIDs are among the most widely used class of medications. Peptic ulcers develop in 15 to 30 percent of individuals using these drugs on a regular basis for the treatment of arthritic conditions.

Ulcers may develop within a week or after many months of treatment. Each year more than 100,000 people are hospitalized and more than 16,000 die from NSAID-related ulcers and bleeding. The risk of this problem may be lower with the NSAID selective COX-2 inhibitor celecoxib (Celebrex).

Misoprostol is used to prevent peptic ulcers caused by long-term use of NSAIDs. It works by reducing acid secretion and increasing the protective barriers against acid.

Up to 30 percent of misoprostol users experience diarrhea, which may be associated with abdominal pain and cramps.

Misoprostol should not be used by pregnant women. It can increase contractions of the uterus leading to a spontaneous abortion.

Patients at high risk of NSAID-related ulcers would be advised to take PPIs, which are safer and just as effective.

Antibacterial Drugs

Several different drug combinations have been proposed for the eradication of Helicobacter pylori, when this microbe is associated with peptic ulcer conditions. These three- or four-drug combinations typically contain an acid reducer (either a PPI or histamine-2 blocker) and two or three antibacterial drugs; bismuth is sometimes included as the fourth drug.

In this section, we talk about the preferred antibacterial drugs. These are bismuth subsalicylate, clarithromycin, amoxicillin, tetracycline, and metronidazole. The best-documented results are obtained when these specific antibacterial drugs are used. All acid reducers are equally effective.

Bismuth Subsalicylate

Bismuth subsalicylate (BSS) has been a familiar occupant of medicine cabinets since the early years of the twentieth century. Pepto-Bismol has been used by generations as an OTC medication for the treatment of indigestion and diarrhea.

Its use in peptic ulcer disease is based on its antibacterial effects and by providing a protective coating on the stomach lining.

BSS may cause a harmless black coloration of the tongue and stools.

Clarithromycin

Clarithromycin is a member of the erythromycin (a.k.a. macrolides) class of antibiotics. When two antibacterial drugs are used for Heliobacter pylori eradication, clarithromycin is invariably one of these.

Clarithromycin is taken twice daily, and can be taken with or independent of meals.

Side effects are few and include nausea, diarrhea, and a strange taste. Clarithromycin is much better tolerated and works for a longer period of time than doses of erythromycin.

Amoxicillin

Amoxicillin is a penicillin-like drug that is highly effective after being taken by mouth. It is among the most commonly prescribed of all drugs.

Diarrhea is the most common side effect, and this occurs less frequently than with other oral penicillins, such as ampicillin.

Name hint: generic names of penicillins end in "cillin."

Whereas amoxicillin and other penicillins are very safe drugs, their use poses a risk of causing an allergic reaction. Signs of an allergic response may vary in severity from a slight rash to a rare but life-threatening inability to breathe and a sudden drop in blood pressure.

Individuals allergic to one penicillin are likely to be allergic to all other penicillins.

Warning!

If you are allergic to penicillin, you should wear a bracelet or have another form of identification that alerts healthcare workers of your condition. All doctors, dentists, pharmacists, and nurses with whom you interact should be notified of your allergy, and this should be entered on the medical records they maintain for you.

Tetracycline

Tetracycline is only used when two other antibacterial drugs are also included in the four-drug combination.

Name hint: generic names of tetracycline-like drugs end in "cycline."

The most common side effects are gastrointestinal disturbances, including indigestion, nausea, and diarrhea.

Tetracycline binds to calcium, magnesium, aluminum, and iron, interfering with its absorption into the bloodstream. Antibiotic levels in the blood are lowered, reducing its antibacterial

Warning!

Tetracycline should never be taken if it is outdated, has changed color or taste, looks different, or if it has been stored in a setting that is too warm or too damp. Such medication should be discarded. Tetracycline can decompose into chemicals that may cause serious adverse effects, including kidney damage.

effectiveness. Because of this, calcium supplements, most antacids, and iron supplements should be taken one hour before or two hours after tetracycline.

Milk and other calcium-rich dairy products and food interfere with tetracycline absorption and lower its blood levels. Take tetracycline one hour before or two hours after meals and with a full glass of water.

Warning!

Avoid alcoholic beverages when taking metronidazole. The combination may cause nausea, vomiting, facial flushing, palpitations of the heart, and a marked drop in blood pressure.

Metronidazole

Metronidazole is effective against Heliobacter pylori, but the development of resistant strains present a problem.

Common side effects include nausea, headache, dry mouth, and a metallic taste. The urine may darken after taking this drug, but this is of no concern.

The Least You Need to Know

◆ Peptic ulcer disease and acid reflux are caused by stomach acid erosion of the digestive system.

◆ Occasional discomfort from peptic ulcer disease, heartburn, and acid reflux can be rapidly relieved with antacids, while frequent episodes are effectively prevented and treated with acid-reducing drugs, namely histamine-2 blockers and proton pump inhibitors (PPIs).

◆ Acid-reducing drugs include namely histamine-2 blockers and PPIs.

◆ Peptic ulcer disease is associated with Heliobacter pylori infection and can be eradicated using a combination of antibacterial drugs and acid reducers.

◆ Antibacterial drugs include bismuth subsalicylate, clarithromycin, amoxicillin, tetracycline, and metronidazole.

◆ Recurrence of peptic ulcers after a course of drug therapy is not an infrequent occurrence and may require continuous drug therapy.

Drugs Used to Treat Heartburn and Peptic Ulcers

Generic Name	Trade Name	Generic Available
Acid-Reducing Drugs		
Histamine-2 Blockers ("tidine" endings)		
Cimetidine	Tagamet	Yes
Famotidine	Pepcid	Yes
Nizatidine	Axid	No
Ranitidine	Zantac	Yes
Proton Pump Inhibitors ("prazole")		
Esomeprazole	Nexium	No
Lansoprazole	Prevacid	No
Omeprazole	Prilosec	Yes
Pantoprazole	Protonix	No
Rabeprazole	Aciphex	No
Antibacterial Drugs		
Amoxicillin	Omnipen, Principen, Totacillin	Yes
Bismuth subsalicylate	Pepto-Bismol	Yes
Clarithromycin	Biaxin	No
Metronidazole	Flagyl, Metizol	Yes
Tetracycline	Sumycin	Yes
Miscellaneous Drugs		
Misoprostol	Cytotec	Yes
Sucralfate	Carafate	Yes

Herpes

Herpes infections are caused by the herpes simplex virus (HSV). There are two types of HSV: HSV-1 primarily affects the mouth, causing "fever blisters" or "cold sores." HSV-2 mainly causes genital herpes involving the penis, vulva, and rectum. Each HSV type can cause sores in both locations.

Did You Know That ...?

More than 40 million Americans suffer from herpes infections. Because many don't have symptoms, they are unaware of it. Genital herpes doesn't usually cause major problems in healthy adults. Oral and genital herpes are contagious, spread by person-to-person contact, even when symptoms are absent.

After being infected, symptoms appear within 2 to 10 days and last for several weeks. Following infection but before the outbreak, telltale sensations frequently forewarn eruptions. Symptoms include itching, burning, pain, swelling, and tenderness at the site of contact. Blisters appear, which progressively become red, swollen, and filled with fluid. They burst and leave sores, which heal within 7 to 10 days.

The herpes virus remains dormant in nerves, with recurring episodes occurring periodically over a lifetime. These episodes are milder and last for shorter periods than the initial episode.

Antiherpes Drugs: An Overview

Acyclovir and related antiviral drugs do not cure herpes. Rather, they ease the discomfort somewhat and shorten the time an episode persists. These drugs are used to treat the primary episode and recurring ones, when they are present. These drugs are effective in treating infections caused by both HSV-1 and HSV-2.

In addition, these drugs may be taken daily by individuals who experience more than six recurrences per year to reduce the frequency and severity of such attacks. Mild recurring episodes don't need drug treatment.

Women having their first episode while pregnant may deliver a premature baby. Infected babies may die or suffer from nerve damage. Babies may have other problems affecting their eyes, skin, or brain, a risk that may be reduced by drugs.

Acyclovir-Like Drugs

Acyclovir is the preferred drug for the treatment of most herpes infections. It works by preventing the reproduction of viruses. It causes few serious side effects and can be used topically, intravenously, or orally.

Oral acyclovir is preferred for the treatment and prevention of both genital and oral episodes. When used chronically, it reduces the severity and duration of recurring episodes by 70 to 90 percent. Intravenous injections are generally reserved for very severe cases or those in patients with impaired immune function, such as AIDS.

Name hint: most generic names end in "cyclovir" or "ciclovir."

Oral acyclovir can cause nausea, vomiting, diarrhea, dizziness, and headache. Intravenous administration may cause inflammation of the veins. A less common, but more serious, side effect is kidney toxicity.

The Least You Need to Know

- Herpes simplex virus (HSV) infections of the mouth and genitals are recurring conditions.
- Acyclovir and related drugs are used to treat initial or recurring episodes when they occur or are taken on a chronic basis to reduce the frequency of recurring episodes.

Drugs Used to Treat Herpes

Generic Name	Trade Name	Generic Available
Acyclovir	Zovirax	Yes
Famciclovir	Famvir	No
Foscarnet	Foscavir	No
Penciclovir	Denavir	No
Valacyclovir	Valtrex	No

High Blood Pressure (Hypertension)

Before delving into a discussion of high blood pressure, we need to understand how blood pressure works. Each time the heart beats, blood is forcefully propelled into the arteries. This force pushes against the elastic walls of the arteries and causes them to expand. As we age, the walls of our arteries become less elastic and blood pressure tends to increase.

Blood pressure values are expressed as two numbers, such as 120/80, which we say as "120 over 80." A blood pressure of 120/80 is considered to be normal. The upper number, or systolic pressure, is the pressure against the walls of the arteries when the heart beats. The lower number, or diastolic pressure, is the pressure when the heart is relaxed, immediately before the next beat.

If your systolic blood pressure is either 140 or above or your diastolic pressure is 90 or above, you have high blood pressure, which is referred to as hypertension.

Did You Know That ...?

More than 50 million Americans have high blood pressure (are hypertensive), but only 2 out of every 3 know it. Until blood pressure becomes very markedly elevated, most people experience no symptoms and are unaware of its presence.

Three out of four individuals with high blood pressure are either not being treated or are not receiving adequate benefit from their medicines.

Sometimes we know what causes high blood pressure, but usually we don't. The cause can only be identified in 5 to 10 percent of individuals, who are hypertensive as the result of another condition or from drugs. This is called secondary hypertension and can often be cured by treating the underlying cause.

In most cases, we don't know why elevated blood pressure occurs—this is called primary or essential hypertension. Essential hypertension can be controlled but cannot be cured. When a decision is made to control hypertension with medicines (antihypertensives), these drugs must be taken for a lifetime.

Warning!

Hypertension has been called "the silent killer." If not controlled or if inadequately managed, in time the persistent elevation in blood pressure will increase the risk of diseases to vital organs. These include the heart (causing angina, heart attack, heart failure), brain (stroke), kidneys (kidney failure), and eyes (blindness). These conditions can cut life expectancy by 10 to 20 years.

Sorting Out Medicines That Lower Blood Pressure

More than six dozen blood pressure medications are on the market. Based on how they work—which accounts for both the good and bad effects they produce—they have been placed into seven primary classes:

- Diuretics ("water pills")

- Beta-blockers

- Calcium antagonists (calcium channel blockers, CCBs)

- ACE inhibitors

- Angiotensin-receptor blockers (ARBs)

- Direct vasodilators (artery wideners)

- Centrally acting drugs

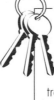

Did You Know That ...?

Blood pressure medications are also used to rid the body of excess salt and water, prevent migraine headaches, reduce tremors, calm aggressive behavior, relieve anxiety, and treat baldness.

Medicine-Patient Matchmaking

Because all these drugs lower high blood pressure, why is it important that we go into detail about these drug classes? Learning a bit about these drugs will make you more savvy in understanding how these drugs are used safely and effectively. Here are some facts to keep in mind:

- Most individuals use more than one medicine to effectively lower blood pressure. These drugs are selected from different drug classes.

- The results of recent studies tell us that, based on our race, age, and the degree to which blood pressure is increased, some drugs are better than others.

◆ Other medical conditions, such as diabetes, high cholesterol levels, or asthma, must be considered because some drugs may worsen such problems.

◆ Each drug class causes a different assortment of side effects, which may be more troubling to some individuals than others.

Treatment Game Plan

The most appropriate drugs and their doses are customized to fit each patient. Commonly doctors prescribe more than one drug to treat high blood pressure. Why? Because these drugs work in very different ways, they have a greater likelihood of being more effective. More important, using lower doses of individual drugs may reduce the likelihood or severity of their side effects.

Nevertheless, physicians generally follow similar step-wise approaches after determining that blood pressure needs to be lowered:

1. Drugs may not be needed for individuals with only modest increases in blood pressure. Nondrug approaches should be tried first to get blood pressure to return to normal levels.

   These nondrug approaches include changes in diet, including cutting back on salt (sodium) intake in the diet; exercising or increasing physical activity and losing weight; quitting smoking and moderating alcohol consumption. If these do not produce satisfactory results, medication begins.

2. Medication typically starts with a low dose of a single drug, usually a water pill (diuretic) or, less often, a beta-blocker. A trial period of several weeks determines if the dose is adequate. If necessary, the dose is increased, though this is done gradually to minimize side effects.

3. If a reasonably high dose of the first drug fails to reduce blood pressure, the health-care provider has one of two choices: (1) Drop the first drug and try another drug from a different class; or (2) continue the first drug and add a second drug and, if necessary, a third drug, selected from a different class.

Maximizing Your Medicine

Blood pressure medications all cause side effects. If excessively troublesome, some patients may be tempted to stop taking their drugs, especially if they don't have symptoms caused by their elevated blood pressure. Don't do it! Instead, ask your doctor to change the dose or prescribe another drug.

Diuretics ("Water Pills")

Diuretics are usually the first class of medications selected when treating elevated blood pressure. They are effective and inexpensive. When several drugs are used in combination, water pills—in particular hydrochlorothiazide or HCT—are most commonly included as members of the blood-pressure-lowering team.

Water pills increase the excretion of salt (sodium) and water in the urine. This loss of fluid from the bloodstream reduces blood pressure in the arteries.

In addition to reducing blood pressure, water pills are also used to rid excessive fluids seen in heart failure.

Preferred Patient Groups

Elderly folks, blacks, obese persons, and those with heart failure generally respond particularly well to water pills.

Cautions

Use cautiously if you have diabetes or gout. Women who are pregnant or nursing should use water pills only when they are absolutely essential. Potential undesirable drug interactions may occur when some water pills are taken with digoxin and lithium.

Some drugs, such as water pills, may cause excessive potassium loss in the urine. This may result in feelings of fatigue or muscle cramps. To prevent this problem, a potassium supplement can be taken or include bananas in the diet—a rich natural source of potassium. When taking water pills, blood levels of potassium should be checked regularly.

To reduce the likelihood that sleep will be disturbed because of the urge to urinate, these drugs should be taken early in the day.

Beta-Blockers

Beta-blockers are among the most widely used group of drugs for high blood pressure. They reduce the force of each heartbeat and decrease the rate at which the heart beats. Users of beta-blockers drugs have a slow heart beat, which is difficult to elevate when exercising.

def•i•ni•tion

Beta-blockers block the neurotransmitters noradrenaline (norepinephrine) and adrenaline (epinephrine). Older beta-blockers, such as propranolol, act on beta receptors located on both the heart (a good thing) and on the lungs (a bad thing, because it interferes with breathing). Newer beta-blockers, such as metoprolol, act much more selectively on the heart without acting on the lungs.

Name hint: Generic names for beta-blockers all end in "lol" and most in "olol."

Preferred Patient Groups

These drugs are most effective in younger people, whites, and individuals who have had heart attacks, rapid heartbeats, or angina. Beta-blockers are often combined with diuretics.

Beta-blockers are a very popular class of medicines. In addition to reducing high blood pressure, they are used for the treatment of such heart conditions as heart failure, irregular heart rhythms, angina, and heart attacks.

They also prevent migraine headaches, reduce tremors, calm aggressive behavior and relieve anxiety, and slow the heart in overactive thyroid disease (hyperthyroidism). Eye drops containing this drug class are used to treat glaucoma.

Maximizing Your Medicine

Because high blood pressure medications are usually taken for a lifetime, their cost becomes a major consideration. Not only do major differences in cost exist among the different classes of drugs, there are even extreme differences within a single class.

Take the beta-blockers, for example. A month's supply of a single drug may vary in cost from $10 to more than $250. Look for generic products. They are just as effective as the trade-name medicines in their class at only a fraction of the cost.

Cautions

Common side effects include slowing of the heartbeat and reduction of good cholesterol (HDL) levels in the blood. In addition, beta-blockers may cause breathing difficulties, sleep disturbances, and erectile dysfunction.

Warning!

Beta-blockers should not be used by patients with certain slow heartbeats (sinus bradycardia) or heart block.

Nonselective beta-blockers should be used with great care by individuals with asthma, bronchitis, emphysema, or a history of severe allergic reactions. They may mask the signs of low blood sugar in diabetics. Beta-blockers may worsen the mood of persons with depression.

Beta-blockers should never be abruptly discontinued, because a rebound rapid and irregular heartbeat may occur. This is a particular risk for angina patients.

Calcium Channel Blockers

With each beat, blood is carried from the heart into arteries, the smallest branch of which are called arterioles. Arterioles can widen (dilate or increase their diameter) or constrict (decrease their diameter).

When arterioles are constricted, it takes more pressure to move blood through these blood vessels. This increases blood pressure. Widening the diameter of arterioles increases the flow of blood and decreases blood pressure.

Most calcium channel blockers or CCBs, also called calcium antagonists, block the movement of calcium in blood vessels, causing arterioles to widen. This makes it easier for blood to flow through these very fine blood vessels, reducing blood pressure.

Preferred Patient Groups

Patients who respond best to the calcium channel blockers include older persons, blacks, and individuals with angina, a rapid heartbeat, or migraine headaches.

In addition to reducing blood pressure, calcium antagonists are also used to treat angina and abnormal heart rhythms.

Cautions

Common side effects include constipation, headache, swelling of the feet and ankles, and inflammation of the gums.

Calcium channel blockers should be avoided in patients with heart failure.

ACE Inhibitors and Angiotensin-Receptor Blockers (ARBs)

ACE inhibitors and ARBs lower blood pressure by widening the diameter of arterioles. Their action involves *angiotensin II*.

def•i•ni•tion

Angiotensin II is an important naturally occurring protein that is very powerful in its ability to constrict arterioles, which results in increased blood pressure.

There are two approaches to reducing angiotensin's effects on blood pressure:

◆ Angiotensin-converting enzyme (ACE) inhibitors prevent angiotensin from forming in blood vessels.

◆ Angiotensin-receptor blockers (ARBs) prevent angiotensin from causing constriction of arterioles.

Name hint: The generic names of ACE inhibitors end in "pril." ARBs end in "sartan."

Preferred Patient Groups

ACE inhibitors and ARBs are particularly useful for young patients, whites, and individuals with angina, heart failure, chronic kidney disease, or kidney disease associated with diabetes.

When used alone, ACE inhibitors and ARBs are less effective in blacks. Addition of a water pill greatly increases their effectiveness in such individuals.

When using ACE inhibitors, patients with high blood pressure and heart failure show improvements in their symptoms of heart failure. They have a reduced risk of future hospitalizations, future heart attacks, or death caused by heart failure.

Cautions

A dry, nonproductive cough is seen in 5 to 10 percent of persons using ACE inhibitors. This is more often seen in women than men and is the most common reason why people stop using these medications.

For ARBs, dizziness is sometimes seen, but it doesn't produce a cough or an allergic reaction.

Warning!

Pregnant women should not take ACE inhibitors or ARBs. Their use during months four to nine—the second and third trimester of pregnancy—may have harmful effects on the developing fetus.

ACE inhibitors can cause an allergic reaction, which is initially seen as a sudden swelling of the lips, face, and cheeks. If such symptoms appear, drug use should be stopped and medical assistance should be sought.

Direct-Acting Vasodilators (Artery Wideners)

Direct-acting vasodilators lower blood pressure by widening arteries but are rarely used any longer. Safer and more effective blood pressure-lowering drugs, which have been previously discussed, have replaced such artery wideners as hydralazine (Apresoline) and minoxidil (Loniten).

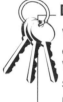

Did You Know That ...?

Within weeks, four out of five persons taking minoxidil experience an unusual side effect. Hair begins to grow on their face and later on their arms, legs, and back. When minoxidil solution (Rogaine) is applied for several months to the scalp, it may slow hair loss and stimulate hair growth. It only works in one third of balding users, more specifically those with male-pattern and female-pattern baldness.

Centrally Acting Drugs

Centrally acting drugs reduce blood pressure by acting on the lower brain (brain stem). These drugs, including clonidine and methyldopa, commonly cause drowsiness, and are infrequently used. If clonidine is abruptly discontinued, blood pressure can significantly rebound upward.

Methyldopa is the preferred drug for the treatment of chronic high blood pressure in pregnant women. A clonidine patch can be applied to the skin and replaced at weekly intervals. This product has fewer side effects than oral clonidine and is generally taken with other blood pressure-lowering drugs.

The Least You Need to Know

♦ High blood pressure often has no symptoms. If inadequately treated, it can increase the risk of diseases affecting the heart, brain, kidneys, and eyes, and can shorten life expectancy.

♦ Although medicines are highly effective in controlling blood pressure and reducing the risk of these complications, they are not cures and must be taken for a lifetime.

♦ Usually several drugs are used to treat elevated blood pressure. The choice of drugs and their doses should be tailored to the person's individual needs. Choices are based on their age, race, other medical conditions, and undesirable side effects.

♦ Water pills and beta-blockers are common first-drug choices. They are effective, and many are available as generic products.

♦ Some prescribers use ACE inhibitors, calcium antagonists, and even angiotensin-receptor blockers as their first choice.

Drugs Used for Hypertension

Generic Name	Trade Name(s)	Generic Available
Diuretics		
Thiazide-Related Diuretics		
Chlorthalidone	Hygroton, Thalitone	Yes
Hydrochlorothiazide (HCT)	HydroDIURIL	Yes
Indapamide	Lozol	Yes
Metolazone	Mykrox, Zaroxolyn	Yes
Loop Diuretics		
Bumetanide	Bumex	Yes
Ethacrynic acid	Edecrin	No
Furosemide	Lasix	Yes
Torsemide	Demadex	Yes

Generic Name	Trade Name(s)	Generic Available
Potassium-Sparing Diuretics		
Amiloride	Midamor	Yes
Spironolactone	Aldactone	Yes
Triamterene	Dyrenium	Yes
Beta-Blockers ("lol" or "olol")		
Acts on Heart and Lungs		
Carvedilol	Coreg	No
Labetalol	Normodyne, Trandale	Yes
Nadolol	Corgard	Yes
Propranolol	Inderal	Yes
Acts on Heart Selectively		
Acebutolol	Sectral	Yes
Atenolol	Tenormin	Yes
Bisoprolol	Zebeta	Yes
Metoprolol	Lopressor, Toprol	Yes
Calcium Channel Blockers		
Amlopidipine	Norvasc	No
Diltiazem	Cardizem, Dilacor	Yes
Felodipine	Plendil	No
Nifedipine	Adalat, Procardia	Yes
Verapamil	Calan, Isoptin, Verelan	Yes
ACE Inhibitors ("prils")		
Captopril	Capoten	Yes
Enalapril	Vasotec	Yes
Lisinopril	Prinivil, Zestril	Yes
Perindopril	Aceon	No
Quinapril	Accupril	No
Ramipril	Altace	No

continues

Drugs Used for Hypertension (continued)

Generic Name	Trade Name(s)	Generic Available
ARBs ("sartans")		
Candesartan	Atacand	No
Eprosartan	Teveten	No
Irbesartan	Avapro	No
Losartan	Cozaar	No
Telmisartan	Micardis	No
Valsartan	Diovan	No
Centrally Acting Drugs		
Clonidine	Catapres	Yes
Methyldopa	Aldomet	Yes

Infertility

Infertility refers to the decreased ability of a couple to achieve pregnancy after repeated efforts. Some 15 to 20 percent of couples are infertile. (Sterility is the inability to become pregnant.) Infertility may result from problems arising from either the male or the female partner or both.

In men, when erectile dysfunction is responsible for infertility, Viagra-like drugs are highly effective at correcting the problem (see "Erectile Dysfunction" for more on Viagra-like drugs). However, drugs are not available that reliably increase the number of sperm or their mobility or quality, which is the most common cause of male infertility.

Infertility in women can occur because eggs are not released from the ovaries. Drugs can promote ovulation. In other cases, infertility can result from blocked or abnormal fallopian tubes. This prevents eggs from being fertilized by sperm in the fallopian tube. The fertilized egg travels to the uterus (womb), where it is implanted and grows. Drugs are not useful here, and the woman might consider the options of surgical correction or in-vitro fertilization to become pregnant. Endometriosis (see "Endometriosis") has been associated with infertility.

The primary drugs used to stimulate the release of eggs are clomiphene and menotropins.

Clomiphene

Often called the "fertility pill," clomiphene (Clomid) is extremely effective in promoting ovulation in 75 to 90 percent of properly selected women. About 40 percent of these women become pregnant. About 10 to 25 percent of these pregnancies are multiple births, usually twins.

Clomiphene is taken by mouth for five consecutive days. Ovulation generally occurs 5 to 10 days after the last dose. If ovulation has not occurred, this 5-day cycle can be repeated at 30-day intervals. Doses are determined by the woman's ability to ovulate.

Common side effects include hot flashes, nausea, bloating, breast swelling, headaches, and sometimes visual disturbances.

Enlargement of the ovaries may occur, which can have serious consequences. This can cause abdominal distention and discomfort and a 5 to 10 lb. weight gain. Treatment should be stopped in either case.

Menotropins

If clomiphene does not cause ovulation, *menotropins* can be tried. When given to pre-selected women, this hormonal preparation induces ovulation in virtually all women. Some 50 to 75 percent become pregnant, with about 20 percent having multiple births.

Menotropins is given once daily by intramuscular injection for 8 to 12 days. To assess the status of ovulation, treatment is monitored by measuring estrogen levels or by ultrasound.

Excessive enlargement of the ovaries occurs in about 20 percent of women receiving menotropins. In most cases, there is little reason for concern, because it corrects itself after treatment is stopped. If enlargement occurs rapidly, with a collection of fluid in the abdomen causing pain, the woman should be hospitalized and treated without delay because this side effect can be life-threatening.

def•i•ni•tion

Menotropins is also referred to as human menopausal gonado-tropin or HMG. This name is highly descriptive because HMG consists of natural hormones that have been extracted from the urine of postmenopausal women.

Unlike clomiphene, which is relatively inexpensive, a single cycle of menotropins treatment can cost more than $1,000 for drug costs alone. To this must be added doctor and laboratory costs. If pregnancy does not occur, cycles may be repeated several times.

The Least You Need to Know

◆ Effective drugs are not available to safely and reliably increase the number or quality of sperm.

◆ Clomiphine and menotropins successfully induce ovulation in a large proportion of preselected women, with about half becoming pregnant.

Drugs Used for Infertility

Generic Name	Trade Name	Generic Available
Clomiphene	Clomid, Serophene	Yes
Menotropins	Pergonal, Repronex	No

Inflammation

Inflammation is a major defensive response to infection or injury. Fluids, chemicals, and white blood cells rapidly travel to the affected area, trapping, inactivating, and removing the source of infection. Inflammation gradually dissipates, injured tissues are removed, and the healing and repair processes are set into motion.

Regardless of the cause of the inflammatory reaction, the body's protective response is similar. At the site of an injury or infection, chemicals are released, causing …

 ◆ Pain.

 ◆ Increased blood flow, redness, and warmth.

 ◆ Fluid movement into the area, leading to swelling and tenderness.

 ◆ Specialized cell movement into the area.

Types of Inflammatory Reactions

The inflammatory reaction may be short-lived (acute) or long-lasting (chronic).

Acute inflammation provides protection, prevents additional foreign invasion or tissue injury, and promotes healing. Examples include sore throat and skin reactions to a burn or insect bite, and often an early sign of an infection. Symptoms of acute inflammation usually abate within one to two weeks.

The acute inflammatory reaction is not always sufficient to control microbes or tissue injury. Occasionally, chronic inflammation slowly develops and can persist for weeks, months, or even years. Over time, tissues become damaged, pain continues, and the patient becomes debilitated. Bodily function may be impaired (e.g., joint performance in rheumatoid arthritis).

Did You Know That …?

A growing body of evidence suggests that chronic inflammation may disrupt cholesterol plaques in the arteries in the heart, which causes heart attack and stroke. Chronic inflammation has also been implicated in Alzheimer's disease and colon cancer.

Examples of chronic inflammatory conditions include inflammatory bowel disease (ulcerative colitis and Crohn's disease), tuberculosis, gout, arthritis, and asthma, to name a few.

The beneficial protective effects of inflammation may be accompanied by undesirable, unpleasant effects. Lymph nodes in the neck, under arms, and in the groin may become swollen after trapping foreign materials. Fever, loss of appetite, and fatigue may accompany the inflammatory process.

Anti-inflammatory medicines may be given to alleviate these distressing symptoms. Antibiotics also may be required to combat infectious diseases.

Drug Treatment of Inflammation: An Overview

Drugs used to combat a harmful inflammatory response, called anti-inflammatory drugs, decrease redness, pain, and swelling, and improve function. There are two primary groups of drugs used to treat inflammation: nonsteroidal anti-inflammatory drugs (NSAIDs) and steroids. Apart from reducing the inflammatory response, these drug classes are very different in all other respects.

Nonsteroidal Anti-Inflammatory Drugs (NSAIDs)

NSAIDs relieve pain and, at higher doses, have anti-inflammatory effects. They are useful for the treatment of both acute and chronic inflammation.

Aspirin was the original NSAID. It is a very effective drug for rheumatoid arthritis and other inflammatory conditions affecting the joints but can cause stomach distress and promote bleeding at the higher doses needed.

Did You Know That ...?

Desirable and undesirable effects of NSAIDs result from their interfering with two types of COX enzymes. When COX-2 is blocked by NSAIDs, good things happen—pain, fever, and inflammation are relieved. When COX-1 is blocked, bad things happen— stomach ulceration, bleeding tendencies, and kidney problems. The selective COX-2 inhibitor celecoxib is promoted as not causing these latter bad effects. It does appear to increase the risk of heart attack and stroke, however.

More than a dozen NSAIDs are on the market. All, with the possible exception of the selective COX-2 inhibitor celecoxib (Celebrex), produce the same general effects. There may be individual differences in how we favorably or unfavorably respond to these drugs. Moreover, some drugs act for longer periods of time and require fewer daily doses.

NSAID Cautions

Do not take an NSAID if you are sensitive to aspirin. Symptoms of sensitivity include a running nose, hives, breathing difficulties, and shock. This risk is greater in persons with nasal polyps.

Use NSAIDs cautiously if you have peptic ulcer disease. Long-term NSAID use can cause stomach ulceration and bleeding, which can worsen an existing ulcer condition. Taking an acid-blocking drug, such as omeprazole (Prilosec) or famotidine (Pepcid), can prevent ulcers. Misoprostol (Cytotec) is specifically used to prevent gastric ulcers caused by long-term use of NSAIDs.

NSAIDs interfere with platelet function, which leads to bleeding tendencies. They should be used with extreme caution, if at all, by persons with bleeding disorders.

Maximizing Your Medicine

Rheumatoid arthritis requires drug treatment for a lifetime. Monthly costs of prescription NSAIDs range from $20 to $100, and selective COX-2 inhibitors are particularly expensive. You can save some very big bucks by noting that most NSAIDs are available as generic products. Moreover, a few (ibuprofen, ketoprofen, naproxen) can be purchased OTC at half strength. Make sure that you take the correct dose of these OTCs.

The elderly or individuals with a history of kidney disorders, high blood pressure, or heart disorders, should use NSAIDs under a doctor's supervision. These drugs may cause kidney toxicity in susceptible persons.

NSAIDs and more particularly, COX-2 inhibitors, when used over extended periods, may increase the risk of high blood pressure, heart attack, and stroke. In some instances, this has led to a fatal outcome.

Use NSAIDs with great caution when also taking the blood thinner (anticoagulant) warfarin.

Aspirin, and to a somewhat lesser degree all other NSAIDs, upset the stomach, causing heartburn, indigestion, nausea, bloating, and diarrhea. Take these drugs with food or water to reduce this distress.

Steroids

Steroids can dramatically relieve the inflammatory response. They act by inhibiting the manufacture of chemical mediators of inflammation and interfering with the movement of white blood cells to the site of injury or infection. Steroids don't usually cure the underlying cause of inflammation.

How Given

Steroids can be given by many routes of administration, using a wide array of dosage forms. For example, they can be …

Did You Know That …?

Steroids act like cortisol, a hormone produced by the adrenal gland, which sits atop the kidney. These drugs have profound effects on the body's sugars, proteins, and fats. They are widely used to treat hormone deficiencies and, as we will see, many nonhormonal conditions.

- Given by mouth or injection for systemic inflammatory conditions.

- Injected directly into the site of inflammation, such as for bursitis and tendinitis (e.g., tennis elbow, swimmer's shoulder).

- Inhaled as aerosols for asthma.

- Applied topically as creams, lotions, and ointments to relieve itching, swelling, and redness in wide variety of skin conditions, such as psoriasis and poison ivy.

- Applied as suspensions, solutions, and ointments to treat a variety of eye disorders, such as conjunctivitis (pink eye).

Steroid Cautions

When properly used, steroids can be life-saving drugs. When improperly used, their adverse effects can affect organs throughout the body. In general, steroids should be taken at the lowest effective doses for the shortest period of time. Some major problems associated with their use include …

◆ Adrenal insufficiency. High steroid doses cause the adrenal glands to shut down and become unable to release natural steroids when the body is confronted with stress.

◆ Bone loss, osteoporosis, and bone fractures.

◆ Increased susceptibility to infections.

◆ Loss of control of sugar levels in diabetics.

◆ Muscle weakness.

◆ Salt and water retention, causing high blood pressure.

◆ Suppression of growth in children.

◆ Behavioral and mood changes, such as depression or a high feeling (euphoria).

◆ Cataracts and glaucoma.

◆ Peptic ulcer disease.

Steroids should not be used by people with systemic fungal infections or those receiving live-virus vaccines.

Steroids should be used cautiously in children and pregnant or nursing women, as well as by people with high blood pressure, heart failure, kidney disease, peptic ulcers, diabetes, osteoporosis, and infections resistant to treatment.

The Least You Need to Know

◆ Classic signs of inflammation include pain, redness, warmth, swelling, and—in joints—loss of function.

◆ Acute and chronic inflammation can be managed with nonsteroidal anti-inflammatory drugs (NSAIDs) and steroids.

◆ Steroids are given by many routes of administration for a wide range of inflammatory conditions.

Drugs Used for Inflammation

Generic Name	Trade Name	How Taken: Topical (T), Inhaled (Ih), Injection (I), Oral (O)	Generic Available
Nonsteroidal Anti-Inflammatory Drugs (NSAIDs)			
Celecoxib	Celebrex	O	No
Diclofenac	Cataflam, Voltaren	O	Yes
Diflunisal	Dolobid	O	Yes
Fenoprofen	Nalfon	O	Yes
Flurbiprofen	Ansaid	O	Yes
Ibuprofen	Advil, Motrin	O	Yes
Indomethacin	Indocin	O	Yes
Ketoprofen	Orudis, Oruvail	O	Yes
Meloxicam	Mobic	O	No
Nabumetone	Relafen	O	Yes
Naproxen	Aleve, Naprosyn	O	Yes
Oxaprozin	Daypro	O	Yes
Piroxicam	Feldene	O	Yes
Sulindac	Clinoril	O	Yes
Tolmetin	Tolectin	O	Yes
Steroids			
Alclometasone	Aclovate	T	No
Amcinonide	Cyclocort	T	Yes
Beclomethasone	Beclovent	Ih	Yes
[Beclometasone]	Vanceril	Ih	
Betamethasone	Celestone, Diprolene, Diprosone, Valisone	Ih/I/O/T	Yes
Budesonide	Pulmicort, Rhinocort	In	Yes
Clobetasol	Temovate	T	Yes
Desonide	DesOwen, Tridesilon	T	Yes
Desoximetasone	Topicort	T	Yes
Dexamethasone	Decadron, Hexadrol	Ih/I/O,T	Yes

Generic Name	Trade Name	How Taken: Topical (T), Inhaled (Ih), Injection (I), Oral (O)	Generic Available
Fluocinolone	Synalar	T	Yes
Fluocinonide	Lidex	T	Yes
Flurandrenolide	Cordran	T	Yes
Fluticasone	Flovent	Ih	No
Halcinonide	Halog	T	No
Hydrocortisone	Cortaid, Cortizone, Hytone	I/O/T	Yes
Methylprednisolone	Medrol	Ih/O	Yes
	Depo-Medrol	I	Yes
Prednisolone	Delta-Cortef	Ih/I/O	Yes
Prednisone	Deltasone, Meticorten	O	Yes
Triamcinolone	Aristocort, Kenalog	Ih/I/O/T	Yes

Inflammatory Bowel Disorders: Ulcerative Colitis and Crohn's Disease

Several different types of inflammatory bowel disease (IBD) exist. Two important forms are ulcerative colitis and Crohn's disease. These conditions have similarities, the most obvious being chronic and recurring diarrhea as a major common symptom. Complications may affect the joints (with arthritis-like symptoms), liver, eyes, and skin.

Ulcerative colitis is an inflammatory condition that is limited to the inner linings of the rectum and colon. Bloody stools are highly characteristic of this condition. Severe attacks with violent abdominal cramping may occur. Distention of the large intestine may lead to its rupture, with massive bleeding and a possible fatal outcome. The risk of colon cancer is much higher in individuals with ulcerative colitis.

In Crohn's disease, by contrast, the inflammatory condition may affect any part of the gastrointestinal tract, from the mouth to the anus. Stools may be watery but infrequently contain blood. Fever, fatigue, feelings of sickness, intestinal obstructions, vitamin and other nutritional deficiencies, and weight loss are common. Even in the absence of treatment, the patient may be free of symptoms.

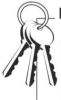

Did You Know That ...?

Although the exact cause of IBD has not been determined, common links appear to be involved in causing ulcerative colitis and Crohn's disease. Contemporary theories suggest that they result from genetic factors, infectious microbes, and an abnormal immune response. The immune response may be one in which the immune system launches an attack against its own tissues (an auto-immune disorder).

Treatment of IBD: An Overview

Drugs do not cure IBD. Realistic goals of drug therapy include reduction of inflammation, relief of symptoms, stabilization of these diseases, and prevention of their return. Preventing the recurrence of symptoms is much more difficult with Crohn's disease than ulcerative colitis.

Drugs used to treat IBD include the following:

♦ Anti-inflammatory drugs (e.g., sulfasalazine and steroids)

♦ Modulators of the immune system (a.k.a. immunomodulators; e.g., azathioprine)

♦ Antimicrobial drugs (e.g., metronidazole and ciprofloxacin for Crohn's disease)

Sulfasalazine

Sulfasalazine and related drugs are taken orally to relieve inflammation in mild to moderate IBD and, ideally, to suppress active symptoms for extended periods of time. Better results have been obtained with ulcerative colitis than with Crohn's disease.

Common side effects include nausea, vomiting, loss of appetite, joint pain, and headaches. Less common, but more severe effects include allergic reactions, with rash, fever, and disorders of the blood, liver, and pancreas.

Steroids

For moderate to severe cases, steroids such as prednisone (orally or by injection) or budesonide (orally) are used on a short-term basis to control IBD acute attacks. Steroids can dramatically and rapidly relieve the redness and swelling associated with the active symptoms. They also act by modulating the response of the immune system. When symptoms are controlled, steroid dosage must be reduced slowly over a three- to four-week period.

Steroids cannot be used over extended periods to prevent recurrences because they cause adverse effects on organs throughout the body. In general, steroids should be taken at the lowest effective doses for the shortest period of time. Some major problems with steroid use include …

♦ Adrenal insufficiency. High steroid doses cause the adrenal glands to shut down and become unable to release natural steroids when the body is confronted with stress.

♦ Bone loss, osteoporosis, and bone fractures.

♦ Increased susceptibility to infections.

- Loss of control of sugar levels in diabetics.

- Muscle weakness.

- Salt and water retention, causing high blood pressure.

- Suppression of growth in children.

- Behavioral and mood changes, such as depression or a high feeling (euphoria).

- Cataracts and glaucoma.

- Peptic ulcer disease.

Steroids should not be used by people with systemic fungal infections or those receiving live-virus vaccines.

Steroids should be used cautiously in children and pregnant or nursing women (also by people with high blood pressure, heart failure, kidney disease, peptic ulcers, diabetes, osteoporosis, and infections resistant to treatment).

Immunomodulators

For patients with moderate to severe cases of Crohn's disease, who fail to benefit from steroids, drugs such as azathioprine and mercaptopurine are used to suppress the immune system. These drugs are taken to treat the active symptoms and also for extended periods of time to prevent recurrences of Crohn's disease.

Did You Know That ...?

Smokers are more prone to developing Crohn's disease, whereas the risk of ulcerative colitis is considerably lower in smokers than in nonsmokers. In preliminary studies, nicotine patches were found to reduce symptoms of mild to moderate ulcerative colitis. This treatment approach is not recommended at this time.

Severe attacks of ulcerative colitis can be treated intravenously with cyclosporine for 7 to 10 days before switching to oral therapy. Azathioprine, when taken for four to six months, prevents relapses of ulcerative colitis for periods of up to two years.

The monoclonal antibody drug infliximab, given intravenously at eight-week intervals, over extended periods of time, controls the acute symptoms of severe ulcerative colitis and also prevents the recurrence of this condition. This very effective and expensive new drug is reserved for patients who fail to benefit from other safer drugs.

Azathioprine and mercaptopurine can cause adverse effects to the pancreas, lower white blood cell counts (increasing the susceptibility to infections), and may cause allergic reactions.

Infliximab injections can cause a number of adverse effects including fever, chills, itching, hives, changes in blood pressure, and breathing difficulties. Patients may become more susceptible to infections.

Antimicrobial Drugs

Microbes are thought to be involved in the inflammation seen in Crohn's disease, but not ulcerative colitis. Metronidazole is the most commonly used antimicrobial drug, particularly when inflammation is in the area of the anus. Ciprofloxacin is also used.

Common side effects with metronidazole include nausea, headache, dry mouth, and a metallic taste. When taken over an extended period, nerve disorders can result, causing a pins-and-needles sensation. The urine may darken after taking metronidazole, but this is of no concern.

Side effects with ciprofloxacin are mild and infrequent and include nausea, vomiting, and diarrhea, as well as dizziness and nervousness.

Absorption of ciprofloxacin into the blood is reduced by antacids containing aluminum or magnesium, and by iron and zinc salts, and milk and other dairy products. These interactions reduce its antibacterial effectiveness.

Ciprofloxacin can increase the blood levels and the intensity of the effects of theophylline and warfarin. To avoid the risk of adverse effects, the doses of theophylline and warfarin may have to be reduced.

The Least You Need to Know

◆ Ulcerative colitis and Crohn's disease—the two major types of inflammatory bowel disorders—are chronic and recurring conditions affecting the gastrointestinal tract, causing pronounced diarrhea and often systemic complications.

◆ Drugs control the active symptoms of IBD and prevent the recurrence of active symptoms, but do not cure IBD.

◆ Sulfasalazine and steroids are used to suppress active IBD symptoms.

♦ Sulfasalazine and the immunomodulators azathioprine and infliximab are used to control the active symptoms of Crohn's disease and prevent its recurrence.

♦ Metronidazole and ciprofloxacin are used to combat the microbes thought to be involved in the inflammatory response in Crohn's disease.

Drugs Used in Inflammatory Bowel Diseases

Generic Name	Trade Name	How Given: Injection (I), Oral (O), Rectal (R)	Generic Available
Anti-Inflammatory Drugs			
Balsalazide	Colazal	O	No
Mesalamine [Aminosalicylic acid]	Asacol, Pentasa, Rowasa	O/R	Yes
Olsalazine	Dipentum	O	No
Sulfasalazine	Azulfidine	O	Yes
Steroids			
Budesonide	Entocort EC	O	No
Prednisone	Deltasone, Meticorten	I/O	Yes
Immunomodulators			
Azathioprine	Immuran	I/O	Yes
Cyclosporine	Neoral	I/O	Yes
Infliximab	Remicade	I	No
Mercaptopurine	Purinethol	O	No
Methotrexate	Abitrexate	I	Yes
Antimicrobial Drugs			
Ciprofloxacin	Cipro	I/O	Yes
Metronidazole	Flagyl	O	Yes

Influenza

Influenza, commonly called the flu, is a viral infection of the lungs and airways. Symptoms include fever, running nose, sore throat, cough, and muscle aches and pains. There are two major flu types: A and B. The strain of virus causing flu changes each year, and this has made it difficult to develop a flu vaccine.

It's far easier to prevent the flu than to treat it. Vaccines prevent the flu, and this is the most desirable approach, because the flu is highly contagious. A number of drugs are available for flu treatment, but none provide impressive benefits.

Flu Prevention: Vaccine

Although there are several live flu vaccines, most flu vaccines are composed of inactivated (killed) flu viruses. Several weeks after injection into a muscle, the vaccine begins to provide protection. This lasts for four to six months. Vaccination is very strongly recommended for people likely to become very sick, with possible pneumonia, if infected.

The most common side effect is soreness at the injection site. The vaccine should not be given to people who are allergic to eggs or egg products.

Very recently, a flu vaccine given as a nasal spray (FluMist) has become available. Its use is limited to all healthy people ages 5 to 49. The most common side effects include a running or stuffy nose and cough. This live vaccine should not be given to pregnant women or health-care workers or those caring for patients with impaired immune function (such as HIV/AIDS patients). This vaccine should not be given to people who are allergic to eggs or egg products.

Maximizing Your Medicine

High-flu-risk individuals or those at high risk of complications from the flu include all people 50 and over; nursing home residents; people with chronic heart or lung disease (such as asthma, chronic bronchitis, emphysema), kidney disease, diabetes, or immune deficiencies; women in their second or third trimester of pregnancy; and health-care workers likely to come into contact with high-risk patients.

Flu Treatment: Drugs

Amantadine and rimantadine are taken by mouth and are used for the prevention and treatment of type A flu. They are not highly active and resistance rapidly develops to them.

Common side effects: amantadine causes dizziness, nervousness, insomnia, and difficulty in concentrating. Rimantadine causes similar effects but far less frequently.

Oseltamivir (Tamiflu, by mouth) and zanamivir (Relenza, inhaled) are used for the treatment of both types A and B flu. These drugs are only effective when given within two days after the start of symptoms. They modestly reduce the severity of flu symptoms and the length of time the symptoms continue but may reduce the complications of the flu in high-risk individuals. Both these drugs show signs of being effective in treating avian (bird) flu.

The Least You Need to Know

- ◆ Vaccines for injection and as a nasal spray prevent the flu.
- ◆ Oseltamivir (by mouth) and zanamivir (inhaled) reduce, somewhat, the severity and duration of flu symptoms caused by types A and B. They may be effective in treating avian (bird) flu.

Drugs Used for Influenza

Generic Name	Trade Name	How Taken: Injection (I), Oral (O), Inhaled (Ih)	Generic Available
Flu Prevention			
Influenza virus vaccine	Fluzone, Fluvirin	I	No
	FluMist	Ih	No
Flu Treatment			
Amantadine	Symmetrel	O	Yes
Rimantadine	Flumadine	O	No
Oseltamivir	Tamiflu	O	No
Zanamivir	Relenza	Ih	No

Insomnia

Sleep problems are common, and for many of us, a chronic problem. Insomnia includes having difficulty falling asleep, remaining asleep, or enjoying a good, restful night of sleep.

Causes of insomnia are many and include depression or anxiety; medical problems, such as pain or breathing difficulties; jet lag, day-time napping, exercising too close to bedtime; and the use of coffee and other stimulants, and alcohol.

Drug Treatment of Insomnia: An Overview

Try nondrug alternatives, such as going to sleep at the same time each night and arising each morning at the same time, to deal with insomnia before resorting to medications. Drugs are intended to be a short term solution to insomnia. The best drugs produce a state resembling natural sleep without causing morning-after drowsiness. Commonly used medications include OTC sleep aids, Halcion and related benzodiazepines, and newer Ambien-like drugs.

OTC Alternatives

OTC sleep aids are antihistamines that cause sedation and include diphenhydramine (Compoz, Nytol, Sominex) and doxylamine (Unisom). They should not be used longer than 7 to 10 days. Antihistamines commonly cause such side effects such as dry mouth, blurred vision, constipation, and difficulty in urinating. Individuals with glaucoma or prostate gland enlargement should not take these drugs. Older persons sometimes become nervous or agitated after their use.

The dietary supplement melatonin is purportedly effective for the prevention and/or treatment of insomnia and jet lag.

Halcion-Like Benzodiazepines

Prescription Halcion-like benzodiazepines are effective drugs for treating insomnia. They speed the time needed to fall asleep, reduce unintended awakenings during the night, and increase the total time spent sleeping.

Benzodiazepines specifically recommended for persons having difficulty falling asleep include triazolam (Halcion) and temazepam (Restoril). If they are abruptly discontinued after being taken for extended periods of time, temporary periods of sleep disturbances may result.

Flurazepam (Dalmane) is used for those insomniacs who wake up during the night and can't get back to sleep. It produces sedation over an extended period of time and may cause morning-after drowsiness, particularly in elderly individuals.

Halcion-like benzodiazepines cautions:

- **Common side effects.** Drowsiness, dizziness, and impairment of driving may occur.

- **Drug dependence.** Individuals who have a history of abusing alcohol or other drugs are the most likely candidates to also abuse benzodiazepines. Using these drugs, even at normal doses for periods of four to six weeks, can lead to dependence on them.

- **Drug withdrawal.** Taking benzodiazepines for several months and then suddenly not taking them can result in real signs of withdrawal. These include nervousness, sleep disturbances, and tremors. To avoid these problems, reduce doses gradually.

Warning!

When taken alone, even in high doses, benzodiazepines are virtually "suicide-proof." However, their potential for harm is much greater when they are taken with alcohol or other drugs that produce reduced mental or physical functioning.

Benzodiazepines have been reported to cause fetal abnormalities when taken during the first trimester of pregnancy. These drugs should not be used during pregnancy or by nursing mothers.

Ambien-Like Drugs

Zolpidem (Ambien) and eszopiclone (Lunesta) are widely used drugs that shorten the time needed to fall asleep and increase the total time spent sleeping. Zaleplon (Sonata) is intended for use by those having difficulty in falling asleep, rather than persons who can't stay asleep. Generic products are not available for any of these drugs.

These drugs produce a state that resembles natural sleep and cause no sleep disturbances when discontinued. Their most common side effects include dizziness and drowsiness but cause rather little morning-after sedation.

Antidepressants

Some 40 percent of all individuals with insomnia have a psychiatric condition, such as depression, anxiety, and substance abuse. In many instances, the condition may be the cause of chronic insomnia.

Antidepressants that cause sedation, such as trazodone, are used to treat the underlying depression and promote sleep. Because these drugs are not subject to abuse, and tolerance doesn't develop to their sleep-producing effects, they are particularly useful for individuals with chronic insomnia who are subject to substance abuse.

Side effects with trazodone include daytime sedation and a sudden drop in blood pressure when rapidly sitting upright or standing (orthostatic hypotension). Rarely, this drug causes a persistent erection (priapism), which if not treated, can cause permanent erectile dysfunction (impotence).

The Least You Need to Know

- Before any drugs are used, an attempt should be made to determine the cause of the insomnia. Nondrug approaches to its treatment should be tried first.

- Antihistamine-containing OTC sleep aids and melatonin may be helpful for the short-term relief of insomnia.

- Sleep-inducing Halcion-like benzodiapepines and Ambien-like drugs are effective for the treatment of insomnia and produce states that more resemble natural sleep.

- Antidepressants, such as trazodone, are used for the treatment of chronic insomnia in individuals with a history of psychiatric illnesses.

Drugs Used to Treat Insomnia

Generic Name	Trade Name	Generic Available
Benzodiapepines ("epam" or "olam")		
Estazolam	ProSom	Yes
Flurazepam	Dalmane	Yes
Quazepam	Doral	No
Temazepam	Restoril	Yes
Triazolam	Halcion	Yes
Antidepressants		
Amitriptyline	Elavil	Yes
Amoxapine	Asendin	Yes
Doxepin	Sinequan	Yes
Nortriptyline	Aventyl, Pamelor	Yes
Trazodone	Desyrel	Yes
Others		
Chloral hydrate	—	Yes
Eszopiclone	Lunesta	No
Zaleplon	Sonata	No
Zolpidem	Ambien	No

Intestinal Infections

Intestinal tract infections are caused by a variety of bacteria, viruses, single-celled protozoan parasites, and worms, and are almost always are associated with diarrhea. The severity of diarrhea may vary from being rather mild and merely troublesome to a life-threatening condition. In addition to diarrhea, abdominal cramping, loss of appetite, nausea, and vomiting may be present. These intestinal infections are often termed gastroenteritis.

Severe diarrhea results in the loss of excessive amounts of body water and salts. This causes a marked drop in blood pressure and shock, leading to damage to such critical organs as the kidneys, liver, and brain. Worldwide, intestinal infections are the second-leading cause of disease and death, particularly affecting infants and children younger than five.

Did You Know That ...?

"Food poisoning" results from the ingestion of contaminated food or water. Of international travelers, 20 to 50 percent may experience traveler's diarrhea (a.k.a. turista), caused by ingesting bacteria in drinking water or improperly cooked foods. Giardia is a pear-shaped single-celled organism that is the most common parasitic cause of diarrhea throughout the world, including the United States.

Treatment Overview

Mild to moderate cases of diarrhea should not be treated with antibiotics or other antimicrobial medicines. These drugs can, in some cases, worsen the problem in infections. Some of these same drugs can cause diarrhea, which doesn't help the problem. By contrast, the appropriate use of such drugs in severe intestinal infections, such as cholera, may be lifesaving.

Similarly, with the exception of traveler's diarrhea, the use of antidiarrheal drugs such as loperamide (Imodium) should not be used. These drugs slow the removal of bacterially produced toxins that invade and damage the inner walls of the intestines and cause diarrhea.

OTC Alternatives

Drugs are not recommended for intestinal infections causing mild to moderate diarrhea. Lost body water, sodium and potassium salts, and glucose (sugar) can be replenished using oral rehydration therapy (ORT). ORT is highly effective for all diarrheal disorders, is universally available, and is very inexpensive. ORT does not reduce diarrhea but prevents dehydration, the major cause of death.

Antimicrobial Medicines

If diarrhea persists for more than 48 hours, its cause should be determined and appropriate treatment started. Antimicrobial drugs should not be used to treat viral infections. A wide range of drugs is available to treat bacterial or protozoan causes of severe intestinal infections. They reduce the duration of the illness and may be lifesaving.

Antibacterial drugs, typically given orally for three to five days, include erythromycin; quinolones, such as ciprofloxacin or norfloxacin; tetracyclines, such as doxycycline or tetracycline; and trimethoprim-sulfamethoxazole. Metronidazole is the preferred treatment for the parasitic intestinal infections.

Erythromycins

Erythromycins (a.k.a. macrolides), such as erythromycin, azithromycin, and clarithromycin, are used as the first-choice medicines for the treatment of Campylobacter intestinal infections.

Name hint: most generic names end in "mycin."

Erythromycins are best taken on an empty stomach (one hour before meals or two hours after) with a full glass of water.

Common side effects include indigestion, nausea, vomiting, and diarrhea. These adverse effects can be minimized by taking the drug with meals.

Individuals should notify their doctor if they have severe abdominal pain, yellow coloration of the eyes or skin, or dark urine. These are signs of drug-caused liver toxicity. Individuals with a history of liver disease should not take these drugs.

Metronidazole

Metronidazole is the first choice for the treatment of giardiasis and amoebiasis (amoebic dysentery), tropical diseases caused by protozoan parasites.

It is taken by mouth for 5 to 10 days.

Common side effects include nausea, headache, dry mouth, and a metallic taste. The urine may darken after taking this drug, but this is of no concern.

Warning!

Avoid alcoholic beverages when taking metronidazole. The combination may cause nausea, vomiting, facial flushing, palpitations of the heart, and a marked drop in blood pressure.

Quinolones

Quinolones, such as ciprofloxacin and norfloxacin, are used for the treatment of a range of intestinal infections caused by Escherichia coli, Salmonella, and traveler's diarrhea.

Name hint: generic names usually end in "floxacin."

Side effects are mild and infrequent and include nausea, vomiting, and diarrhea, as well as dizziness and nervousness.

The absorption of quinolones into the blood is reduced by antacids containing aluminum or magnesium, and by iron and zinc salts, and milk and other dairy products. These interactions may result in a reduction in their antibacterial effectiveness.

Quinolones can increase blood levels and the intensity of the effects of theophylline and the blood thinner warfarin. To avoid the risk of adverse effects, the doses of theophylline and warfarin may have to be reduced.

Tetracyclines

Tetracyclines, such as doxycycline and tetracycline, are used to treat Vibrio cholerae, the bacterium causing cholera.

Name hint: generic names end in "cycline."

Gastrointestinal disturbances are the most common side effect, and these include indigestion, nausea, and diarrhea, which can be potentially dangerous.

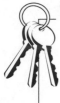

Did You Know That ...?

Cholera is most commonly spread by fecal contamination of drinking water. Multiple epidemics have occurred in the past half century, primarily in Southeast Asia, and also Africa and Latin America. Death can occur within hours after "rice-water stools" appear, with a mortality rate of over 50 percent if untreated. With treatment, oral rehydration therapy and drugs, deaths are reduced to less than 1 percent.

These drugs increase sensitivity to the sun, with a greater risk of severe sunburn. Individuals, particularly those with fair skin, taking tetracyclines should limit their exposure to sun and use sunscreen and wear protective clothing.

Warning!

Tetracyclines should never be taken if they are outdated, have changed color or taste, look different, or if they have been stored in a setting that is too warm or too damp. Such medication should be discarded. Under such circumstances, tetracyclines can decompose into chemicals that may cause serious adverse effects, including kidney damage.

Tetracyclines bind to metals such as calcium, magnesium, aluminum, and iron, which interfere with their absorption into the bloodstream. Antibiotic levels in the blood are reduced, reducing their antibacterial effectiveness. Hence, calcium supplements, most antacids, and iron supplements should be taken one hour before or two hours after tetracyclines.

Milk and other calcium-rich dairy products interfere with tetracycline absorption and lower their blood levels. Food interferes with the absorption of all tetracyclines, except doxycycline and minocycline. Other tetracyclines should be taken one hour before or two hours after meals and with a full glass of water.

Trimethoprim-Sulfamethoxazole

The sulfa drug sulfamethoxazole, in combination with the antibacterial drug trimethoprim (TMP-SMZ), is used to treat intestinal infections caused by Shigella and Salmonella and to prevent and treat traveler's diarrhea.

The most common side effects with TMP-SMZ are nausea, vomiting, and skin rash.

The Least You Need to Know

◆ If diarrhea continues for more than 48 hours, its cause should be determined and appropriate treatment started.

◆ Effective drugs are available for the treatment of intestinal infections caused by bacteria and parasites but not for viruses.

◆ Selection of the most appropriate drugs may vary depending on the local availability of drugs and the relative sensitivity of different microbial strains in different parts of the world.

◆ Antibacterial drugs include erythromycin, quinolones, tetracyclines, and trimethoprim-sulfamethoxazole.

◆ Metronidazole is the preferred drug for most intestinal parasitic infections.

Drugs Used to Treat Intestinal Infections

Generic Name	Trade Name	Generic Available
Erythromycins (Macrolides) ("mycin")		
Azithromycin	Zithromax	Yes
Clarithromycin	Biaxin	No
Erythromycin	E-Mycin, Ery-Tab, Erythrocin, Ilosone	Yes
Quinolones ("floxacin")		
Ciprofloxacin	Cipro	Yes
Norfloxacin	Noroxin	No
Tetracyclines ("cycline")		
Doxycycline	Vibramycin	Yes
Tetracycline	Sumycin	Yes
Miscellaneous		
Metronidazole	Flagyl, Metizol	Yes
Trimethoprim + sulfisoxazole [Co-Trimoxazole, TMP-SMZ]	Bactrim, Septra	Yes

Lyme Disease and Other Tick-Borne Disorders

Tick-borne diseases include Lyme disease, ehrlichioses, and Rocky Mountain spotted fever (RMSF). In each, an infectious microbe is transmitted to humans by the bite of an infected tick. Each disorder is caused by different microbes.

Preventive Measures

Ticks inhabit wooded areas and are picked up by hikers and gardeners. If you plan to travel or work in such areas, an insect repellant, such as DEET, should be applied.

Note that pets often brings ticks home, facilitating the transmission of infections to their human owners, individuals who may rarely actually venture into wooded areas or even their own yards.

At the conclusion of a day in the woods, the body should be carefully inspected for the presence of ticks. If found, a pair of tweezers should be used to remove them.

OTC Alternatives

DEET is the term used for diethyltoluamide and is the most widely used and effective repellant against ticks, mosquitoes, and biting flies. It can be applied to skin or clothing. Under ideal conditions, it works for up to five hours. Because of the risk of nerve toxicity, DEET should not be used in children under age 2.

Treatment

The microbes responsible for these tick-borne diseases readily respond to treatment with common, readily available, oral antibiotics, many of which are relatively safe.

Lyme Disease

Lyme disease has three stages. During the first stage, a large red spot may appear at the site of the tick bite. When present, the spot is generally 6 inches across, has a clear center (bull's eye), and doesn't itch. This stage is followed by flu-like symptoms, which may continue for weeks. Within months and even years after being infected, untreated Lyme disease may develop into a late stage with chronic arthritis.

Early Lyme disease is effectively treated with the doxycycline (a tetracycline) or amoxicillin (a penicillin) for three to four weeks. For pregnant women, for whom tetracyclines cannot be used, or patients allergic to tetracyclines or penicillins, cefuroxime or erythromycin can be given.

Later treatment requires intravenous dosing of ceftriaxone or penicillin for four weeks or longer, depending on the severity of the disease. Hospitalization may be required.

Ehrlichioses and Rocky Mountain Spotted Fever

Ehrlichioses and RMSF have similar symptoms, namely a severe headache and fever, and may be mistaken for the flu. Small purple spots are present with RMSF.

Both are severe disorders, difficult to specifically diagnose without a specialized laboratory test, and often require hospitalization. Fatalities may occur in the absence of prompt treatment. When symptoms suggest that these diseases may be present, doxycycline is given immediately, even before they are confirmed by laboratory studies.

Doxycycline or another tetracycline is given for at least 5 to 10 days. This treatment is so reliable that, if fever doesn't drop within 24 to 72 hours, these diseases may not be present. For patients who can't take tetracyclines, rifampin is used for ehrlichioses and chloramphenicol for RMSF.

The Least You Need to Know

◆ Lyme disease, ehrlichioses, and RMSF are tick-borne diseases caused by bacteria and related microbes (rickettsiae).

◆ Doxycycline is highly effective in curing these disorders.

Drug Treatment of Tick-Borne Disorders

Generic Name	Trade Name	Antibiotic Class	Generic Available
Amoxicillin	Amoxil, Trimox	Penicillin	Yes
Ceftriaxone	Rocephin	Cephalosporin	No
Cefuroxime	Ceftin, Kefurox, Zinicef	Cephalosporin	Yes
Chloramphenicol	Chloromycetin	—	Yes
Doxycycline	Vibramycin	Tetracycline	Yes
Erythromycin	E-Mycin, E.E.S., Erythrocin, Ilosone	Macrolide	Yes
Rifampin	Rifadin, Rimactane	Anti-TB	Yes

Malaria

Malaria is most often contracted after being bitten by an infected female *Anopheles* mosquito. While biting, the mosquito injects saliva containing malaria-causing parasites (*Plasmodium*, a protozoan) into the body of her victim.

Symptoms of malaria may appear while traveling or even months after returning from a malaria-risk area. Common recurring symptoms are high fever, shaking chills, sweating, headache, and nausea.

Malaria is a disorder that affects red blood cells. The disease is confirmed by the presence of the parasite in the patient's blood, as seen under a microscope.

Did You Know That ...?

More people are affected worldwide by malaria than any other disorder. There are 300 to 500 million new infections each year, with 1 to 2 million deaths, mostly in children under 5. Of the 1,300 annual cases in the United States, most are in immigrants from affected areas, American travelers, and less commonly, from blood transfusions or contaminated needles.

Drug Treatment of Malaria: An Overview

Antimalarial drugs are used to either prevent malaria or to treat it. There are no universally effective drugs. The Centers for Disease Control and Prevention provides authoritative, current, and detailed information on the preferred treatments and prevention strategies in different regions of the globe. Contact www.cdc.gov/travel/regionalmalaria/index.htm or the toll-free number 1-877-FYI-TRIP.

The choice of prescription drugs is based on the type of malaria, the malaria-risk area visited, the disease history of the traveler, pregnancy status, and age.

Prevention of Malaria

To prevent malaria, drugs are taken in each of the following three periods: one or two days to one week before arriving in the area; once daily to once weekly while in the area; and one to four weeks after leaving the area.

An OTC mosquito insect repellent containing DEET should be used. For both adults and children, chloroquine (Aralen) is the preferred drug for the prevention of malaria.

In those geographic areas where chloroquine-resistant strains of malaria exist, mefloquine (Lariam), doxycycline (Vibramycin), or atovaquone plus proguanil (Malarone) can be used. Each drug, taken by mouth, has its own distinctive directions for use, side effects, and precautions.

Antimalarial drugs must be taken as prescribed at the doses recommended. Inadequate doses can fail to prevent malaria, and overdoses can cause potentially serious side effects and toxicity.

Each of these antimalarial drugs has unique side effects. Several of these medications cause stomach pain, nausea, vomiting, and headache. In addition, doxycycline may cause increased sensitivity to the sun causing sunburn, and mefloquine has been known to cause anxiety, vivid dreams, and visual disturbances.

Maximizing Your Medicine

Although antimalarial drugs are far cheaper abroad, get your prescription filled at home. Drugs purchased in malaria-risk areas may be counterfeit or of substandard quality. Because there is little local demand for these drugs, your local pharmacy may not have them in stock. So don't try getting your prescription filled at the last minute.

Research laboratories around the world are working to develop a vaccine that effectively prevents malaria.

Do not take if ...

- **Mefloquine.** The patient has epilepsy, history of severe mental disorder, or irregular heartbeat.

- **Doxycycline.** The patient is pregnant or under the age of 8.

- **Atovaquone plus proguanil.** If the patient is pregnant, nursing an infant who weighs less than 24 lbs., or has severe kidney disease.

- **Primaquine.** If you are pregnant or have a G6PD enzyme deficiency.

Treatment of Malaria

All types of malaria can make the individual feel very sick and, in some cases if not treated promptly, lead to death. Some 90 percent of all deaths occur in sub-Saharan Africa.

Chloroquine is the preferred drug for treating acute attacks in simple cases. Severe cases are treated with oral quinine or injected quinidine.

Common side effects include visual disturbances, itching, headache, nausea, and diarrhea.

The Least You Need to Know

- ◆ Take an antimalarial drug before traveling to malaria-risk areas, while there, and after leaving these areas.
- ◆ Chloroquine is the preferred drug for the prevention and treatment of malaria.

Drugs Used to Treat Malaria

Generic Name	Trade Name	Generic Available
Atovaquone + proguanil	Malarone	No
Chloroquine	Aralen	Yes
Doxycycline	Vibramycin	Yes
Hydroxychloroquine	Plaquenil	Yes
Mefloquine	Lariam	Yes
Primaquine	—	Yes
Quinidine gluconate	Quinaglute	Yes
Quinine	—	Yes
Sulfadoxine + pyrimethamine	Fansidar	No

Menopause

The woman's monthly cycle and ovulation are controlled by the female hormones estrogen and progesterone. When many women approach the age of 50, their ovaries become less regular. Eventually ovulation stops. Periods end for good, and 12 months later, at about the age of 51, menopause begins.

For many women, the early years of menopause can be extremely unpleasant. Many women commonly experience hot flashes (also called hot flushes or vasomotor symptoms). Other symptoms may include fatigue, anxiety, irritability, depression, emotional disturbances, decreased sexual desire, and sleep disturbances, which are aggravated by night sweats. Vaginal dryness may cause pain during sexual intercourse, and a decrease in bone mass increases the risk of osteoporosis.

To improve women's quality of life and health, for decades prior to 2002, doctors routinely prescribed hormone replacement therapy (HRT). This is typically an oral estrogen (e.g., Premarin) or an estrogen plus progesterone-like drug combination (e.g., Prempro). These drugs are highly effective in relieving the signs of menopause and preventing or greatly slowing bone loss.

HRT Benefits vs. Risks

Thinking abruptly changed in 2002. Several studies found that women taking estrogen or Prempro for an average of five years had increased risks of heart disease, breast cancer, stroke, clot formation in the lung arteries (pulmonary embolism), and Alzheimer's disease. These same studies found a decreased risk of bone fractures and colorectal cancer, the second leading cause of cancer deaths in the United States.

Warning!

The Women's Health Initiative was a long-term research study started in 1993 and involved 16,000 women. It anticipated seeing the benefits of HRT in protecting women against heart disease and cancer. The study prematurely ended in 2002. Subjects taking HRT for an average of five years had increased risks of developing heart disease, breast cancer, stroke, clotting disorders, and Alzheimer's disease.

The decision whether to take HRT is a difficult one, with no single correct answer for all women. It is generally agreed that estrogen is very effective in relieving hot flashes and other menopausal symptoms. Moreover, its use may be strongly considered when the distressing symptoms of menopause clearly outweigh the potential hazards of HRT. However, before starting HRT, the doctor should fully and clearly explain to women the benefits and potential risks of such drugs. If a decision is made to use them, drugs should be taken at the lowest effective dose for the shortest possible time.

Did You Know That ...?

Why use estrogen plus progestin rather than only estrogen for the relief of menopausal symptoms? Estrogen-only increases the risk of endometrial cancer (lining of the uterus) 4 to 14 times. Addition of a progestin eliminates this risk. For women who have had their uterus surgically removed (hysterectomized), endometrial cancer is not a risk, and estrogen-only can be used.

HRT Products

Medicines with estrogen-like properties may be natural or laboratory prepared. None are better or safer than others.

Estrogen-only products can be taken in many different forms based on the woman's preference. The most commonly used forms are oral tablets, skin patches, vaginal products as creams, tablets, or rings, and skin emulsions and gels.

Common Side Effects with Estrogen

Nausea, headache, breast tenderness, and heavy bleeding. These problems are reduced with products applied to the vagina.

Addition of a progestin prevents the risk of estrogen-associated endometrial cancer. A variety of estrogen plus progestin dosing approaches are used. The estrogen plus progesterone combination may be taken every day. Early during the therapy, unpredictable bleeding or spotting may occur. Alternatively, progestin may be added to estrogen for the last 12 to 14 days on 28-day cycle. With this approach, monthly bleeding occurs.

Common Side Effects with Progestin

Irritability, headache, and depression. Some women experience premenstrual-like symptoms.

Bone-Mass Protectors

Raloxifene (Evista) selectively prevents bone loss. It is used for the prevention and treatment of osteoporosis in postmenopausal women. It has no effects on the uterus nor does it benefit hot flashes and may even worsen them. This drug reduces the risk of breast cancer in high-risk women after menopause.

The Least You Need to Know

◆ Hormone replacement therapy consists of an estrogen or an estrogen plus progestin combination.

◆ HRT effectively relieves such menopausal symptoms as hot flashes, sleep disturbances, and vaginal dryness; it also slows bone loss.

◆ Women using HRT for extended periods have a greater risk of heart disease, breast cancer, stroke, clot formation in the lungs, and Alzheimer's disease, but a lower risk of colorectal cancer and bone fractures.

◆ Estrogen products are available as oral tablets, skin patches, and vaginal and skin products.

Hormone Replacement Products

Form	Trade Names
Estrogen-Only	
Tablet	Cenestin, Estrace, Menest, Ogen, Premarin
Skin patch	Alora, Climara, Estraderm, Vivelle
Skin emulsion	Estrasorb
Vaginal tablets	Vagifem
Vaginal cream/gel	Estrace Vaginal, Estrogel, Ogen Vaginal, Premarin Vaginal
Vaginal ring	Estring
Estrogen + Progestin	
Tablets	Activella, Estratest, Premphase, Prempro
Patch	CombiPatch

Migraine and Other Severe Headaches

Headaches may range from being an annoyance to being totally disabling and incapacitating. Some headaches have an identifiable cause, such as very high blood pressure, tumors, head injuries, and brain infections. Headaches are also common during caffeine withdrawal. If the cause is known, it should be treated. Migraine, cluster, and tension headaches have no identifiable cause.

Migraine Headache

A migraine is a recurring, throbbing headache, causing moderate to severe pain. It is usually on one side of the head and continues for several hours to days. Attacks may be accompanied by nausea and vomiting. Some 20 to 25 percent of migraine sufferers (referred to as migraineurs) experience a visual sensation (aura) prior to an attack.

In the United States, 18 percent of women and 6 percent of men are migraineurs, and it runs in families. Migraine attacks are triggered by estrogen, the female hormone.

Many theories have been proposed to explain what causes migraines. One of these suggests that blood vessels in the brain widen and pulsate, and that these effects involve the neurotransmitter serotonin.

Drugs used for migraine treatment either stop an attack in progress or prevent it from occurring.

Did You Know That ...?

If you are a migraineur, you are in very distinguished company. Among those known or believed to have migraines include Alexander Graham Bell, Julius Caesar, Lewis Carroll, Charles Darwin, Sigmund Freud, Thomas Jefferson, Stephen King, Robert E. Lee, Edgar Allan Poe, Elvis Presley, George Bernard Shaw, and Woodrow Wilson.

Stopping Migraine Headaches

Medicines most effectively stop an attack when taken at its earliest signs. If the headache is of mild intensity, a nonsteroidal anti-inflammatory drug (NSAID) may be sufficient.

OTC Alternatives

For mild to moderate migraine headaches, an OTC NSAID may effectively relieve pain. Such drugs include aspirin, ibuprofen (Motrin), or naproxen (Aleve). The combination of aspirin, acetaminophen, and caffeine (Excedrin Migraine) is specifically used for treating migraines.

Severe headache pain can be relieved using opioids (narcotics) such as meperidine (Demerol), oxycodone (OxyContin), and butorphanol (Stadol) nasal spray. Regular use may produce a drug dependency state.

Migraines of greater severity are usually treated first with a triptan or, as a backup, an ergot-like drug. Ergot-like drugs and the triptans are thought to act by constricting widened blood vessels in the brain and reducing their pulsations. These drugs work by acting like the neurotransmitter serotonin.

With the exception of the triptans, taking any of these drugs on a daily basis can cause a rebound headache, i.e., headaches that start when the medication is abruptly stopped.

Ergot-Like Drugs

Ergotamine and dihydroergotamine (DHE) effectively stop moderate to severe migraines. Ergotamine is taken orally, under the tongue, and rectally.

Warning!

Pregnant women should not use ergotamine or DHE because it may cause contractions of the uterus, resulting in harm to the fetus or an abortion. Similarly, persons with liver, kidney, or heart disease or circulation problems in their extremities should not use ergotamine or DHE.

Ergotamine cautions:

◆ **Common side effects.** One in 10 persons experience nausea and vomiting after taking ergotamine.

◆ **Overdosage.** Severe ergot toxicity (ergotism) can result when excessive doses are taken. Constriction of small blood vessels in the hands and feet reduce blood circulation, which may cause gangrene.

◆ **Drug dependency.** Regular use of ergotamine, even at prescribed doses, can lead to a drug-dependent state. If ergotamine use is stopped abruptly, migraine-like symptoms, (e.g., a rebound headache, nausea, vomiting, restlessness) can occur.

Did You Know That …?

During the Middle Ages, there were strange epidemics in which people suffered from gangrene of the hands and feet and pregnant women miscarried. The disease, called St. Anthony's fire, was caused by ergot, a fungus that contaminated rye and other grains. Sporadic outbreaks of ergot poisoning have been reported in Europe during the twentieth century.

Dihydroergotamine (DHE), taken by injection or nasal spray, works like ergotamine. It does not constrict blood vessels in the hands and feet, nor does it cause nausea and vomiting or drug dependency. Diarrhea commonly occurs.

Triptans

Triptans (such as Imitrex) are the first choice for stopping headaches. Triptans work rapidly, a tremendous benefit when an attack is looming, and they help a very high proportion of treated persons. They are far more selective in their serotonin-like effects than ergot-like drugs and cause far fewer side effects.

The many available triptans are all effective. They are taken by mouth, injection, or as a nasal spray. They differ with respect to how quickly and how long they work and in their incidence of side effects.

The generic names of all triptans end in "triptan."

Triptan cautions:

◆ **Common side effects.** Generally mild and short-lasting and include tingling in the extremities, fatigue, dizziness, flushing, and feelings of warmth in the upper body. Chest pressure (but not pain) is a commonly experienced side effect.

◆ **Drug interactions.** Triptans should not be taken less than 24 hours after ergot-like drugs or within 2 weeks of monoamine oxidase inhibitors (MAOIs) used to treat depression.

Warning!

Pregnant women or people who have had angina, heart disease, stroke, or high blood pressure that is not controlled should not use triptans.

Preventing Migraine Attacks

When attacks occur more often than twice weekly, or if medicines intended to stop attacks don't do so effectively enough, other drugs may be taken to prevent attacks. To do the job, they must be taken daily. These include selected beta-blockers, antidepressants, and antiseizure medications.

Did You Know That ...?

Beta-blockers are a very popular class of medicines. In addition to preventing migraine headaches, they are also used to reduce high blood pressure and treat such heart conditions as heart failure, irregular heart rhythms, angina, and heart attacks.

Maximizing Your Medicine

A month's supply of a single drug may vary in cost from $10 to more than $250. Look for generic products. They are just as effective as the trade-name medicines in their class at only a fraction of the cost.

Beta-Blockers

Beta-blockers, in particular propranolol (Inderal), are the most widely used medicines for preventing migraines. They reduce the frequency of attacks by one-half in most people.

Not all beta-blockers work. Other effective ones include atenolol, metoprolol, nadolol, and timolol.

Note the "olol" ending of the generic names.

Beta-blocker cautions:

- **Common side effects.** Slowing of the heartbeat; reduction of good cholesterol (HDL) levels in the blood; may cause breathing difficulties, sleep disturbances, and erectile dysfunction.

- **Drug withdrawal.** Beta-blockers should never be abruptly discontinued, because a rebound rapid and irregular heartbeat may occur. This is a particular risk for angina patients.

Warning!

Beta-blockers should not be used by patients with certain slow heartbeats (sinus bradycardia) or heart blockage.

Nonselective beta-blockers should be used with great care by individuals with asthma, bronchitis, emphysema, or a history of severe allergic reactions. They may mask the signs of low blood sugar in diabetics. Beta-blockers may worsen the mood of persons with depression.

Antidepressants

Certain drugs used to treat depression may also prevent migraine attacks. Of these, amitriptyline (Elavil) is the most widely used.

Antidepressant cautions:

◆ **Common side effects.** Dry mouth, blurred vision, constipation, difficulty in urinating, sedation, dizziness, increased heart rate, impairment of memory, weight gain, impairment of sexual function. Side effects may be more pronounced in the elderly.

◆ **Overdoses.** These drugs are potentially dangerous, even deadly, when taken in excessive doses. They interfere with normal heart rhythms.

◆ **Drug withdrawal.** Don't stop using drugs abruptly. Dizziness, nausea, diarrhea, sleep difficulties, and nervousness may result.

Antiseizure Drugs

Valproic acid and divalproex, drugs originally developed to treat epilepsy, also effectively prevent migraines. Common side effects include weight gain, hair loss, tremors, and feelings of fatigue. They should not be used in pregnant women or persons with diseases of the liver or pancreas.

Ergot-Like Drug

Methysergide (Sansert) is very effective in preventing migraines but causes serious side effects that greatly limit its use to a medicine of last resort.

Cluster Headaches

Cluster headaches are a series or cluster of severe headaches, each lasting from 15 minutes to several hours, and occurring one or more times a day. Pain is on one side of the head, in the eye, or around it. Attacks continue for weeks or even months. Each cluster attack may be separated by attack-free periods of months or years. Cluster headaches are relatively rare, seen in 4 of 1,000 men, which is 4 to 7 times more often than in women.

Medicines stop and prevent cluster headaches. Emphasis is on prevention—reducing how long the headache lasts, as well as how often attacks occur and their severity. Drug therapy begins early during the headache and continues on a daily basis until the patient is headache-free for two weeks.

Treatments to stop cluster headaches include inhaled oxygen, ergot-like drugs, and the triptans.

Of the calcium antagonists (a.k.a. calcium channel blockers), verapamil is the preferred drug for the prevention of attacks. Common side effects include constipation, headache, swelling of the feet and ankles, and inflammation of the gums.

Other cluster prevention drugs include lithium, ergotamine, methysergide, and steroids.

Tension Headaches

This is the most common type of headache. It causes moderate pain around the head in the "hatband" area and does not throb. OTC NSAIDs such as Advil are highly effective in their treatment.

The Least You Need to Know

- ◆ Medicines are available to stop and prevent migraine and cluster headaches.

- ◆ Triptans are highly effective and are the most widely used drugs to stop migraines, and the beta-blocker propranolol is preferred to prevent attacks.

- ◆ Ergot-like drugs are effective in stopping migraine attacks but excessive doses can produce serious adverse effects on blood circulation.

Drugs to Stop Migraines

Generic Name	Trade Name	Generic Available
Ergot-Like Drugs		
Dihydroergotamine (DHE)	D.H.E. 45, Migranal	No
Ergotamine	Ergomar, Ergostat	Yes
Ergotamine	Cafergot, Wigraine	Yes

Generic Name	Trade Name	Generic Available
Triptans		
Almotriptan	Axert	No
Eletriptan	Relpax	No
Frovatriptan	Frova	No
Naratriptan	Amerge	No
Rizatriptan	Maxalt	No
Sumatriptan	Imitrex	No
Zolmitriptan	Zomig	No

Drugs to Prevent Migraine and Cluster Headaches

Generic Name	Trade Name	Generic Available
Beta-Blockers ("lol" or "olol")		
Atenolol	Tenormin	Yes
Metoprolol	Lopressor, Toprol	Yes
Nadolol	Corgard	Yes
Propranolol	Inderal	Yes
Timolol	Blocarden	Yes
Tricyclic Antidepressants		
Amitriptyline	Elavil	Yes
Doxepin	Sinequan	Yes
Imipramine	Tofranil	Yes
Nortriptyline	Aventyl, Pamelor	Yes
Protriptyline	Vivactil	Yes
Antiseizure Drugs		
Divalproex	Depakote	No
Valproic acid	Depakene	Yes

continues

Drugs to Prevent Migraine and Cluster Headaches (continued)

Generic Name	Trade Name	Generic Available
Ergot-Like Drug		
Methysergide	Sansert	No
Calcium Antagonists		
Verapamil	Calan, Isoptin, Verelan	Yes

Obesity

In recent years, society's interest in weight control has shifted in emphasis from our appearance to our health. One in three adults is now obese, and a similar proportion is overweight, and these numbers are increasing. Because of the health hazards associated with obesity, this condition in children is of growing concern to health-care workers.

Obese people are at greater risk of developing diabetes mellitus (type 2 diabetes), certain cancers, coronary artery disease potentially leading to heart attack and stroke, high blood pressure, and elevated cholesterol levels.

The old Metropolitan Life Insurance Company tables of normal weight ranges have been replaced by the body mass index (BMI), a measure of relative weight based on height. With increasing BMI values (i.e., body weight), the relative risk of death from weight-related conditions increases.

Drug Treatment of Obesity: An Overview

Currently there are two different drug approaches to treating obesity:

◆ **Drugs that reduce appetite.** Amphetamine-like drugs (appetite suppressants) reduce feelings of hunger, so less is eaten and fewer calories are consumed. They act on brain centers that signal us to stop eating.

◆ **Drugs that interfere with the absorption of fats.** For calories to count, food, including fats, must be absorbed from the intestines into the blood. Before being absorbed, fats must be broken down into smaller units. Orlistat prevents this fat breakdown.

Amphetamine-Like Appetite Suppressants

Appetite suppressants are intended for the short-term treatment of obesity, when nondrug alternatives have proved ineffective. When combined with exercise and a change in eating behavior, users of these drugs can lose weight.

Warning!

Use of amphetamine-like drugs for extended periods or at high doses may lead to drug dependency. Individuals feeling a strong need or desire to continue to take these drugs should consult their doctor. Drug use should not be stopped abruptly.

Amphetamine-like drugs are generally safe and effective in suppressing appetite and increasing weight loss for up to 12 weeks. Thereafter, they become less effective. To restore their effectiveness, users sometimes increase their drug dosage without consulting their doctor. This may result in undesirable side effects or drug dependency.

Amphetamine's stimulating effects on the brain may cause irritability, nervousness, sleep disturbances, and headache. Its effects on the heart and blood vessels may cause heart palpitations, increased heart rate, and an increase in blood pressure.

Rimonabant (Accomplia), a recently introduced non-amphtamine, reduces the desire to eat. It also reduces cravings for nicotine and is used to promote smoking cessation.

Drugs That Interfere with Fat Absorption

Orlistat (Xenical) acts in the intestines to reduce fat absorption from foods. Unfortunately, absorption of beta-carotene and the fat-soluble vitamins A, D, and E are also decreased. This drug is modestly effective in facilitating weight loss when used for extended periods of time.

Common side effects include pain in the abdomen, diarrhea, urge to defecate, intestinal gas, and fatty and oily stools.

The Least You Need to Know

◆ Successful weight reduction programs combine dietary modification, increased physical activity, and permanent changes in eating attitudes and patterns.

◆ Amphetamine-like appetite suppressants should only be used for short periods and only after nondrug approaches have been tried and have not been successful.

◆ Orlistat interferes with the absorption of fats in the diet that serve as a source of calories.

Drugs Used for Obesity

Generic Name	Trade Name	Generic Available
Amphetamine-Like Appetite Suppressants		
Benzphetamine	Didrex	No
Dextroamphetamine	Dexedrine	Yes
Diethylpropion	Tenuate	Yes
Methamphetamine	Desoxyn	No
Phendimetrazine	Bontril, Prelu-2	Yes
Phentermine	Adipex-P, Ionamin	Yes
Sibutramine	Meridia	No
Non-Amphetamine Appetite Suppressants		
Rimonabant	Accomplia	No
Fat-Absorption Interference		
Orlistat	Xenical	No

Osteoarthritis

Osteoarthritis, also called degenerative joint disease, is a chronic disease that affects joints and causes pain, stiffness, and loss of motion. It is the most common joint disease, affecting more than half of us by 65 and virtually all people over 75. Osteoarthritis (OA) is second only to cardiovascular disease as a cause of disability.

Cartilage covers the ends of bones, permitting them to move smoothly. Over time, cartilage wears down so that bone rubs against bone at the joint. OA most commonly occurs in the hips, knees, fingers, and spine.

The most important factors contributing to the development of OA are increased body weight, repetitive motion, disease, injury, and genetic influences.

Treatment of OA: An Overview

The most common symptom of OA is pain, which leads to loss of motion and function. Medicines are primarily used to relieve pain. Weight loss, exercise, and physical therapy are nondrug components of OA treatment plans.

Medications generally start with acetaminophen (Tylenol) followed by such nonsteroidal anti-inflammatory drugs (NSAIDs) as ibuprofen (Motrin) and naproxen (Aleve). The dietary supplements glucosamine and chondroitin may also be helpful. When other treatments fail to provide pain relief, injections of steroids or hyaluronic acid may be tried. If drugs don't help or there is an unacceptable loss of function, joint replacement surgery may be the last option.

OTC Alternatives

Experts recommend acetaminophen (also known as paracetamol) as their first choice for OA pain relief. It is safe, effective, and inexpensive, but it does not improve inflammation. Acetaminophen is available as a generic product, and far more expensively as Tylenol, Anacin Aspirin Free, and many other trade names. Daily doses must not exceed 4 grams. Overdoses may cause liver damage, and overindulgence in alcohol must be avoided.

NSAIDs

One of a great many NSAIDs may be selected if acetaminophen fails to provide adequate pain relief. NSAIDs are also effective anti-inflammatory medicines.

Aspirin was the original NSAID. It is a good drug for relieving OA pain but causes stomach distress and can promote bleeding. Crushing aspirin and placing it in water or taking aspirin with food can reduce these problems.

There are more than a dozen highly effective NSAIDs on the market. All, with the possible exception of the selective COX-2 inhibitor celecoxib (Celebrex), produce the same general effects. There may be individual differences in how we respond, both favorably and unfavorably. Some drugs require fewer daily doses.

Warning!

Desirable and undesirable effects of NSAIDs result from their interfering with two types of COX enzymes. When COX-2 is blocked by NSAIDs, good things happen—pain, fever, and inflammation are relieved. When COX-1 is blocked, bad things happen—stomach ulceration, bleeding tendencies, kidney problems. Selective COX-2 inhibitors, such as Celebrex, are not supposed to cause these latter bad effects but may increase the risk of stroke and heart attack.

No NSAID is best at relieving pain—and that includes Celebrex. Comparable relief of mild to moderate OA pain is produced when using equivalent doses of acetaminophen, aspirin, ibuprofen, and naproxen. Some NSAIDs prove to be more effective for some persons and cause fewer side effects.

Do not take an NSAID if you are sensitive to aspirin. Symptoms of sensitivity include a running nose, hives, breathing difficulties, and shock. This risk is greater in persons with nasal polyps.

Maximizing Your Medicine

Monthly costs of prescription NSAIDs range from $20 to $100, and selective COX-2 inhibitors (such as Celebrex) are particularly expensive. You can save some big bucks by noting that most NSAIDs are available as generic products. Moreover, a few (ibuprofen, ketoprofen, naproxen) are available OTC at half strength. Make sure that you take the correct dose of these OTCs.

Use cautiously if you have peptic ulcer disease. Long-term NSAID use can cause ulceration of the stomach and bleeding, which can worsen an existing ulcer condition. Taking an acid-blocking drug, such as omeprazole (Prilosec) or famotidine (Pepcid), can prevent ulcers. Misoprostol (Cytotec) is specifically used to prevent gastric ulcers caused by long-term use of NSAIDs.

Celebrex has been aggressively marketed based on its ability to cause a lower risk of stomach ulcers than other NSAIDs. This claim may not be completely valid.

NSAIDs interfere with platelet function, which leads to bleeding tendencies. They should be used with extreme caution, if at all, by persons with bleeding disorders.

The elderly or individuals with a history of kidney disorders, high blood pressure, or heart disorders, should use NSAIDs under a doctor's supervision. These drugs may cause kidney toxicity in susceptible persons.

NSAIDs and more particularly, COX-2 inhibitors, when used over extended periods, may increase the risk of stroke and high blood pressure.

Use NSAIDs with great caution when also taking the blood thinner (anticoagulant) warfarin.

Aspirin, and to a somewhat lesser degree all other NSAIDS, upset the stomach causing heartburn, indigestion, nausea, bloating, and diarrhea. Take these drugs with food or water to reduce this distress.

OTC Alternatives

NSAIDs effectively relieve OA pain after taking a few doses, but they don't correct or slow the deterioration of cartilage between joints. The dietary supplement glucosamine is thought to both reduce the loss of cartilage and stimulate its formation after being taken for several months. Glucosamine may relieve pain, improve motion, and reduce the need for joint replacement surgery. Evidence supporting the effectiveness of condroitin is not convincing.

Steroid and Hyaluronic Acid Injections

Injection of steroids directly into the joint can produce relief of pain and stiffness. To prevent adverse effects in other parts of the body, these injections should not be repeated more often than three to four times per year.

Because their benefits have not been proven and their adverse effects are well known, steroid injections are not recommended for the treatment of OA. The risk of damage to cartilage has not been fully determined.

Hyaluronic acid is a natural component of cartilage and has lubricating and shock-absorbing properties. Typically, injections are given once weekly for three or five weeks. Treatments are expensive, and their effectiveness in OA has not been clearly proven. Hyaluronic acid should be reserved for those persons not responding to other drugs.

The Least You Need to Know

- Osteoarthritis is a common, chronic joint disease that causes pain, stiffness, and loss of motion.

- Acetaminophen is the first choice recommended by experts to relieve OA pain.

- There is a wide choice of relatively safe and highly effective prescription and nonprescription NSAIDS, which differ significantly in cost and in their desirable and undesirable effects among individuals.

- Stomach distress is the most common side effect of NSAIDs. Stomach ulceration a major potential risk, and selective COX-2 inhibitors are supposed to reduce this risk.

- Other treatment approaches include glucosamine, an OTC dietary supplement, and injections of steroids and hyaluronic acid.

Drugs Used for Osteoarthritis

Generic Name	Trade Name	Generic Available	Rx/OTC
Nonsteroidal Anti-Inflammatory Drugs (NSAIDs)			
Celecoxib	Celebrex	No	Rx
Diclofenac	Cataflam, Voltaren	Yes	Rx
Diflunisal	Dolobid	Yes	Rx
Endolac	Lodine	Yes	Rx
Fenoprofen	Nalfon	Yes	Rx
Flurbiprofen	Ansaid	Yes	Rx

continues

Drugs Used for Osteoarthritis   (continued)

Generic Name	Trade Name	Generic Available	Rx/OTC
Ibuprofen	Advil, Motrin	Yes	Rx/OTC
Indomethacin	Indocin	Yes	Rx
Ketoprofen	Orudis, Oruvail	Yes	Rx/OTC
Meloxicam	Mobic	No	Rx
Nabumetone	Relafen	Yes	Rx
Naproxen	Aleve, Naprosyn	Yes	Rx/OTC
Oxaprozin	Daypro	Yes	Rx
Piroxicam	Feldene	Yes	Rx
Sulindac	Clinoril	Yes	Rx
Tolmetin	Tolectin	Yes	Rx
Injectable Steroids			
Betamethasone	Celestone	No	Rx
Dexamethasone	Decadron, Hexadrol	Yes	Rx
Methylprednisolone	Depo-Medrol	Yes	Rx
Triamcinolone	Kenalog	Yes	Rx
Hyaluronic Acid			
Hyaluronic acid	Hyalgan, Orthovisc, Synvisc	No	Rx

Osteoporosis

In osteoporosis, bones are thin and more susceptible to fracture. This is a common problem facing 10 million Americans, 80 percent of whom are elderly women. This is also a problem for men. Osteoporosis is largely responsible for the 300,000 hip fractures Americans suffer each year, leading to the death of 50,000.

Bones provide structure and protect the organs, which they encase. Calcium is responsible for the strength and density (together making up the mass) of bones. For men and women, old bone tissue is constantly broken down and replaced by new bones. Weight-bearing exercises, such as walking, stimulate bone formation. During our first 30 years, bone density is built up faster than its breakdown.

Breakdown is faster and occurs at a constant rate for men for the remainder of their lives. By contrast, in women, estrogen slows the breakdown of bone. During menopause, estrogen release stops. Bone density is then rapidly lost for about five years, before returning to a gradual decline.

Did You Know That ...?

As bones become thinner (have lower bone mineral density or BMD), the risk of bone fractures increases. BMD is measured with an x-ray-like machine called DEXA. BMD values less than −1 mean that you have or are on your way to developing osteoporosis and require treatment.

Drugs and Osteoporosis: An Overview

OTC drugs can be used to prevent osteoporosis. Prescription medicines are used to both prevent and treat it.

OTC Alternatives

Calcium and vitamin D maintain bone mass and prevent osteoporosis. Daily calcium doses of 1000–1500 mg are required, and this can be provided by OTC high-calcium products. Calcium is present as a salt—e.g., carbonate (Caltrate, Tums), citrate (Citracal), tribasic phosphate (Posture). Look on the label for the amount of "elemental calcium" in each tablet. Some products also contain vitamin D.

Prescription drugs for osteoporosis work in one of two ways: most slow the rate at which bone is broken down (e.g., Fosamax-like drugs, Evista, estrogen, and calcitonin). Forteo, by contrast, increases bone formation.

Fosamax-Like Drugs

Alendronate (Fosamax), risedronate (Actonel), and ibandronate (Boniva) are biphosphonates. They prevent and treat postmenopausal osteoporosis and osteoporosis caused by long-term steroid use. Bone density is increased and the risk of fractures is reduced by one half.

After being taken orally, only a very small fraction of the dose enters the blood. If taken with foods or juices, even less drug is absorbed.

To increase the amount absorbed and decrease the risk of injury to the esophagus, take these drugs at least 30 minutes before breakfast or any drinks. Only take with a full glass of tap water. Remain upright, i.e., seated or standing. Persons who cannot swallow or remain upright for 30 minutes should not take these drugs. Fosamax and Actonel are available as tablets that can be taken only once weekly while Boniva can be taken once monthly.

Common side effects include nausea and abdominal pain and upset. Inflammation and ulceration of the esophagus (esophagitis) are potential dangers.

Estrogens and Evista

Estrogen prevents bone breakdown and can be used to prevent osteoporosis and treat it after menopause. Because it increases the risk of breast and uterine cancers, as well as heart disease, estrogen is not recommended. (For more on its effects, *see* "Menopause.")

Raloxifene (Evista) selectively produces some estrogen effects but not others. It prevents bone breakdown but has no effects on the breast or uterus. It is referred to as a selective estrogen receptor modulator (SERM).

When taken daily by mouth, Evista increases bone density and decreases the risk of spinal fractures, but not hip fractures.

The most common side effect is hot flashes.

Like estrogen, Evista increases the risk of clot formation in the veins, a risk increased by extended periods of inactivity. Women should stop taking Evista at least 72 hours prior to extended bed rest or surgery.

Recent studies have shown that Evista reduces the risk of breast cancer in high-risk women when taken after menopause.

Calcitonin

Calcitonin (Miacalcin) is used as a nasal spray and as an injectable product for the treatment but not prevention of postmenopausal osteoporosis. It is much less effective in decreasing bone loss or reducing the risk of fractures.

Forteo

Teriparatide (Forteo) stimulates bone formation. It increases bone density and reduces the risk of bone fractures in men and women. Because of its side effects, need for daily injections, and high cost, its use is limited to persons who are at high risk of fractures.

The Least You Need to Know

- ◆ Drugs used to prevent or treat osteoporosis either slow the rate of bone breakdown (Fosamax-like drugs, Evista, and calcitonin) or increase bone formation (Forteo).

- ◆ Fosamax, the most effective and widely used of these medicines, must be taken with water in an upright position.

- ◆ Evista has estrogen-like effects on bone without increasing the risk of cancer.

Drugs Used for Osteoporosis

Generic Name	Trade Name	Prevent (P)/Treat (T)	Generic Available
Alendronate	Fosamax	P/T	No
Ibandronate	Boniva	P/T	No
Risedronate	Actonel	P/T	No
Raloxifene	Evista	P/T	No
Calcitonin	Miacalcin	T	No
Teriparatide	Forteo	T	No

Pain

Pain is a protective mechanism telling us that we are in danger of injury or that a body part has been injured and needs time to recover or be healed. But some types of pain persist for extended periods of time. They provide no protective function, but may cause disability and unhappiness.

There are two primary components typical with pain: tissue injury and an emotion, with the latter component having an important impact on how pain is experienced.

The Different Faces of Pain

There is no single type of pain. Pain can be acute or chronic. Acute pain arises from an injury, illness, or surgery. It is generally relieved by drugs, and after its underlying cause has run its course, the pain passes.

Chronic pain continues for many months, long after the healing process has ended. There are strong emotional or behavioral components associated with chronic pain, and traditional pain relievers are not always effective.

Pain arises from different parts of the body and causes different symptoms. Somatic pain originates in muscles, bones, tendons, ligaments, or the skin. The patient can pinpoint where the pain comes from and may describe it as being sharp, stabbing, or throbbing. Such pain can vary in severity from being mild to extreme (the worst possible) and can be effectively managed with appropriate doses of most pain-relieving medications, called analgesics.

Visceral pains come from the stomach, intestines, liver, or other internal organs. These pains are dull or aching, and their site of origin is more diffuse and vague. This pain is more effectively treated with opioid, morphine-like drugs.

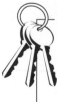

Did You Know That ...?

Pain may come from tissues or nerves. Pain resulting from injury to tissues includes somatic and visceral pains. These can be relieved with opioids and often nonopioid pain relievers (a.k.a. analgesics), such as aspirin or acetaminophen. Pains that result from injury to nerves give rise to burning or tingling sensations and often respond to helper painkillers (a.k.a. adjuvant analgesics).

Pain Management Overview

There are many nonmedication approaches to managing pain, including acupuncture, the use of electrical nerve stimulation, and biofeedback. Our focus is on medications. The drug(s) selected depend on the type of pain and its severity.

Drugs used for the relief of pain (a.k.a. analgesics) fall into three categories:

♦ Nonopioids (a.k.a. nonnarcotics), which include the nonsteroidal anti-inflammatory drugs (NSAIDs) and acetaminophen, are used for mild to moderate pain.

♦ Opioids (a.k.a. narcotics), which include morphine and related drugs, are used to relieve moderate to severe acute and chronic pain.

♦ Helper pain relievers (a.k.a. adjuvant analgesics) are used in combination with nonopioid and opioid analgesics to assist these drugs in relieving pain. Adjuvant drugs are primarily used to treat other conditions, such as depression and seizures.

Nonopioid Analgesics

Nonopioids (a.k.a. nonnarcotics) include NSAIDs, such as aspirin, ibuprofen, and naproxen, as well as acetaminophen. These drugs all effectively relieve mild to moderate pain. Increasing their doses above the recommended limits will not produce greater pain relief, but will increase the incidence and severity of side effects.

Maximizing Your Medicine

All NSAIDs and acetaminophen relieve mild to moderate pain and reduce fever. Apart from these similarities, these drugs produce a different array of effects, both good and bad. As their name denotes, NSAIDs are anti-inflammatory drugs. Acetaminophen lacks this activity. Individuals who cannot take aspirin can usually take acetaminophen quite safely.

Let's now talk about NSAIDs and acetaminophen and focus on their pain-relieving and undesirable effects.

NSAIDs

There are some 12 NSAIDs used for the relief of pain. All are effective, and none stand out as being better than others. Through trial and error, you will find that some drugs prove to be more effective for you and can be better tolerated than others.

NSAIDs primarily differ with respect to how long they continue to work and, consequently, how many doses need to be taken each day to maintain relief. Aspirin and ibuprofen work for 4 hours and are taken 4 times a day, whereas naproxen remains effective for 12 hours and needs to be taken only twice a day.

Several of these drugs are available OTC, many others require a prescription, and a few are both OTC and prescription. Almost all NSAIDs are effective when taken orally.

Indigestion, bloating, and diarrhea are common side effects with aspirin and occur to a somewhat lower extent with other NSAIDs. Ulcers and stomach and intestinal bleeding may also occur. These effects can be minimized by taking NSAIDs with food, antacids, or drugs that prevent the release of stomach acids.

Do not take an NSAID if you are allergic or sensitive to aspirin. Symptoms of sensitivity include a running nose, hives, breathing difficulties, and shock. The risk of this occurring is greater in persons with nasal polyps or a history of asthma.

Use NSAIDs cautiously if you have peptic ulcer disease. Long-term, high-dose NSAID use can cause ulceration of the stomach and bleeding, which can worsen an existing ulcer condition. Taking an acid-blocking drug, such as omeprazole (Prilosec) or famotidine (Pepcid), can prevent ulcers. Misoprostol (Cytotec) is specifically used to prevent gastric ulcers caused by long-term use of NSAIDs.

> ### Maximizing Your Medicine
>
> There is a 10-fold difference in monthly cost between the most expensive and least expensive NSAID. Almost all these drugs are available as generic equivalents, and many are OTC. Because there are no differences in their effectiveness or in safety, you can save some very big bucks if you look for generic equivalents of such OTC drugs as ibuprofen or naproxen.

> ### Warning!
>
> Recent evidence suggests that all NSAIDs, when used at high doses for long periods of time, may increase the risk of heart attack or stroke. This risk may be greater with celecoxib (Celebrex). There is little reason to believe that risks exist if NSAIDs are used for a short time, at relatively low doses, for the relief of ordinary aches and pains.

NSAIDs interfere with platelet function, which leads to bleeding tendencies. They should be used with extreme caution, if at all, by persons with bleeding disorders.

The elderly or individuals with a history of kidney disorders, high blood pressure, or heart disorders, should use NSAIDs under a doctor's supervision. These drugs may cause kidney toxicity in susceptible persons.

Use NSAIDs with great caution when also taking the blood thinner warfarin.

Acetaminophen

Acetaminophen (Tylenol) is as effective as aspirin and other NSAIDs for the relief of mild to moderate pain. Many experts consider acetaminophen to be the best choice for such pain. It is also used in combination with opioids to treat more severe pain.

Unlike NSAIDs, acetaminophen doesn't have anti-inflammatory effects. Moreover, it doesn't share their side effects or precautions for safe use. In particular, acetaminophen does not have effects on blood clotting, cause adverse effects on the stomach or kidneys, or increase the risk of heart attack or stroke. Acetaminophen can be safely used in patients who are allergic to aspirin.

High doses of acetaminophen can cause serious damage to the liver. This risk is increased in moderate to heavy alcohol drinkers.

Opioid Analgesics

Opioids (a.k.a. narcotics) are the most effective drugs for relief of even the most severe pain, both acute and chronic, regardless of its site of origin. When we think about opioids, we think about and compare all similar drugs to morphine, the first opioid.

Morphine and codeine are naturally occurring chemicals in opium and are responsible for its effects. Other opioids have been manufactured in the laboratory, drugs which share many but not all of morphine's effects. None of these drugs relieves pain better than morphine. However, some are less prone to being abused and are safer when taken in excessive doses.

Did You Know That ...?

Opium was among the oldest drugs recorded in human history, appearing in medical writings of the ancient Greeks and Romans dating back 2,500 years ago. Even up to the early 1800s, opium was one of the few really effective drugs available for treating pain, insomnia, cough, and diarrhea. Morphine, the active ingredient in opium, was isolated from the opium poppy in 1806.

Pain Relief and Abuse Potential

Opioids produce pain relief by interacting with opioid receptors in the brain and spinal cord. They work on the behavioral aspects of pain. Patients report that they can still feel the pain, and are aware of its presence, but it no longer bothers them.

Not all opioids relieve pain of the same severity, have the same potential for abuse, or work as fast or as long.

◆ Morphine, hydromorphone, and fentanyl are strong opioids that are capable of relieving the most severe pain. They have a high potential for abuse.

◆ Codeine and hydrocodone are only effective in relieving mild to moderate pain, and have moderate abuse potential.

◆ Pentazocine and related drugs are newer opioids useful in treating moderate to severe pain and have low abuse potential.

Most opioids relieve pain for about three to four hours after being taken by mouth. Some drugs (such as fentanyl) work for shorter periods of time (two to four hours), whereas others (such as methadone) may be effective for six to eight hours after a single dose. Modifying the nature of the oral product can extend the time morphine acts from 3 to 4 hours up to 12 or even 24 hours.

Common Side Effects

To a greater or lesser extent, all opioids cause such side effects as sedation, depression of breathing, nausea and vomiting, constipation, and urinary retention. With the exception of constipation, these effects become greatly diminished in severity after repeated doses. Let's take a closer look at these side effects:

◆ **Sedation.** At pain-relieving doses, opioids can cause drowsiness, confusion, and impairment of function. Driving or participating in other potentially hazardous activities should be avoided, if these effects are evident.

◆ **Depression of breathing.** Strong opioids such as morphine interfere with breathing. This is a greater problem for the elderly and individuals suffering from such respiratory conditions as asthma and emphysema.

When these drugs are taken in excessive doses, death almost invariably results from their stopping breathing. Naloxone (Narcan) is a very specific and rapid-acting antidote for the treatment of opioid overdose.

◆ **Nausea and vomiting.** The first doses may cause nausea and vomiting, a problem occurring more frequently with ambulatory patients than those who are bed-ridden. This effect is reduced with later doses and can be minimized with anti-nausea drugs.

◆ **Constipation.** One of the persisting problems facing chronic opioid users, especially elderly individuals, is constipation. A stimulant laxative, such as senna (e.g., Senokot) or a stool softener, such as docusate (e.g., Colace) can be used to prevent constipation or manage it once it occurs.

◆ **Dependence.** When taken over extended periods for the management of pain, there is the risk of dependence or addiction. Because of the fear of causing addiction, physicians have undermedicated their patients with opioids. They have prescribed doses that have been too low or given less often than necessary to adequately manage pain.

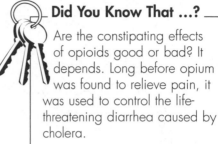

Did You Know That …?

Are the constipating effects of opioids good or bad? It depends. Long before opium was found to relieve pain, it was used to control the life-threatening diarrhea caused by cholera.

There is obvious reason for concern, and these drugs must be used with caution. But there seems little justification for withholding their use in terminal cancer patients experiencing extreme pain. In fact, it is your right as a patient to have your complaint of pain to be taken seriously and treated appropriately.

Let's talk about the development of tolerance and physical dependence to opioids. Within several weeks of their regular use, *tolerance* develops to their undesirable effects. Happily, tolerance occurs more gradually to their effectiveness as a pain reliever but, over time, they do become progressively less effective.

To offset this problem, larger doses must be given or the drug must be taken more often. The use of an analgesic ladder (described later in this chapter) is intended to delay, as long as possible, the decrease in the effectiveness of strong opioids.

Physical dependence refers to a response by the body after a drug taken for an extended period is abruptly discontinued (going "cold turkey") or after a sudden and marked reduction in its dose. The resulting response, called an abstinence syndrome, is evidence that physical dependence has developed with opioids. These

def•i•ni•tion

Tolerance refers to a condition in which a larger dose is required to produce the same effect that was formerly produced by a smaller dose. When tolerance occurs, a given dose produces less effect than it did initially. Tolerance develops to different effects produced by the drug to varying degrees and at different speeds.

possibly intense flu-like responses may be very unpleasant but they are not life-threatening and they do pass.

When an individual has a compulsive desire to continue taking a medication, without regard to the harm it may cause, addiction is said to be present. The best available evidence suggests that medically induced addiction to opioids is extremely rare. Their benefits in relieving pain and suffering far outweigh the potential risks of addiction.

How These Drugs Are Taken

Opioids should be taken by mouth, if at all possible. This method is simple, convenient, doesn't hurt, and is least expensive. A variety of oral products are available—both solid and liquid, immediate acting and long acting—to meet the needs of all patients.

For patients unable to take oral medications, different opioids are available as rectal suppositories, long-acting (72 hour) patches, and by injection. Patient-controlled analgesia (PCA) permits the user to manage pain by controlling (within limits) the amount of opioid received. When activated, a pump delivers the drug under the skin or into the veins through a catheter.

Drug-Drug Interactions

Drugs that have a depressing effect, including anti-anxiety or sleep promoters, alcohol, and sedating antihistamines can intensify the drowsiness and depressed breathing caused by opioids. Drugs with atropine-like effects (e.g., antihistamines and tricyclic antidepressants) can increase opioid-induced constipation and the retention of urine.

Meperidine, an opioid, should never be used in combination with a monoamine oxidase (MAO) inhibitor antidepressant.

Helper Pain-Relievers

Pain arising from nerves (called neuropathic pain) is very different from pain arising from a tissue injury. It is described by the sufferer as being burning, tingling, or shooting.

Helper pain relievers, also called adjuvant analgesics, are useful for treating pain from nerve injuries. These drugs—which include medicines used primarily to treat depression, abnormal heart rhythms, and seizures—have little or no analgesic action when taken alone. They increase pain relief or reduce side effects when given with opioid or nonopioid analgesics. Unlike traditional analgesics, their beneficial effects are not immediate but develop rather gradually. Helper pain relievers are often included in the analgesic ladder.

Analgesic Ladders and Drug Combinations

Unlike the relatively short-lived pain experienced after a bone fracture or an operation, some pains are severe and persist for extended periods and even a lifetime. The pains experienced in some types of terminal cancer are notable examples. In such cases, medications are intended to relieve pain in the absence of disabling side effects, permit the sufferer to enjoy a reasonable quality of life, and continue to function as much as possible.

The World Health Organization has developed a three-level "analgesic ladder" for the management of cancer pain:

1. **Mild to moderate pain.** Use non-opioid analgesic.

2. **More severe pain.** Use a nonopioid analgesic plus a moderate-strength opioid (e.g., codeine, hydrocodone).

3. **Severe pain.** Use a nonopioid analgesic plus a strong opioid (e.g., morphine, fentanyl).

Did You Know That ...?

Pain associated with cancer can result from the cancer or from its treatment. As the cancer grows and spreads, it may compress or block the function of nearby organs, nerves, and muscles. Cancer spread to bones is common and very painful. Pain may also arise from surgery, radiation therapy, and chemotherapy.

Doses of individual analgesics can be increased and helper pain relievers can be added as needed.

Combinations of different classes of drugs are usually more effective in relieving pain than are individual drugs when used alone. Equivalent pain relief may be achieved using lower doses of each component. Lower doses reduce side effects.

The Least You Need to Know

◆ Mild to moderate pain can be managed with nonopioids (e.g., nonsteroidal anti-inflammatory drugs or NSAIDs), whereas moderate to severe pain is effectively controlled with opioid (narcotic) analgesics, such as morphine.

◆ The analgesic ladder, using combinations of nonopioid, opioid, and helper pain relievers, is an effective approach for managing chronic pain, such as is seen in terminal cancer.

◆ NSAIDs, such as aspirin, ibuprofen, and naproxen, can cause indigestion, bleeding tendencies, and stomach ulcers, and these drugs and celecoxib (Celebrex) can increase the risk of stroke and heart attack.

◆ Acetaminophen is a relatively safe aspirin substitute with no anti-inflammatory effects nor does it cause bleeding, stomach ulcers, or increased risk of heart attack and stroke. Liver toxicity can occur.

◆ Chronic use of opioid analgesics for the relief of moderate to severe pain has a very low risk of creating addiction.

◆ Tolerance develops to such common opioid side effects as sedation, depression of breathing, nausea and vomiting, but not to constipation.

◆ Helper pain relievers (a.k.a. adjuvant analgesics), which include selective tricyclic antidepressants, anti-arrhythmic, and anti-seizure drugs, are used with nonopioid and opioid analgesics to treat neuropathic pain (i.e., pain arising from nerves).

Drugs Used for Pain

Generic Name	Trade Name	How Taken: Injection (I), Oral (O), Suppository (S), Topical (T)	Generic Available
Nonopioid Analgesics			
Acetaminophen	Tylenol	O	Yes
Aspirin	Ascriptin, Bufferin	O	Yes
Celecoxib	Celebrex	O	No
Diclofenac	Cataflam, Voltaren	O	Yes
Diflunisal	Dolobid	O	Yes
Etodolac	Lodine	O	Yes
Fenoprofen	Nalfon	O	Yes
Ibuprofen	Advil, Motrin	O	Yes
Ketoprofen	Orudis, Oruvail	O	Yes
Ketorolac	Toradol	I/O	Yes

Generic Name	Trade Name	How Taken: Injection (I), Oral (O), Suppository (S), Topical (T)	Generic Available
Meclofenamate	—	O	Yes
Mefenamic acid	Ponstel	O	No
Naproxen	Aleve, Naprosyn	O	Yes

Opioid Analgesics			

Strong Opioids for Moderate to Severe Pain

Fentanyl	Duragesic, Sublimaze	I/T	Yes
Hydromorphone	Dilaudid	I/O/S	Yes
Levorphanol	Levo-Dromoran	O	Yes
Meperidine (Pethidine)	Demerol	I/O	Yes
Methadone	Dolophine, Methadose	I/O	Yes
Morphine	MS Contin, MSIR, Oramorph, Roxanol	I/O/S	Yes
Oxycodone	OxyContin, Roxicodone	O	Yes
Oxycodone, + acetaminophen	Percocet, Tylox	O	Yes
Oxymorphone	Numorphan	I/S	No

Opioids for Mild to Moderate Pain

Codeine		I/O	Yes
Codeine + acetaminophen	Tylenol w/Codeine	O	Yes
Codeine + aspirin	Empirin w/Codeine	O	Yes
Hydrocodone + acetaminophen	Vicodin	O	Yes
Propoxyphene	Darvon-N	O	Yes
Propoxyphene + acetaminophen	Darvocet-N	O	Yes

continues

Drugs Used for Pain (continued)

Generic Name	Trade Name	How Taken: Injection (I), Oral (O), Suppository (S), Topical (T)	Generic Available
Low-Abuse Potential Opioids for Moderate to High Pain			
Buprenorphine	Buprenex	I	Yes
Butorphanol	Stadol	I	Yes
Nalbuphine	Nubain	I	Yes
Pentazocine	Talwin	I	No
Pentazocine + aspirin	Talwin Compound	O	No
Helper Pain-Relievers (Adjuvant Analgesics)			
Anti-Seizure Drugs			
Carbamazepine	Tegretol	O	Yes
Gabapentin	Neurontin	O	No
Local Anesthetic/Anti-Arrhythmic Drugs			
Lidocaine	Xylocaine	I/T	Yes
Mexiletine	Mexitil	O	No
Steroids			
Dexamethasone	Decadron, Hexadrol	O	Yes
Prednisone	Deltasone, Meticorten	O	Yes
Tricyclic Antidepressants			
Amitriptyline	Elavil	O	Yes
Doxepin	Sinequan	O	Yes
Imipramine	Tofranil	O	Yes
Nortriptyline	Aventyl, Pamelor	O	Yes

Parkinson's Disease

Parkinson's disease is a chronic, progressive nerve disease affecting bodily movements. Common symptoms include rigidity or stiffness of body movements, difficulty in walking and maintaining balance, hand tremors when muscles are resting, facial distortions, difficulty in speaking, and behavioral depression.

An estimated one million people in the United States have Parkinson's disease (PD), and the risk of its development increases with advancing age.

When the cause of Parkinson's disease is unknown, it is called idiopathic Parkinson's disease. Secondary Parkinson's disease can be caused by chemicals, other disorders, head injuries, and drugs. It is commonly caused by certain drugs used to treat schizophrenia and severe nausea and vomiting.

Drug Treatment of PD: An Overview

The basal ganglia region of the brain influences voluntary muscle movements. It communicates with nerves in its neighborhood by releasing the chemical messenger (neurotransmitter) dopamine. In PD, the nerves producing dopamine have deteriorated. Dopamine is not produced in sufficient quantity, which results in problems in movement.

Drug treatment of PD is intended to pump up the activity of the dopamine system in several different ways. Drugs can replace the loss of natural dopamine, prevent dopamine breakdown and loss of activity, or it can imitate the effects of dopamine. Drugs significantly improve the movement problems but do not cure or slow down the progressive loss of functions that occur in PD.

Normal motor control involves a balance between dopamine and acetylcholine, another neurotransmitter. They work in opposite directions, like the gas pedal and brake in your car. Acetylcholine-blocking drugs (anticholinergics) are sometimes used to control PD tremors.

Drugs That Replace Dopamine

If you don't have enough dopamine, it would seem reasonable to simply replace it by taking a dopamine pill. Unfortunately, dopamine does not enter the brain after being taken by mouth. However, when given as a drug, levodopa (Dopar, Larodopa) can enter the brain and is converted to dopamine.

Carbidopa prevents the breakdown of levodopa and increases the amount of levodopa entering the brain. When carbidopa is given with levodopa, a lower dose of levodopa is needed and it causes fewer side effects. The combination of levodopa plus car-bidopa (Sinemet) is the most effective and widely used treatment for PD.

Levodopa is highly effective in controlling PD symptoms for the first few years. After five years, drug benefits lessen, and doses must be given more frequently. In addition, an "on-off" response often occurs, with a sudden return of symptoms that may last for minutes to hours.

Levodopa plus carbidopa cautions:

- ◆ **Common side effects.** Nausea and vomiting, involuntary movements of the head and face, and reduction in blood pressure and feelings of fainting when arising. Major behavioral changes including hallucinations, vivid dreams or nightmares, and confusion are not uncommon.

- ◆ **Drug interactions.** Do not use traditional drugs for schizophrenia (e.g., Thorazine-like, Haldol) with levodopa because they block levodopa's beneficial effects. Resperdal and related newer drugs can be safely used. Use of MAO inhibitor antidepressants (Nardil and Parnate) with levodopa can increase blood pressure to dangerously high levels.

- ◆ **Food interaction.** Avoid high-protein meals because they interfere with the amount of levodopa entering the brain.

Drugs That Prevent Dopamine Breakdown

Some anti-PD drugs, such as selegiline (Eldepryl) and entacapone (Comtan), have no effects themselves. They are used in combination with levodopa to extend the length of time each dose of levodopa works and to decrease the dose of levodopa. They do this by preventing dopamine's breakdown.

Selegiline's most common side effect is insomnia. It can cause dangerous and even potentially life-threatening interactions when used with many other drugs, in particular, with levodopa, meperidine, and fluoxetine. Patients taking selegiline should consult their doctor or pharmacist before starting or discontinuing any other medications.

Fatal liver toxicity has been caused by tolcapone but not encapone.

Drugs That Imitate Dopamine's Effects

These drugs act at the same target site (i.e., receptor site) as dopamine. They can be taken alone during the early stages of PD but are usually used with Sinemet. Common side effects include nausea, dizziness, drowsiness, and behavioral disturbances, such as hallucinations.

Amantadine may work by increasing the release of dopamine from nerves. Common side effects include dry mouth, behavioral disturbances, and mottled discoloration of skin, which slowly disappears after the drug is stopped.

Acetylcholine-Blocking Drugs

These drugs are primarily effective in controlling PD tremors. They are used alone in mild PD, and also with Sinemet.

Common side effects include dry mouth, blurred vision, constipation, an increase in heart rate, and difficulty in urinating. Persons with glaucoma or an enlarged prostate gland should use these drugs with great caution.

The Least You Need to Know

♦ The loss of dopamine-producing nerves and dopamine production and release in the brain is responsible for the voluntary motor problems seen in Parkinson's disease.

♦ Drugs used to treat PD replace dopamine, prevent its breakdown and loss of effectiveness, and imitate its effects. They may also block acetylcholine's effects.

♦ Levodopa plus carbidopa is most effective for PD and is used alone or in combination with other drugs.

Drugs Used for Parkinson's Disease

Generic Name	Trade Name	Generic Available
Dopamine Replacement		
Levodopa	Larodopa, Dopar	No
Levodopa + carbidopa	Sinemet	Yes
Prevent Dopamine Breakdown		
Entacapone	Comtan	No
Selegiline [deprenyl]	Eldepryl	Yes
Tolcapone	Tasmar	No
Imitates Dopamine's Effects		
Amantadine	Symmetrel	Yes
Bromocriptine	Parlodel	Yes
Pergolide	Permax	Yes
Pramipexole	Mirapex	No
Ropinirole	Requip	No
Acetylcholine-Blocking Drugs		
Benztropine	Cogentin	Yes
Diphenhydramine	Benadryl	Yes
Trihexyphenidyl	Artane	Yes

Peripheral Circulatory Disorders

Poor circulation to the arms and legs may result from either a block in blood flow as the result of clogged arteries (e.g., atherosclerosis). Atherosclerosis is caused by fat and cholesterol deposits (plaque) in arteries. Plaques enlarge as additional material is deposited, slowing and reducing the flow of blood. Moreover, these plaques becomes brittle over time and occasionally rupture. This may trigger the formation of a blood clot, which can further narrow or completely close the affected artery. In other instances, there is a temporary narrowing in blood-carrying vessels. Both these conditions are collectively referred to as peripheral artery disease. The causes of each are different, as are the drugs used for their management.

Two drug approaches are taken to relieve the symptoms of leg cramps and other peripheral circulatory disturbances:

◆ Reduce the block to blood flow. If fatty deposits are lining blood vessels, cholesterol levels in the blood can be lowered with statins. If clots are the cause of the block, the tendency for clot formation can be reduced by using antiplatelet drugs, such as aspirin.

◆ Widen small arteries in the extremities using calcium antagonists or cilostazol and pentoxifylline, which modify blood so that it flows more easily.

Blood-Flow Block: Treatment

In atherosclerosis, layers of fatty materials form on the inner walls of arteries, clogging them. This interferes with or even blocks the flow of blood. When blood flow fails to reach the brain or heart, a stroke or heart attack may occur. Blood flow may also be reduced to the arteries in the legs, causing leg cramps. Patients with leg cramps are at higher risk of heart attack and stroke.

The individual with reduced blood flow to the legs experiences tiredness; cramping; or pain or numbness in the buttock, thigh, or calf of the affected leg. Early on, these symptoms occur during exercise or while walking but later even at rest.

Among the major risk factors for developing atherosclerosis are smoking, high blood cholesterol levels, high blood pressure, diabetes, and obesity. Controlling these conditions can prevent or delay the worsening of atherosclerosis and peripheral arterial disease. We talk about the specific management of each of these conditions elsewhere in this book.

In this section, we talk about drugs used to lessen the block of blood flow by reducing clot formation.

Antiplatelet Drugs

During the formation of a clot, platelets clump together. Aspirin and other antiplatelet medicines work by preventing this clumping. Low doses of aspirin reduce the risk of heart attack that results from peripheral arterial disease. However, there is no clear evidence that these drugs prevent or delay the development of peripheral arterial disease.

> **Maximizing Your Medicine**
>
> Experts agree that aspirin is highly effective for preventing blood clotting and heart attacks. The most effective dose has not been determined, although less is probably better. Recommended daily doses range from one children's aspirin (81 mg) to one adult's aspirin (325 mg). Lower doses cause fewer side effects.

At the low recommended doses of aspirin, side effects are few and include an increased risk of stomach ulceration, bleeding, and indigestion. Aspirin-allergic individuals must avoid any dose and should consider taking another antiplatelet drug.

The combination of aspirin and dipyridamole is only slightly more effective than aspirin taken alone. The far more expensive cloidogrel is about as effective as aspirin.

> **Warning!**
>
> Antiplatelet drugs increase the risk of bleeding. Individuals should inform their doctors and dentists that they are taking such medicines before any elective surgery is scheduled.

Dipyridamole, when taken alone, interferes with platelet clumping in a different way than aspirin. A fixed combination of aspirin (25 mg) and dipyridamole (in an extended-release preparation called Aggrenox), taken twice daily, is slightly more effective than when either drug is used alone. Common side effects include headache, indigestion, abdominal pain, and diarrhea.

Clopidogrel (Plavix) is only slightly more effective than aspirin in preventing platelet clumping in patients with a history of ischemic stroke or heart attack. It causes similar side effects, and to the same extent as aspirin, such as abdominal pain, indigestion, diarrhea, and rash.

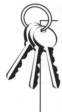

Did You Know That ...?

In Buerger's disease, small- and medium-size blood vessels become inflamed and spastic, and blood flow is blocked. Most commonly, a leg or foot is affected. Pain, cramps, and numbness are followed by ulceration and gangrene. Some 95 percent of affected individuals are men who smoke and who are under the age of 40. Treatment options are simple: give up smoking or face potential gangrene.

Blood Vessel Constriction: Treatment

When subjected to the cold, blood vessels located under the skin normally narrow, a process called vasoconstriction. This response prevents the loss of heat from the body. Sometimes such constriction occurs much more readily and more intensely.

Did You Know That ...?

When exposed to cold, the body responds by acting to both prevent the loss of heat and to produce more heat. One of the first heat-conserving mechanisms that occur is a marked narrowing of blood vessels located directly under the skin. This so-called peripheral vasoconstriction prevents the movement of heat from the core of the body to the skin where it can be lost.

In Raynaud's disease, spasms of the small arteries in the fingers and occasionally the toes temporarily reduce the flow of blood. These episodes can be triggered by a variety of physical, emotional, or environmental conditions, including exposure to the cold and stress. A genetic predisposition appears to play a role in some cases. The affected areas become numb, tingle, and initially become white, and then blue, and finally red. In advanced cases, the skin may become ulcerated.

Calcium antagonists are the most effective drugs available for reducing the frequency and duration of these spasms to the small arteries.

Raynaud's disease may be worsened by nasal decongestants, beta-blockers, and oral contraceptives.

Calcium Antagonists

Calcium antagonists, such as nifedipine, are considered to be the safest and most effective drugs for the treatment of Raynaud's disease and leg cramps. They cause relaxation of the involuntary muscle that lines small arteries. This relaxation widens the diameter of these arteries, thereby increasing blood flow through these very fine blood vessels. The frequency and severity of leg cramp attacks is reduced in two thirds of those treated. These medicines also help the healing of skin ulcers.

Calcium antagonists (a.k.a. calcium channel blockers or CCBs) are also used to reduce high blood pressure and treat angina and abnormal heart rhythms.

Common side effects include constipation, headache, swelling of the feet and ankles, and inflammation of the gums.

Cilostazol and Pentoxifylline

Cilostazol and pentoxifylline are the only drugs that have been approved by the FDA for leg cramps. Neither produces impressive improvements of this condition.

Cilostazol increases the maximum distance subjects can walk and their ability to walk pain-free. It acts by widening small arteries and also as an antiplatelet drug. It should not be used in individuals who have heart disease in addition to their leg cramps.

Common side effects include headache, diarrhea, palpitations of the heart, and dizziness.

Pentoxifylline produces only modest improvements in maximal walking distances. It acts by reducing the thickness of blood, thereby improving its flow through small arteries.

Common side effects include angina (chest pains), rapid or irregular heartbeat, and dizziness.

The Least You Need to Know

- Poor circulation of blood to the extremities, from blockade of blood flow or temporary closing of small arteries, causes peripheral artery disease.
- Blood clot formation can be slowed using antiplatelet drugs such as aspirin.

◆ Calcium antagonists are the safest and most effective drugs for Raynaud's disease.

◆ Cilostazol and pentoxifylline produce some benefit in the management of leg cramps.

Drugs Used for Circulatory Conditions

Generic Name	Trade Name(s)	Generic Available
Antiplatelet Drugs		
Aspirin	Ascriptin	Yes
	Bufferin	
Aspirin + dipyridamole [Extended-release]	Aggrenox	No (Not recommended)
Clopidogrel	Plavix	No
Ticlopidine	Ticlid	No
Calcium Antagonists		
Amlopidipine	Amvaz, Norvasc	No
Diltiazem	Cardizem, Dilacor	Yes
Felodipine	Plendil	No
Isradipine	DynaCirc	No
Nifedipine	Adalat, Procardia	Yes
Verapamil	Calan, Isoptin, Verelan	Yes
Miscellaneous Drugs		
Cilostazol	Pletal	No
Pentoxifylline	Trental	Yes

Premenstrual Syndrome

Premenstrual syndrome (PMS) includes the psychological and physical symptoms that typically occur several days before the start of the menstrual period and end several days after the period begins.

Psychological symptoms include irritability, crying spells, depression, mood swings, and the desire to be left alone. Physical signs include acne, breast tenderness, salt and water retention with weight gain, abdominal swelling, headaches, and appetite disturbances.

The exact cause of PMS is not known. Treatment is based on the relief of symptoms.

Drugs That Treat Depression and Other Psychological Symptoms

Depression and anxiety may be two of the most troubling symptoms of PMS. In some 3 to 5 percent of women, these symptoms may be particularly severe. This condition, called premenstrual dysphoric disorder (PMDD), is thought to be caused by abnormalities in serotonin in the brain.

OTC Alternatives

Studies have shown that calcium carbonate (Tums) reduces such premenstrual symptoms as anxiety, depression, fluid retention, cramps, and food craving. Doses of 600 mg twice per day were used, the same dose that is effective in preventing osteoporosis. This is a safe and very inexpensive treatment approach.

Members of the SSRI (selective serotonin-reuptake inhibitor) class of antidepressant drugs are highly effective in relieving the psychological symptoms of PMDD. These symptoms include premenstrual anxiety, depression, overeating, and weight gain. Many physical symptoms of PMS are also helped. Such Prozac-like drugs must be taken for several days before their benefits are seen.

Common side effects are generally mild and include nausea, vomiting, diarrhea, insomnia, weight gain, and interference with sexual function.

Xanax and Other Anti-Anxiety Drugs

Anti-anxiety drugs, such as Xanax (alprazolam, a benzodiazepine), very rapidly relieve feelings of anxiety, irritability, and tension. Regular use of Xanax may produce a drug-dependent state.

Common side effects include drowsiness and dizziness; impairment of driving may occur.

Individuals who have a history of abusing alcohol or other drugs are the most likely candidates to also abuse benzodiazepines. Using these drugs, even at normal doses for periods of four to six weeks, can lead to dependence on them.

Taking benzodiazepines for several months and then suddenly not taking them can result in real signs of withdrawal. These include nervousness, sleep disturbances, and tremors. To avoid these problems, reduce doses gradually.

Buspirone (BuSpar)

BuSpar is an effective drug for the treatment of the anxiety component of the premenstrual syndrome. Unlike benzodiazepines, it does not cause drowsiness, which may interfere with thinking or operating motor vehicles, nor is it subject to abuse.

BuSpar must be taken for about two weeks before menstruation for its anti-anxiety effects begin. Therefore, it is not a useful drug choice for individuals who need immediate relief.

> **OTC Alternatives**
>
> Headaches and pains can be relieved using OTC nonsteroidal anti-inflammatory drugs (NSAIDs), such as ibuprofen (Advil, Motrin) and naproxen (Aleve).

Water Pills

Water pills (diuretics) increase the elimination of salt and water in the urine, helping reduce fluid retention and bloating. Although there are many diuretic drugs, Aldactone has been found to be most useful in relieving premenstrual weight gain and bloating.

The Least You Need to Know

- ◆ The cause of PMS is not known, and its treatment is based on relieving psychological and physical symptoms.

♦ Premenstrual dysphoric disorder is effectively treated with Prozac-like SSRI antidepressants.

Drugs Used for Premenstrual Syndrome

Generic Name	Trade Name	Generic Available
Anti-Anxiety Drugs		
Alprazolam	Xanax	Yes
Buspirone	BuSpar	Yes
Antidepressant, SSRI		
Fluoxetine	Prozac, Sarafem	Yes
Paroxetine	Paxil	Yes
Sertraline	Zoloft	Yes
Venlafaxine	Effexor	No
Diuretics (Water Pills)		
Spironolactone	Aldactone	Yes

Prenatal Supplements

Many expectant mothers want to enhance their health as well as the health of their unborn babies by taking a vitamin-mineral supplement. Is it necessary? For a woman getting a nutritious diet, probably not. Will it hurt? No. For women with special needs, prenatal supplements are essential.

When we talk about prenatal supplements, we need to focus on three important ingredients: folic acid, calcium, and iron.

Folic Acid, Calcium, Iron

Prenatal vitamin supplements differ from regular vitamin supplements based on the extra amounts of folic acid, calcium, and iron they contain. Of these, folic acid is the most important during the first four weeks of pregnancy.

Folic Acid

Folic acid reduces the risk of the baby being born with the neural tube defect spina bifida. The spine does not close, exposing nerves, which are unprotected. Damage to these nerves may lead to such problems as paralysis and incontinence.

Neural defects develop during the first 28 days of pregnancy, long before many women know they are pregnant. To provide protection, women should take folic acid during this critical 28-day period. All women of childbearing age should get 400 micrograms (0.4 mg) of folic acid a day from their diet or in supplements.

Some women are at higher risk of having a baby with a neural defect. These include mothers having a family history of babies with this condition and mothers taking medication for epilepsy. Doctors generally recommend that these women take 4,000 micrograms (4 mg) a day.

Calcium

The developing baby has priority and takes the calcium it needs from the mother. This can leave the mother short. As the fetus takes calcium for bone growth, the bone density of the mother may be reduced. A calcium supplement can compensate for this loss.

Iron

Hemoglobin in red blood cells carry oxygen to the tissues of the mother and her fetus. Adequate iron is needed for the normal formation of hemoglobin and to prevent the development of iron deficiency anemia. Iron supplements may be of particular importance for women with sickle cell anemia.

Did You Know That ...?

The Food and Nutrition Board of the Institute of Medicine issued Dietary Reference Intake (DRI) recommendations in 2004 for males and females of different ages and during pregnancy. These values differ somewhat from the Recommended Daily Allowances (RDA) issued in 1989.

DRI and RDA recommendations for pregnant women include the following:

	DRI (2004)	RDA (1989)
Folic acid	600 micrograms	400 micrograms
Calcium	1,000 mg	1,200 mg
Iron	27 mg	30 mg

Prescription vs. OTC Dietary Supplements

Many dietary supplement products are available on the market, some OTC and others requiring a prescription. Most prescription and OTC prenatal products contain 200 to 300 mg of calcium and 25 to 65 mg of iron.

Products containing greater than 800 micrograms (0.8 mg) of folic acid require a prescription. No prescription supplement contains over 1,000 micrograms. If your doctor recommends a higher dose (e.g., 4 mg), very inexpensive 1 mg tablets can be obtained with a prescription.

OTC Alternatives

If you are paying for the prenatal supplement, OTC products—containing appropriate levels of folic acid, calcium, and iron—will cost less than comparable ones requiring a prescription. For a quality product, look for "USP" on the label. Also check with your doctor or pharmacist for a recommendation. If swallow-whole tablets nauseate you, try chewable tablets.

It's not a good idea to take more than one prenatal supplement tablet or capsule a day. Too much vitamin A or D can be potentially dangerous to the baby. If you need more of a particular ingredient (such as folic acid), take it separately.

Notwithstanding promotional claims to the contrary, natural vitamins are no safer nor are they more effective than those made in the laboratory. They are more expensive, however.

The Least You Need to Know

- ◆ The only major difference between prenatal supplements and regular vitamins is their higher content of folic acid, calcium, and iron.

- ◆ The primary difference between prescription and OTC prenatal supplements is that prescription products contain more than 800 micrograms of folic acid.

Prostate Enlargement

If you're a man old enough to start collecting Social Security checks, there is a reasonable likelihood that you may have early signs of a noncancerous enlargement of your prostate gland (also called benign prostatic hypertrophy, or BPH).

The prostate gland surrounds the urethra, the canal that carries off urine from the bladder. At about the age of 40, the prostate undergoes a major growth spurt, increasing in size several fold.

As it grows, the prostate compresses the urethra. This interferes with the flow of urine and decreases the force of urine flow. In addition, the bladder cannot fully empty with each voiding. This causes a need to urinate more often, including (and most troubling) at night, which disrupts sleep.

Two very different types of medicines are used to treat the symptoms of BPH: those that relax the muscles of the bladder and prostate, and those that shrink the size of the prostate. Early studies suggest that better results may be obtained when drugs from each class are used in combination.

If drugs do not produce satisfactory results, or if it is necessary to restore urinary flow without delay, surgery is performed to remove all or a portion of the prostate.

Bladder Muscle-Relaxing Drugs

Tamsulosin (Flomax) and similar drugs, called adrenergic blockers, relax bladder muscles. This permits the bladder to expand more fully when it is filling with urine. These drugs also relax the muscles in the prostate, improving the flow of urine.

These drugs are the first choice for the treatment of BPH. Beneficial effects are seen within days. The bladder empties more completely, the force of the urine flow becomes more vigorous, and the need to urinate comes less often, including during sleep time. These drugs do not reduce the size of the prostate gland and only provide relief of BPH as long as they are taken.

Name hint: generic names end in "osin."

Although these side effects do not occur frequently, they could include a drop in blood pressure, fainting, dizziness, sleepiness, and nasal congestion. In addition, retrograde ejaculation may occur, a harmless condition where, during ejaculation, semen moves backward into bladder rather than forward out the penis.

Standing rapidly after lying down or sitting may cause dizziness and a feeling of fainting. Similar problems may occur after drinking alcoholic beverages, standing in place for long periods, exercise, or on hot days.

Did You Know That ...?

Many of the same adrenergic blockers used to treat BPH also relax the involuntary (smooth) muscles in small blood vessels, causing them to widen. This causes a drop in blood pressure. As a matter of fact, these drugs were originally intended to reduce high blood pressure. Tamsulosin selectively acts on muscles in the bladder and does not lower blood pressure.

Prostate-Shrinking Drugs

The male hormone dihydrotestosterone (DHT) is responsible for the enlargement of the prostate we see in men over the age of 40. Finasteride (Proscar) prevents the formation of DHT from testosterone.

Regular use of finasteride and similar drugs cause the slow and gradual shrinkage of the enlarged prostate over a period of 6 to 12 months. As the size of the prostate decreases, the obstruction of the urethra is reduced and urination returns to normal. To retain these benefits, the drug must be taken for a lifetime.

Name hint: generic names end in "steride."

Finasteride appears to reduce the likelihood of developing prostate cancer in men at high risk because of family history and other causes.

Did You Know That ...?

At one fifth the dose, finasteride (Propecia) is also used in pattern baldness in men to stimulate hair growth and prevent additional hair loss.

The drugs are well tolerated. The most common side effects involve problems in sexual function, including a reduction in sex drive. Breast enlargement is sometimes seen.

PSA (prostate-specific antigen) levels are used as a marker for prostate cancer. As finasteride shrinks the prostate, PSA levels also decline from 30 to 50 percent. If levels do not decline, the patient should be checked for prostate cancer.

Standing rapidly after lying down or sitting may cause dizziness and a feeling of fainting. Similar problems may occur after drinking alcoholic beverages, standing in place for long periods, exercise, or on hot days.

OTC Alternatives

Saw palmetto, among the most widely used herbal products (OTC dietary supplement) in the United States, improves urine flow and other beneficial effects in BPH. These benefits approximate finasteride, while causing fewer side effects. Undesirable effects are generally mild and usually involve gastrointestinal upset, which can be minimized by taking saw palmetto with food.

The Least You Need to Know

◆ Enlargement of the prostate gland (benign prostatic hypertrophy or BPH) commonly occurs in men over 60 and interferes with normal urination.

◆ Tamsulosin and related adrenergic blockers relax muscles in the bladder and prostate and produce relief of BPH symptoms within days.

◆ Finasteride relieves BPH symptoms by shrinking the size of the prostate, when given for 6 to 12 months.

◆ Effective relief of BPH requires drug treatment for a lifetime.

◆ Saw palmetto is an herbal dietary supplement that has been shown to be as effective as finasteride while producing fewer side effects.

Drugs Used for Prostate Enlargement

Generic Name	Trade Name	Generic Available
Bladder Muscle-Relaxing Drugs (Adrenergic Blockers) (Generic names end in "osin")		
Alfuzosin	Uroxatral	No
Doxazosin	Cardura	Yes
Tamsulosin	Flomax	No
Terazosin	Hytrin	Yes
Prostate-Shrinking Drugs (Generic names end in "steride")		
Dutasteride	Avodart	No
Finasteride	Proscar	No

Psoriasis

Psoriasis is a chronic skin disorder in which thick patches of irritated skin are covered by large silvery scales. These plaques are most frequently found on the elbows, knees, back, buttocks, and scalp but can occur anywhere on the body including palms, soles, and genitals. Itching is seen in 30 to 70 percent of individuals, and the word psoriasis comes from a Greek word for itch.

This disorder is unpredictable. Some cases are so mild the person may be unaware that they have it. Other cases are severe, and their complications may cause disability and deformity and significant psychological harm.

Attacks may be precipitated by stress, some drugs, and skin irritation; for others, attacks don't have an apparent cause. Conversely, it may suddenly disappear for months or even years. Psoriasis is not contagious, but there appears to be an inherited predisposition to it.

Many treatments may control its signs and symptoms, but there are no cures. Treatment approaches are medications applied to the skin, medicines taken by mouth, and treatment with light. Light therapy may be used in combination with topical or oral medication.

OTC Alternatives
Mild cases of psoriasis can be self-treated with OTC medications applied to the skin. These include skin moisturizers and hydrocortisone (1 percent), a topical steroid. Coal tar shampoos (e.g., Denorex, Neutrogena T, Polytar), which all have a strong, unpleasant odor and stain, are used to remove scales on the scalp or body.

Topical Medicines

Prescription medications applied to the skin include topical steroids, calcipotriene, anthralin, and tarazotene.

Topical Steroids

Topical steroids, such as betamethasone and clobetasol, are the most widely used group of drugs for the treatment of mild psoriasis. Some 20 different prescription-only steroids are available for application to the skin. Most of these products are available in different concentrations and in different dosage forms (e.g., ointments, creams, gels).

Topical steroids should be applied in a thin film and gently rubbed into the skin. They relieve the redness, itching, and scaling.

Some topical preparations are preferred for the treatment of different types of psoriasis. Ointments are the preferred form.

◆ Ointments and creams provide greater moisturizing effects than solutions, lotions, or gels.

◆ Lotions are preferred for oozing rashes.

◆ Solutions, lotions, and gels are easier to apply to hairy areas.

Common adverse effects include skin irritation and thinning of the skin, with stretch marks.

Just because a drug is applied to the skin, it doesn't mean that it can't enter the bloodstream and cause adverse effects in other parts of the body. Don't use these drugs more often or for longer periods than your doctor has recommended.

Calcipotriene

Calcipotriene is used for mild to moderate psoriasis, sometimes in combination with a topical steroid. Its most common side effect after topical use is irritation, and it may also cause a rash.

This vitamin D–related drug should not be applied more often than prescribed. Too much can increase calcium levels in the blood, with potentially dangerous consequences.

Anthralin

Anthralin has been used for some 90 years for the treatment of psoriasis, in particular for thick plaques. It can irritate normal skin and stains everything purple. Avoid contact with the eyes.

Tazarotene

Tazarotene is used for the treatment of mild to moderate psoriasis when topical steroids are not effective. A high percentage of patients favorably respond. Plaques may be controlled for months after the drug is no longer used. This vitamin A–related drug is also used for acne.

Common side effects include itching, stinging, burning, and redness. Tazarotene increases the sensitivity of the skin to sunburn, and users should wear protective clothing and use sunscreen.

Topical tazarotene should never be used by women who are pregnant or who could become pregnant. It is known to cause birth defects in the developing fetus. *See* "Acne" for additional precautions regarding its use.

Oral Medicines

Drugs taken by mouth are reserved for severe cases of psoriasis that have not responded to safer drugs. They include methotrexate, cyclosporine, and acitretin.

Methotrexate

Methotrexate has long been used as an anticancer medicine. In much lower doses, it is also taken to treat severe psoriasis. It works by slowing the growth of skin cells.

Its use is associated with a high incidence of severe adverse effects, including diarrhea and damage to the liver and to red and white blood cells and to platelets, which are required for normal blood clotting.

 Warning!

Women who are pregnant, or who may become pregnant, must never use methotrexate, cyclosporine, and acitretin. Use by pregnant women carries an extremely high risk of causing multiple defects to their developing fetus.

Cyclosporine

When used to treat psoriasis, cyclosporin provides beneficial effects only as long as it is taken. It can cause damage to the kidneys and increases the risk of and dangers associated with infections.

This medicine is primarily used to prevent the rejection of kidney, liver, and heart transplants.

Acitretin

Acitretin is a vitamin A–like drug, also used for acne. It is effective for the treatment of severe psoriasis. Signs of psoriasis return within several months after the medicine is stopped.

Adverse side effects are very common and include loss of hair, peeling of skin, and problems involving bleeding, bones, and joints.

The Least You Need to Know

◆ There are many treatments available to relieve the symptoms of psoriasis, but no cures.

◆ Plaques associated with mild cases can be effectively controlled with a number of topically applied medicines, the most common of which are steroids.

◆ Methotrexate, cyclosporine, and acitretin, drugs taken by mouth to treat severe psoriasis, all cause major adverse side effects. None of these oral drugs, nor topical tazarotene, should be taken by pregnant women.

Drugs Used for Treatment of Psoriasis

Generic Name	Trade Name	Generic Available
Topical Steroids		
Aclometasone	Aclovate	No
Amcinonide	Cyclocort	Yes
Betamethasone	Diprolene, Diprosone, Valisone	Yes
Clobetasol	Temovate	Yes
Desonide	DesOwen, Tridesilon	Yes
Desoximetasone	Topicort	Yes
Fluocinolone	Synalar	Yes
Fluocinonide	Fluonex, Lidex	Yes
Flurandrenolide	Cordran	Yes
Halcinonide	Halog	No
Hydrocortisone	Cortaid, Cortizone, Hytone	Yes
Triamcinolone	Aristocort, Kenalog	Yes

Generic Name	Trade Name	Generic Available
Other Topical Drugs		
Anthralin	Anthraforte, Anthranol, Dritho-Scalp	No
Calcipotriene	Dovonex	No
Tazarotene	Tazorac	No
Oral Drugs		
Acitretin	Soriatane	No
Cyclosporine	Neoral	No
Methotrexate	Trexall	Yes

Rheumatoid Arthritis

Rheumatoid arthritis is the most common whole body (systemic) inflammatory disease. Inflammation primarily affects the joints, but may also involve blood vessels, the eye, skin, nerves, heart, and lungs.

Some 1 percent of the world's adult population has rheumatoid arthritis (RA), and it is seen in women three times more often than men. RA is highly unpredictable, with symptoms slowly progressing over periods of years in some people and rather abruptly in others. Moreover, symptoms may disappear for periods of time and then return.

The small joints of the hands, wrists, and feet are most often affected. Joints are painful, swollen, and warm, which are signs of inflammation, and are affected on both sides of the body. In time, joints may become deformed. An *autoimmune disorder* is responsible for joint destruction.

def•i•ni•tion

> The immune system normally protects us against bacteria, viruses, cancer cells, and foreign substances. Like an efficient defensive military force, it identifies the invading enemy as being foreign (i.e., nonself), attacks, and destroys it. **Autoimmune disorders** are like friendly fire. The immune system mistakes self tissues for foreign ones and attacks them.

Treatment of RA: An Overview

In addition to rest and exercise, a multi-prong effort using medicines is required to treat RA in order to maintain and even improve function. Disease-modifying drugs work slowly to modify the course of the disease, preventing its progression and achieving a state of remission. Biological drugs interfere with chemicals that are responsible for the joint damage caused by the inflammatory process.

Nonsteroidal anti-inflammatory drugs (NSAIDs) and steroids rapidly relieve RA symptoms but don't change the course of the disease. Steroids are used to control severe symptoms.

Disease-Modifying Drugs

Many experts recommend that one or more disease modifiers, called disease-modifying antirheumatic drugs, or DMARDs, be started within months after RA symptoms appear. They are often used in combination with an NSAID or a steroid to provide rapid relief of symptoms.

DMARDs slow and even stop the progression of RA. This prevents additional damage to the joints and decreases pain and swelling. These beneficial effects often require many weeks to several months of drug treatment.

Methotrexate is commonly the first choice of disease modifiers in severe cases of RA. It is the best-studied medicine in this group. It's effective and is low in cost.

Benefits occur rather rapidly, generally within three to six weeks. Adverse effects of methotrexate involve the liver, gastrointestinal tract, blood, and lungs. This drug cannot be used during pregnancy because it can cause fetal abnormalities and death.

Hydroxychloroquine's desired effects take up to six weeks to be seen, with maximum results requiring up to six months. Side effects are generally mild and usually involve skin rashes. Far less commonly, it can cause damage to the retina, with loss of vision and even blindness resulting. Periodic eye exams are strongly recommended.

Did You Know That ...?

Some RA disease-modifying drugs are used for other conditions. These include methotrexate for certain cancers and psoriasis, hydroxychloroquine for malaria, and sulfasalazine for ulcerative colitis.

Biological Drugs

An autoimmune process causes the release of cytokines, chemicals responsible for inflammation and joint damage. One such cytokine is tumor necrosis factor (TNF). Biological drugs work by blocking the effects of TNF and related cytokines and prevent their tissue-destroying effects.

Biological drugs are laboratory-manufactured proteins that can only be used by injection. The long-term safety and effectiveness of these new drugs has not been fully evaluated, but preliminary results are very promising.

Warning!

Biological drugs should not be used by people with tuberculosis or who have been exposed to TB or other serious infections. Treated persons should not receive live vaccines.

They are very expensive (about $12,000 per year) and are generally prescribed only if disease modifiers fail to work. They are sometimes used in combination with disease modifiers.

Several biological drugs should be used cautiously by persons with heart failure. They may increase cancer risk, because TNF plays a natural role in combating cancer.

Common side effects include swelling, redness, pain, and itching at the site of injection.

Nonsteroidal Anti-Inflammatory Drugs (NSAIDs)

NSAIDs are rarely used alone to treat RA. They are often given with disease modifiers to supplement pain relief, or until the maximum benefits of the disease modifiers develop.

Aspirin, ibuprofen (Motrin), naproxen (Naprosyn), and other NSAIDs are used to quickly relieve the pain, stiffness, and inflammation of RA. These relatively safe drugs don't modify joint deformity or the progress of RA. Remember that acetaminophen (Tylenol) relieves pain but is not an NSAID and has no anti-inflammatory properties.

Maximizing Your Medicine

Monthly costs of prescription NSAIDs range from $20 to $100, and the selective COX-2 inhibitor Celebrex is particularly expensive. You can save some big bucks by noting that most NSAIDs are available as generic products. Moreover, a few (ibuprofen, ketoprofen, naproxen) are available OTC at half strength. Make sure that you take the correct dose of these OTCs.

Do not take an NSAID if you are sensitive to aspirin. Symptoms of sensitivity include a running nose, hives, breathing difficulties, and shock. This risk is greater in persons with nasal polyps.

Use NSAIDs cautiously if you have peptic ulcer disease. Long-term NSAID use can cause ulceration of the stomach and bleeding, which can worsen an existing ulcer condition. Taking an acid-blocking drug, such as omeprazole (Prilosec) or famotidine (Pepcid), can prevent ulcers. Misoprostol (Cytotec) is specifically used to prevent gastric ulcers caused by long-term use of NSAIDs.

Celebrex has been aggressively marketed based on its ability to cause a lower risk of stomach ulcers than other NSAIDs, a claim which may not be valid. Avoid the use of

Celebrex if you have risk factors for heart disease or stroke. NSAIDs should be used cautiously, as well. If you are unsure, discuss this with your doctor.

NSAIDs interfere with platelet function, which leads to bleeding tendencies. They should be used with extreme caution, if at all, by persons with bleeding disorders.

The elderly or individuals with a history of kidney disorders, high blood pressure, or heart disorders should use NSAIDs under a doctor's supervision. These drugs may cause kidney toxicity in susceptible persons.

NSAIDs and, more particularly, COX-2 inhibitors may increase the risk of stroke and high blood pressure when used over extended periods.

Warning!

Use NSAIDs with great caution when also taking the blood thinner (anticoagulant) warfarin.

Aspirin, and to a somewhat lesser degree all other NSAIDS, upset the stomach, causing heartburn, indigestion, nausea, bloating, and diarrhea. Take these drugs with food or water to reduce this distress.

Steroids

When taken by mouth or injection, steroids (such as prednisone) can dramatically relieve the inflammatory symptoms of RA. During the early months of therapy with slow-acting disease modifiers, steroids may also be used to provide relief of symptoms.

Low doses of steroids may be given on a long-term basis for patients whose RA symptoms cannot be adequately controlled. Higher doses are used for persons who experience sudden, intense flare-ups in their condition.

Did You Know That ...?

Steroids (also known as glucocorticoids) are also used for the treatment of dozens of conditions, including ulcerative colitis, severe allergic disorders, asthmatic attacks, psoriasis and eczema, blood cancers, allergic and inflammatory eye disorders, multiple sclerosis, and to prevent organ transplant rejection.

When properly used, steroids can be life-saving drugs. When improperly used, their adverse effects can affect organs throughout the body. In general, steroids should be taken at the lowest effective doses for the shortest period of time. Some major problems include …

◆ Adrenal insufficiency. High steroid doses cause the adrenal glands to shut down and become unable to release natural steroids when the body is confronted with stress.

◆ Bone loss, osteoporosis, and bone fractures.

◆ Increased susceptibility to infections.

◆ Loss of control of sugar levels in diabetics.

◆ Muscle weakness.

◆ Salt and water retention, causing high blood pressure.

◆ Suppression of growth in children.

◆ Behavioral and mood changes, such as depression or a high feeling (euphoria).

◆ Cataracts and glaucoma.

◆ Peptic ulcer disease.

Steroids should not be used by people with systemic fungal infections or those receiving live-virus vaccines.

Steroids should be used cautiously in children and pregnant or nursing women—also by people with high blood pressure, heart failure, kidney disease, peptic ulcers, diabetes, osteoporosis, and infections resistant to treatment.

The Least You Need to Know

◆ Rheumatoid arthritis is a chronic systemic inflammatory disease that can cause joint deformities and possible crippling.

◆ RA is generally treated with combinations of drugs.

◆ NSAIDs and steroids are highly effective in rapidly relieving RA symptoms, such as pain, swelling, tenderness, and stiffness of joints.

◆ Low doses of steroids (such as prednisone) should be given for the shortest period of time to avoid serious side effects.

◆ Disease-modifying drugs (such as methotrexate) or biologic drugs (such as Remicade) are given within months after an RA diagnosis to prevent or slow disease progression.

Drugs Used for Treatment of Rheumatoid Arthritis

Generic Name	Trade Name	Generic Available
Disease Modifiers		
Auranofin	Ridaura	No
Aurothioglucose	Solganal	No
Azathioprine	Immuran	Yes
Cyclophosphamide	Cytoxin	Yes
Gold sodium thiomalate	Aurolate, Myochrysine	Yes
Hydroxychloroquine	Plaquenil	Yes
Leflunomide	Arava	No
Methotrexate	Rheumatrex	Yes
Penicillamine	Cuprimine, Depen	No
Sulfasalazine	Azulfidine	Yes
Biological Drugs		
Adalimimab	Humira	No
Anakinra	Kineret	No
Etanercept	Enbrel	No
Infliximab	Remicade	No
Nonsteroidal Anti-Inflammatory Drugs (NSAIDs)		
Celecoxib	Celebrex	No
Diclofenac	Cataflam, Voltaren	Yes
Diflunisal	Dolobid	Yes
Fenoprofen	Nalfon	Yes
Flurbiprofen	Ansaid	Yes
Ibuprofen	Advil, Motrin	Yes
Indomethacin	Indocin	Yes
Ketoprofen	Orudis, Oruvail	Yes
Meloxicam	Mobic	No
Nabumetone	Relafen	Yes
Naproxen	Aleve, Naprosyn	Yes

continues

Drugs Used for Treatment of Rheumatoid Arthritis (continued)

Generic Name	Trade Name	Generic Available
Oxaprozin	Daypro	Yes
Piroxicam	Feldene	Yes
Sulindac	Clinoril	Yes
Tolmetin	Tolectin	Yes
Steroids		
Betamethasone	Celestone	Yes
Dexamethasone	Decadron, Hexadrol	Yes
Methylprednisolone	Medrol	Yes
Prednisolone	Delta-Cortef	Yes
Prednisone	Deltasone, Meticorten	Yes
Triamcinolone	Aristocort, Kenalog	Yes

Sexually Transmitted Diseases

Sexually transmitted diseases (STDs) are infections that are transferred by sexual contact. More than 10 million Americans contract STDs each year. The majority of these infections occur in sexually active teenagers or individuals in their early 20s.

Because many STDs cause minimal or no symptoms, some cases go undetected and, therefore, untreated. Effective treatment of an STD with an antibiotic does not protect against re-infection.

STDs can be caused by ...

- ◆ **Bacteria.** Syphilis, gonorrhea, chylamydia

- ◆ **Viruses.** Genital herpes, genital warts, AIDS/HIV

- ◆ **Parasites.** Trichomoniasis

Did You Know That ...?

In addition to preventing unwanted pregnancy, a condom can prevent the transmission of syphilis, gonorrhea, chlamydia, trichomoniasis, and HIV/AIDS. Condoms can reduce the risk of genital herpes and genital warts, as well. Infected areas must, of course, be covered to prevent the spread of these viral infections.

Syphilis

Syphilis is caused by the bacterium Treponema pallidum and is spread through contact with a syphilis sore during genital, anal, or oral sex.

There was a total of 32,000 cases of syphilis in the United States in 2002, 412 of which were new cases. This STD is three and a half times more common in men, and rates are increasing from man-to-man sexual contact.

Signs and Symptoms

Symptoms of syphilis may not appear for years after being infected, but if untreated, the individual is at risk for the long-term severe complications. Syphilis has been called "the great imitator" because its signs and symptoms resemble many other diseases. In the absence of treatment, syphilis progresses through the following three stages:

◆ **Primary stage.** One or more sores (chancres) appear 10 to 90 days after infection, last for 3 to 6 weeks, and then disappear.

◆ **Secondary stage.** Skin rash and mucous membrane lesions. Also red spots on the palms and soles of feet, fever, swollen glands, sore throat, fever, muscle aches, and fatigue.

◆ **Late stage.** Muscle disorders, paralysis, blindness, dementia, and even death.

Mothers infected during pregnancy have a high rate of stillborns or babies who die shortly after birth. Surviving infants may be developmentally delayed, have seizures, or die.

Individuals with syphilis have an increased risk of HIV/AIDS infection, if exposed to the virus. The open sores of syphilis are thought to make it easier for the HIV virus to enter the body.

Treatment

Syphilis is easy to cure during its early stages. For individuals infected for less than one year, a single injection of penicillin G benzathine into the muscles is effective. Infections untreated for longer than one year require multiple injections of this medicine.

Although treatment cures syphilis, it does not reverse the damage caused, nor does it prevent re-infection.

Doxycycline and tetracycline are useful alternative medicines for the treatment of syphilis in penicillin-allergic patients. These drugs are given orally several times daily for two to four weeks.

Maximizing Your Medicine

Injections of penicillin G must be given every 8 to 12 hours to be effective. Penicillin G benzathine, by contrast, slowly leaks out of muscle and continues to provide antibacterial penicillin blood levels for one to four weeks.

Penicillins

Penicillins were the first class of antibiotics to be discovered and continue to be among the most effective antibiotics and least toxic of all medicines. Since the time of its discovery in the early 1940s, penicillin G has remained the first choice for the treatment of syphilis.

Name hint: generic names end in "cillin."

Whereas penicillins are very safe drugs, their use poses a risk of causing an allergic reaction. Somewhere between 1 to 10 percent of all individuals are allergic to penicillin.

Signs of allergic response may vary in severity from a slight rash to a rare but life-threatening inability to breath and a sudden drop in blood pressure. In such cases, emergency treatment involves an injection of epinephrine, in addition to mechanical support of breathing.

Warning!

If you are allergic to penicillin, you should alert health-care workers of your condition. All doctors, dentists, pharmacists, and nurses with whom you interact should be notified of your allergy, and this should be entered on the medical records they maintain for you.

Individuals allergic to one penicillin are likely to be allergic to all other penicillins. If a severe penicillin-allergic reaction is experienced, no penicillin-, cephalosporin- or carbapenem-like drugs should be taken.

Tetracyclines

Doxycycline and tetracycline are used for the treatment of syphilis in penicillin-allergic patients.

Name hint: generic names end in "cycline."

Gastrointestinal disturbances, such as indigestion, nausea, and diarrhea are the most common side effects.

Tetracyclines readily bind to calcium in newly formed teeth, including those of the fetus. This can lead to yellow-brown discoloration of teeth. Tetracyclines should not be given to pregnant women.

Warning!

Tetracyclines should never be taken if they are outdated, have changed color or taste, look different, or if they have been stored in a setting that is too warm or too damp. Such medication should be discarded. Under such circumstances, tetracyclines can decompose into chemicals that may cause serious adverse effects, including kidney damage.

These drugs increase sensitivity to the sun, with a greater risk of severe sunburn. Individuals, particularly those with fair skin, taking tetracyclines should limit their exposure to sun, use sunscreen, and wear protective clothing.

Tetracyclines bind to metals such as calcium, magnesium, aluminum, and iron, which interfere with their absorption into the bloodstream.

Antibiotic levels in the blood are reduced, reducing their antibacterial effectiveness. As a consequence, calcium supplements, most antacids, and iron supplements should be taken one hour before or two hours after tetracyclines.

Milk and other calcium-rich dairy products and foods interfere with tetracycline (but not doxycycline) absorption and lower its blood levels. Tetracycline should be taken one hour before or two hours after meals with a full glass of water.

Gonorrhea

Gonorrhea is caused by the bacterium Neisseria gonorrhoeae. If a condom is not used, there is a high risk of infection after intercourse with an individual with the disease. Some 700,000 individuals are newly infected in the United States each year, with a far greater number going undiagnosed.

Signs and Symptoms

Infected men typically have no disease symptoms. In others, some 2 to 5 days after being infected and for up to 30 days, they may experience a burning sensation when urinating and may have a white, yellow, or light green discharge from the penis.

Most women don't experience symptoms. Mild symptoms, when present, are nonspecific and may be similar to bladder or vaginal infections. No symptoms are generally present when there are infections of the rectum or throat. Untreated gonorrhea in women can cause pelvic inflammatory disease and indirectly result in infertility. In both sexes, it can also lead to skin disorders, arthritis-like symptoms, and infections of the inner lining of the heart.

Babies delivered from infected mothers through the birth canal may become blind or have joint or blood infections.

Treatment

Gonorrhea is becoming more difficult to treat because of the development of antibiotic-resistant strains of bacteria. Preferred treatment is with a single dose of cephalosporins, either oral (cef ixime) or by injection (ceftriaxone) or with oral quinolones (ciprofloxacin or ofloxacin).

Individuals with gonorrhea often also have chlamidial infections, and both are treated at the same time.

To protect against gonorrhea-induced blindness in newborns, most states require that topical antimicrobial eye drops be placed in each eye immediately after delivery. Such drugs include silver nitrate, tetracycline, or erythromycin.

Cephalosporins

Cephalosporins, the most widely used class of antibiotics, cause relatively little toxicity, and can be given by mouth or injection.

Name hint: most generic names start with "cef" or "ceph."

In general, the cephalosporins are among the safest antimicrobial medicines, with diarrhea a common side effect.

Cephalosporins chemically resemble penicillin. The allergic skin reactions they produce are similar to those produced by penicillin. If a patient experiences difficulties in breathing when taking these drugs, the doctor should be contacted immediately.

Warning!

About 10 percent of penicillin-allergic patients may be also allergic to cephalosporins. Individuals exhibiting mild penicillin-allergic reactions can probably use cephalosporins safely. Those with a history of severe penicillin-allergic reactions should never be given cephalosporins.

Quinolones

Quinolones, such as ciprofloxacin and ofloxacin, taken by mouth, are effective for the treatment of gonorrhea.

Name hint: generic names usually end in "floxacin."

Side effects are mild and infrequent and include nausea, vomiting, and diarrhea, as well as dizziness and nervousness.

Quinolones should not be used to treat pregnant patients.

The absorption of quinolones into the blood is reduced by antacids containing aluminum or magnesium, and by iron and zinc salts, and milk and other dairy products. This interaction may result in a reduction in their antibacterial effectiveness.

Chlamydia

Chlamydial infection, caused by Chlamydia trachomatis, is the most frequently reported bacterial STD in the United States, and its occurrence is increasing. In 2002, 835,000 new cases were reported, and it is estimated that 2.8 million individuals are infected each year. Sexually active teenage girls and young women are at highest risk.

Signs and Symptoms

Symptoms are usually absent—three-fourths of women and one-half of men have either no symptoms or only mild ones.

Symptoms in women include an abnormal vaginal discharge or a burning sensation when urinating. Pain may be experienced in the lower abdomen or lower back and during intercourse.

When symptoms occur in men, they typically include discharges from the penis and burning and itching at the opening of the penis.

Complications rarely occur in men. Untreated chlamidial infections in women may cause pelvic inflammatory disease, a chronic pelvic disease that may result in infertility.

Women infected with chlamidia are five times more likely to be infected with HIV if exposed to the virus.

Babies born of chlamidia-infected mothers may develop infections of their eyes, causing pink eye (a.k.a. conjunctivitis), or lungs, causing early infant pneumonia.

Treatment

It is easy to treat and cure chlamidial infections with a single dose of azithromycin (an erythromycin-like antibiotic) or doxycycline, given twice daily for seven days. Both drugs are taken by mouth.

Azithromycin

Azithromycin is a long-acting erythromycin-like drug that acts against the same types of bacteria as penicillin.

Name hint: most generic names of erythromycin-like drugs end in "mycin."

Azithromycin is best taken on an empty stomach one hour before meals or two hours after with a full glass of water.

Common side effects include indigestion and diarrhea.

Genital Herpes

Most cases of genital herpes are caused by herpes simplex virus type 2 (HSV-2). Genital herpes is common—45 million Americans 12 years and older have had a genital HSV infection.

Signs and Symptoms

Most individuals experience no symptoms or have very small blister clusters on or around the genitals or rectum. After the blisters break, the resulting sores take two to four weeks to heal.

The virus remains in the body for a lifetime, and painful sores typically reappear one or several times a year.

Although rare, potentially fatal HSV-2 infections may occur in newborns. If the infected mother is experiencing an active genital herpes recurrence at the time of delivery, a cesarean delivery is performed.

Genital herpes increases the susceptibility to HIV infections and increases the infectiousness of the HIV-infected person.

Treatment

Antiviral drugs do not cure HSV infections. Rather these drugs reduce the severity of the symptoms and the frequency of their recurrences. Specific treatment approaches differ depending on whether: it is a first episode; a recurring attack; or whether the drug is given on a regular basis to reduce the severity and recurrence of frequently recurring episodes.

An oral dose of an antiviral drug, such as acyclovir, famciclovir, or valacyclovir, is given several times daily for 7 to 10 days for a first episode or 3 to 5 days for recurring episodes. These drugs reduce the severity of the symptoms and reduce the time for healing.

When more than six episodes occur per year, famciclovir or valacyclovir are given on a continuous basis. The frequency and severity of recurrences are reduced by 70 to 90 percent.

Acyclovir-Like Drugs

Acyclovir is the preferred drug for the treatment and prevention of genital herpes episodes. It causes few serious side effects.

Name hint: most generic names end in "cyclovir" or "ciclovir."

Oral acyclovir can cause nausea, vomiting, diarrhea, dizziness, and headache.

Genital and Anal Warts

Genital and anal warts, caused by human papillomaviruses (HPVs) infection, are quite common. Twenty million Americans are currently infected, and more than 6 million new infections occur each year.

There are no signs, symptoms, or complications associated with this condition. The infection usually resolves on its own in the absence of treatment. HPV also causes cervical cancer, and HPV infection increases the risk of cervical cancer.

Surgery, freezing (cryotherapy), or drugs administered by a health professional are used to remove or destroy these warts. Common drugs include podophyllin, trichloro-acetic acid, or bichloroacetic acid, which are applied at weekly intervals.

Trichomoniasis

Trichomoniasis is caused by the single-celled protozoan parasite Trichomonas vaginitis. There are 7.4 million new cases of trichomoniasis each year.

Trichomoniasis causes few if any symptoms in men. The most common sign in women is a yellow-green vaginal discharge with a strong odor. It appears 5 to 28 days after being infected.

Trichomoniasis increases the susceptibility to HIV infections, if exposed to the virus. Babies born of mothers with this condition may be born early or have a low birth weight (less than 5 lbs).

Of all the STDs, trichomoniasis is most easily treated and cured. A single oral dose of metronidazole is used. To be most effective, both sex partners should be treated at the same time. This same drug can be used safely in pregnant women.

Metronidazole

Common side effects of metronidazole include nausea, headache, dry mouth, and a metallic taste. The urine may darken after taking this drug, but this is of no concern.

> **Warning!**
> Avoid alcoholic beverages when taking metronidazole. The combination may cause nausea, vomiting, facial flushing, palpitations of the heart, and a marked drop in blood pressure.

The Least You Need to Know

- Sexually active teenagers and individuals in their early 20s, who have multiple partners and engage in unprotected sex, are at greatest risk of contracting STDs.

- In its early stages, syphilis can be readily cured with penicillin or tetracycline but, if untreated, can cause severe, potentially life-threatening complications.

- Gonorrhea can be cured with a single dose of a cephalosporin or quinolone.

- Chlamydia, the most common bacterial STD, is the easiest to cure using azithromycin or doxycycline.

- Genital herpes cannot be cured but its symptoms can be relieved using acyclovir and related antiviral drugs.

- Trichomoniasis, caused by a protozoan parasite, can be easily cured with metronidazole.

Drugs Used to Treat Sexually Transmitted Diseases

Generic Name	Trade Name	How Taken: Oral (O), Injection (I)	Generic Available
Acyclovir	Zovirax	O	Yes
Azithromycin	Zithromax	O	Yes
Cefixime	Suprax	O	No
Ceftriaxone	Rocephin	I	No
Ciprofloxacin	Cipro	O	Yes

continues

Drugs Used to Treat Sexually Transmitted Diseases (continued)

Generic Name	Trade Name	How Taken: Oral (O), Injection (I)	Generic Available
Doxycycline	Vibramycin	O	Yes
Famciclovir	Famvir	O	No
Metronidazole	Flagyl	O	Yes
Ofloxacin	Floxin	O	No
Penicillin G Benzathine	Bicillin L-A, Permapen	I	Yes
Tetracycline	Sumycin	O	Yes
Valacyclovir	Valtrex	O	No

Stroke

Stroke is the third leading cause of death in North America—after cardiovascular diseases and all cancers—and represents the leading cause of disabilities in adults.

Causes and Consequences of Stroke

Stroke, also called cerebrovascular accident, is the sudden death of brain cells and is caused by an interference with blood flow in the brain. This hindrance can result from either a block in the blood supply to the brain or from a rupture of an artery, causing bleeding within the brain. Each has a different treatment.

The parts of the body disabled after a stroke and the degree of disability depend on those areas of the brain affected and how long and to what extent the injury occurs.

In most instances (80 to 90 percent), stroke is caused by a block in an artery that supplies blood to the brain. This is called an *ischemic stroke*. Oxygen and sugar (glucose), which is required as a source of energy for the brain, do not reach brain cells, leading to their death. In a full-blown stroke, this block lasts for more than 24 hours.

When this block is only of brief duration, usually less than 30 minutes, no permanent damage results. This is called a transient ischemic attack (TIA) and is of concern because it may be followed by a full-blown stroke.

Atherosclerosis is a major risk factor in ischemic stroke. With this disease, fatty deposits (plaques) build up in the walls of the carotid arteries (the main vessels carrying blood to each side of the brain) and reduce the blood flow. The problem is aggravated when a plaque ruptures and a blood clot forms, blocking blood flow altogether. In other cases, a clot formed elsewhere in the body becomes dislodged and travels up to and blocks the carotid artery. Without blood flow, the involved area of the brain is starved of oxygen and quickly dies.

The other type of stroke (10 to 20 percent), called *hemorrhagic stroke*, results from the rupture of a blood vessel within or around the brain. Blood is released and causes damage to the surrounding brain tissue. The main cause of hemorrhagic stroke is high blood pressure. Although hemorrhagic stroke is less common than ischemic stroke, it is far more dangerous.

def•i•ni•tion

There are two primary types of stroke:

◆ **Ischemic stroke** is caused by the sudden block of a blood vessel supplying blood to the brain.

◆ **Hemorrhagic stroke** results from the bursting of a blood vessel in the brain and causes bleeding into or around the brain.

Drug Treatment of Stroke: An Overview

Before starting treatment, the doctor must first determine whether the stroke has been caused by blockage or by bleeding. A CAT scan or MRI is used to make this critical distinction.

Hemorrhagic strokes are treated surgically. If blood pressure is markedly elevated, drugs are sometimes given to reduce the pressure, but generally after a seven-day wait.

Medicines play an essential role in the treatment of an acute ischemic stroke in progress as well as to prevent future strokes from occurring.

Acute ischemic stroke is treated with a clot-buster such as alteplase (tPA) and with aspirin.

Medicines used to prevent recurring ischemic strokes may include …

◆ Antiplatelet drugs, which prevent platelet clumping, such as aspirin, aspirin and dipyridamole, and clopidogrel.

◆ Blood thinners, such as warfarin.

◆ Antihypertensives, which reduce high blood pressure, such as an ACB or ACE inhibitor, and sometimes with a diuretic (water pill).

◆ A cholesterol-lowering drug, most often a statin.

Alteplase (tPA)

Alteplase is highly effective in dissolving blood clots and significantly reducing disability caused by ischemic strokes. This clot-buster drug, tissue plasminogen activator (tPA), is identical to the enzyme the body uses to dispose of unneeded clots.

To be effective, tPA must be administered intravenously no later than three hours after the symptoms of a stroke start. A strict set of criteria has been established to determine which patients are eligible to receive tPA. The decision to use this potentially dangerous drug, which can increase the risk of bleeding within the brain, is not taken lightly.

Among the most important of these many criteria include determining that a block, and not bleeding, has caused the stroke; that the stroke has occurred within the past three hours; and the patient has not recently used blood thinners (warfarin or heparin), which increase bleeding tendencies.

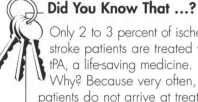

Did You Know That ...?

Only 2 to 3 percent of ischemic stroke patients are treated with tPA, a life-saving medicine. Why? Because very often, patients do not arrive at treatment facilities that can safely administer tPA within the first three hours after the stroke begins. Alteplase is also used for acute heart attacks.

Antiplatelet Drugs

During the formation of a clot, platelets clump together. Aspirin and other antiplatelet medicines work by preventing this clumping.

Aspirin

Aspirin is a time-honored drug for the relief of pain, reduction of fever, and the treatment of inflammatory disorders such as rheumatoid arthritis. Here we only talk about its beneficial effects on clots in stroke.

Aspirin is effective in reducing death and disability when used within 48 hours after the onset of stroke symptoms. It can also reduce the risk of stroke recurrence when taken regularly.

Maximizing Your Medicine

Experts agree that aspirin is highly effective when taken at the first signs of a stroke (or heart attack) and prevent both. The most effective dose has not been determined, although less is better. A lower dose works more effectively and causes fewer side effects. One children's aspirin (81 mg) or half an adult's aspirin (160 mg), taken daily, is effective.

At the first signs of a possible stroke, experts recommend chewing an aspirin tablet and then immediately getting to an emergency room. The antiplatelet effects start working within 60 minutes.

At the low recommended doses of aspirin, side effects are few. They include an increased risk of bleeding and indigestion. Aspirin-allergic individuals must avoid any dose and should consider taking another antiplatelet drug.

Aspirin should never be given within 24 hours of tPA, because tPA increases the risk of bleeding.

Aspirin + Dipyridamole (Aggrenox)

Dipyridamole, when taken alone, interferes with platelet clumping in a different way than aspirin. A fixed combination of aspirin (25 mg) and dipyridamole (in an extended-release preparation), taken twice daily, is more effective in preventing ischemic stroke than when either drug is used alone. The combination is recommended for individuals who have a history of TIAs or an ischemic stroke.

Common side effects include headache, indigestion, abdominal pain, and diarrhea.

Maximizing Your Medicine
A month's supply of Aggrenox costs about $120. To save money, you might be tempted to use aspirin and a generic preparation of immediate-acting (not extended-release) dipyridamole. This ad hoc combination has not been proven to be effective and should not be substituted for Aggrenox.

Clopidogrel

Clopidogrel (Plavix) is used to prevent platelet clumping in patients with a history of ischemic stroke or heart attack. It is only slightly more effective than aspirin. The combination of clopidogrel and aspirin is no more effective in preventing stroke than is clopidogrel used alone.

It causes similar side effects, and to the same extent as aspirin, such as abdominal pain, indigestion, diarrhea, and rash.

At a monthly cost of $115 to $130, and with no apparent advantages over aspirin, Plavix is most appropriate for those who cannot take aspirin or who do not benefit from it.

Unlike clopidogrel, the use of the chemically related ticlopidine (Ticlid) more often causes diarrhea and has been associated with some life-threatening blood disorders.

Warning!

Antiplatelet drugs increase the risk of bleeding. People should inform their doctors and dentists that they are taking such medicines before any elective surgery is scheduled.

Blood Thinners (Warfarin)

Atrial fibrillation is an irregular heart rhythm in which the heart beats very rapidly but not efficiently. This condition increases the risk of dislodging a clot, which may travel to the brain and cause an ischemic stroke. This risk is particularly high when individuals have a recent history of TIAs or stroke.

The blood thinner warfarin is the most effective medicine taken orally for the prevention of stroke in patients with atrial fibrillation.

Warfarin (Coumadin) prevents clot formation. It works by antagonizing the effects of vitamin K, a vitamin essential for the manufacture of clotting factors. It often takes several days to work, and it continues working for several days after drug therapy has been discontinued.

Maximizing Your Medicine

How much warfarin? If the dose is too low, there is a tendency for clot formation to continue. Too much drug, by contrast, increases the risk of bleeding, which can be life-threatening.

Missed Doses

If a dose is missed, it should be taken as soon as possible, and the regular dosing schedule resumed. If the missed dose is not realized until the following day, forget the missed dose. Don't double the next dose, which may increase the risk of bleeding. Just return to the regular schedule.

Overdoses

Bleeding is the major problem caused by excessive doses of warfarin. Patients using anticoagulants should know the signs of overdoses and, if they appear, contact their

Warning! _____

Make sure your doctor, dentist, and pharmacist know that you are taking warfarin. This drug should not be used for several days prior to elective surgical procedures. Carry or wear identification indicating that you are using warfarin. Consult your doctor or pharmacist before starting or stopping any other medicine.

doctor immediately. These signs include bleeding from the gums when brushing teeth, sudden nosebleeds, skin bruising or purplish blotching of the skin, unusually heavy bleeding from cuts or wounds or during menstrual bleeding.

Signs of internal bleeding include abdominal or stomach pain or swelling; backaches; blood in the urine; bloody or tarry stools; coughing up or vomiting blood; constipation; severe and long-lasting headaches; joint pain, swelling, or stiffness.

Bleeding caused by excessive doses of warfarin can be stopped with vitamin K_1 (phytonadione), which can be taken by mouth or injection.

Common Side Effects

Warfarin should not be used by pregnant women or people with a vitamin K deficiency, liver disease, alcoholism, deficiency of platelets (thrombocytopenia), or uncontrollable bleeding. Warfarin should not be used during or immediately after surgery of the brain, spinal cord, or eye, or by patients having a lumbar puncture (spinal tap) or regional anesthesia.

It should be used with great caution in people with gastrointestinal ulcers and severe high blood pressure.

Drug-Drug and -Food Interactions

A large number of medicines—both prescription and OTC—may increase or decrease the effects of blood thinners. Check with your doctor or pharmacist before taking any new drugs or discontinuing old ones.

Drugs that may increase the effects of warfarin and increase the risk of bleeding include acetaminophen, alcohol, antibiotics (oral), aspirin, cimetidine, clofibrate, disulfiram, heparin, phenylbutazone, and sulfa drugs.

Drugs and dietary supplements that may decrease the effects of warfarin and increase the risk of clotting include barbiturates, cholestyramine, ginseng, green tea, griseofulvin, rifampin, St. John's wort, and vitamin K.

Foods that may decrease the effects of warfarin and increase clotting risks include green, leafy vegetables that are rich in vitamin K.

Blood Pressure Reducers: ARBs and ACE Inhibitors

Elevated blood pressure is commonly seen in ischemic stroke and may be a major risk factor. Reduction in blood pressure has been associated with a reduction in the recurrence of stroke.

Studies have shown that several angiotensin-receptor blockers (ARBs) reduce blood pressure and also reduce stroke risk. These ARBs include losartan and eprosartan. The ACE inhibitor perindopril has produced similarly favorably results.

A dry, nonproductive cough is seen in 5 to 10 percent of persons using ACE inhibitors. This is more often seen in women than men and is the most frequent reason why people stop using these medications.

With ACE inhibitors, far less common, but far more serious, is the possibility of kidney damage.

With ARBs, dizziness sometimes occurs.

Warning!

If pregnant, do not take ACE inhibitors or ARBs. Their use during the second and third trimester of pregnancy may cause harmful effects to the developing fetus.

Cholesterol Reducers: Statins

Elevated cholesterol levels are the major risk factor for atherosclerosis, where arteries are clogged and blood flow may be reduced to the brain and heart. This may lead to ischemic stroke and to coronary artery disease, including angina.

Statins are the most widely used drugs for reducing cholesterol levels. They have been shown to decrease the risk of stroke in individuals with coronary artery disease, and who have both elevated and normal cholesterol levels. These statins include lovastatin, pravastatin, and simvastatin.

Some have proposed that statins, which are relatively safe drugs, be used to prevent stroke and heart attacks in all individuals at risk. Moreover, several pharmaceutical manufacturers have formally attempted, but without success yet, to have prescription-only statin drugs moved to an OTC status.

Side effects are generally uncommon and mild and include intestinal upset, rashes, and headache.

Warning! _____

Pregnant women should not take statins. Their use during the second and third trimester of pregnancy may cause injury and death to the developing fetus.

Liver toxicity and muscle injury are rare but very serious. Individuals with liver disease and who consume excessive amounts of alcohol are at greater risk for liver toxicity. Muscle aches, pains, and tenderness can progress to inflammation and breakdown of muscle, which, in turn, has been associated with kidney failure.

The Least You Need to Know

♦ Strokes result from either a block in blood flow supplying blood to the brain (ischemic stroke) or a bursting blood vessel causing bleeding in or around the brain (hemorrhagic stroke).

♦ Aspirin, an antiplatelet drug, is used to prevent and treat ischemic stroke.

♦ Alteplase (tPA), a clot buster, when used in selected patients within three hours after the start of stroke symptoms, can be highly effective in dissolving clots responsible for ischemic stroke.

♦ Warfarin, a blood thinner (anticoagulant), is used to prevent clot development in patients with atrial fibrillation.

♦ Warfarin doses must be adjusted for each patient to prevent clot formation without exposing the patient to an increased risk of bleeding.

♦ Many drugs and food supplements have been found to increase or decrease the effectiveness of warfarin.

♦ Drugs are used to reduce high blood pressure and prevent the development of atherosclerosis, major risk factors for ischemic strokes.

Drugs Used to Treat and Prevent Stroke

Generic Name	Trade Name	Generic Available
Treatment of Stroke		
Alteplase (tPA)	Activase	No
Aspirin		Yes
Prevention of Stroke		
Antiplatelet Drugs		
Aspirin + dipyridamole [extended-release]	Aggrenox	No (Not recommended)
Clopidogrel	Plavix	No
Ticlopidine	Ticlid	No
Blood Thinner (Anticoagulant)		
Warfarin	Coumadin	Yes
Blood Pressure Reducers: ARBs ("sartans") and ACE Inhibitors ("prils")		
Eprosartan	Teveten	No
Losartan	Cozaar	No
Perindopril	Aceon	No
Cholesterol Reducers ("statins")		
Lovastatin	Mevacor	Yes
Pravastatin	Pravachol	Yes
Simvastatin	Zocor	Yes

Thyroid Gland Conditions

The thyroid gland has a butterfly shape and is located directly under the skin in the neck, below the Adam's apple. Simply stated, the gland controls the rate at which chemical reactions occur in the body. When the thyroid gland is not working right, it affects such things as heart rate, body temperature, breathing rate, bowel function, skin texture, and alertness.

def•i•ni•tion

Mild cases of hormone deficiency are called **hypothyroidism**. In adults, severe cases are termed myxedema; in infants, they are called cretinism.

In children, thyroid function is essential for normal growth and development. If inadequate thyroid gland function is not detected in newborns, permanent mental retardation can result.

Thyroid gland effects are carried out by two hormones, T_4 (thyroxine) and T_3 (triiodothyronine). Iodine is essential for the manufacture of these hormones. Thyroid gland disorders result from conditions in which these hormones are deficient (*hypothyroidism*) or excessive (hyperthyroidism).

Underactive Thyroid Activity (Hypothyroidism)

The typical hypothyroid person has dry skin, is very sensitive to cold, is overweight, suffers from constipation, feels tired, and has lost energy and drive. It affects about 7 to 10 women for every 1 man.

Levothyroxine and Other Replacement Drugs

Drug treatment can be described in a single word: replacement. A variety of thyroid preparations are available to replace the hormone deficiency. Most experts prefer levothyroxine, a manufactured form of T_4. In addition, natural hormones from beef or pork and synthetic T_3 and T_3 plus T_4 products are available.

Successful treatment of hypothyroidism requires fine-tuning the dose of a specific thyroid product so that it is neither too low nor too high. This takes several months. Initial drug benefits are seen within weeks. Lifetime replacement therapy is required.

Maximizing Your Medicine

Subtle differences exist among the different kinds of thyroid preparations and even among the different brands of each drug. When you and your doctor have decided on a single drug source (generic or brand name), plan to stick to it for a lifetime. By far, Synthroid is the most expensive brand of levothyroxine. Consider another less-expensive brand that's just as good.

When the appropriate dose has been determined, side effects are few. Too much can cause an increase in heart rate, chest pain (angina), nervousness, insomnia, and sweating. When such symptoms occur, your doctor should be contacted and adjustments in dosage should be made.

A number of drugs interfere with levothyroxine absorption, and they should be taken four hours after levothyroxine: e.g., antacids, cholesterol-lowering resins (cholestyramine). Levothyroxine may increase the effects and potential hazards of warfarin, a blood thinner. Close monitoring of bleeding time is required.

Overactive Thyroid Activity (Hyperthyroidism)

Common signs of hyperthyroidism include weight loss in spite of increased appetite, palpitations, nervousness, tremors, muscle weakness, and intolerance to heat. Most hyperthyroid persons have an enlarged thyroid gland (goiter), and many have protrusions of the eyeballs.

The rapid heart rate, tremors, and anxiety can be controlled with a beta-blocker, such as propranolol (Inderal). This drug provides temporary relief until thyroid function is reduced by drugs or surgery.

Unlike sluggish thyroid function, problems of overactive thyroids can be cured or significantly brought under control using a number of different approaches. These include the following:

◆ Surgical removal of the gland. Lugol's solution (strong iodine solution) is given several weeks before the operation to reduce thyroid function. Thyroid replacement medicines will be required for a lifetime.

◆ Destruction of the thyroid with radioactive iodine.

◆ Depressing the manufacture of thyroid hormones with drugs.

Radioactive Iodine

Radioactive iodine (sodium iodide I 131) is tasteless and odorless and is taken by mouth. Treatment is inexpensive and avoids the need for surgery to depress thyroid function.

During the first several months after radioactive iodine, the enlarged gland is reduced in size, and thyroid function becomes normal. Often, the dose proves to be too high. The destructive process slowly continues for years until the thyroid has been so reduced that the patient requires replacement thyroid medicine.

Radioactive iodine doesn't cause cancer. This drug should not be given to pregnant or nursing women because of its potentially harmful effects on the thyroid gland of the fetus or infant.

Warning!

During the first few months of therapy, PTU has the potential to cause a rare but potentially fatal blood disorder called agranulocytosis. If fever or sore throat develops while taking PTU, patients should immediately notify their doctor.

Antithyroid Drugs

Propylthiouracil (PTU), the most important antithyroid drug, works by preventing the manufacture of a new hormone supply by the thyroid gland. Because existing stores of hormones exist in the gland, it takes several weeks before depression of thyroid effects become evident.

PTU should not be used by nursing mothers and should be used cautiously during pregnancy.

The Least You Need to Know

◆ Thyroid gland disorders cause significant body-wide consequences.

◆ Hypothyroidism is effectively treated with levothyroxine and other thyroid hormone products, which are required for a lifetime.

◆ Hyperthyroidism can be cured or effectively controlled by radioactive iodine or antithyroid drugs.

Drugs for Thyroid Conditions

Generic Name	What Is It?	Trade Name	Generic Available
Drugs for Hypothyroid Conditions			
Levothyroxine	Synthetic T_4	Levothroid, Synthroid, Levoxyl	Yes
Thyroid	Dried natural thyroid gland	Armour Thyroid	Yes
Liothyronine	Synthetic T_3	Cytomel, Triostat	Yes
Liotrix	Synthetic $T_4 + T_3$	Thyrolar	No
Drugs for Hyperthyroid Conditions			
Sodium Iodide I 131	Radioactive iodine	Iodotope	No
Propylthiouracil (PTU)			Yes
Methimazole	—	Tapazole	No
Lugol's Solution	Strong iodine solution	—	Yes

Tuberculosis

One in three people worldwide are infected with tuberculosis (TB). This is the world's number one infectious disease killer, responsible for the deaths of 2 to 3 million people each year. In the United States, there are 15,000 new cases of active TB each year and 1,500 deaths. In spite of these ominous statistics, when drugs are taken as directed, its cure rate is almost 100 percent.

Did You Know That ...?

References to TB go back to writings from ancient Babylon, Egypt, and China. "Consumption," so-called because of significant weight loss, was a major cause of death during the nineteenth century. Among its victims were writers John Keats, Robert Louis Stevenson, Emily and Charlotte Bronte, Anton Checkov, and Franz Kafka, and the composer Frederick Chopin.

def•i•ni•tion

The routine screen for TB involves the **tuberculin skin test** or PPD (purified protein derivative). An injection of PPD is given under the skin. Some 48 to 72 hours later, the skin at the site of the injection is checked for the size of the area of hardness. If this test proves positive, more specific tests for TB are performed.

TB is caused by the bacterium Mycobacterium tuberculosis (also called *tubercle bacillus*) that is transmitted person-to-person by coughing and sneezing. In up to 10 percent of infected individuals, the disease becomes active and capable of being spread. This generally occurs within two years. The risk of active TB is greatly increased in individuals with depressed immune function, as in HIV/AIDS.

The disease primarily attacks the lungs, but can attack any part of the body such as the kidney, spine, and brain. If not treated properly, TB disease can be fatal. Not everyone infected with TB bacteria becomes sick, however. Some people develop latent infections that have no symptoms, and do not spread TB to others. Some people with latent infection will ultimately develop the active form of the disease, experience symptoms, and become contagious. Both latent and active infections must be treated.

In its active form, TB causes a cough that brings up phlegm and blood. Other symptoms include weight loss, fatigue, fever, and night sweats. The latent form shows a positive *tuberculin skin test* but no other symptoms.

Drug Treatment: An Overview

Drug treatment of active TB is intended to control the symptoms, make the individual noninfectious, and cure the disease. Successful treatment takes anywhere from six months to two to three years.

A minimum of two oral drugs (isoniazid and rifampin) are used to treat active TB, but usually three or four are used. Multiple drugs are used to prevent the development of drug-resistant microbial strains and to reduce the risk of patient relapse. In addition, multiple drugs reduce the treatment time.

During the initial two-month phase of treatment, four drugs are used to kill the actively multiplying bacteria. These are isoniazid, rifampin, pyrazinamide, and ethambutol. If treatment goes well, isoniazid and rifampin are continued for four additional months to eliminate any remaining bacteria.

Successful treatment of latent TB reduces the risk of the disease becoming active and spreading to others. For latent TB, isoniazid is used alone for nine months or with rifampin for four months.

The first-line choices of drugs in the treatment of TB are isoniazid, rifampin, pyrazinamide, and ethanbutol. Second-line choice drugs are less effective and often cause more serious side effects. These include streptomycin, para-aminosalicylic acid, capreomycin, cycloserine, and ethionamide.

> ### Maximizing Your Medicine
>
> Successful treatment of TB is a lengthy process involving the use of multiple drugs. Anti-TB medicines must be taken as prescribed for the entire period recommended. Patients often feel better within weeks after starting drugs and so stop taking their medication. This increases the risk of relapse.

Isoniazid

Isoniazid (a.k.a. INH) is the most-effective and least-toxic drug for the treatment of active and latent TB. It also prevents TB infection in individuals who come in direct contact with active TB carriers.

Side effects typically affect the nerves, causing tingling, numbness, burning, and pain in the

> **Warning!**
>
> Isoniazid can produce liver toxicity, a risk that increases with age. This drug should not be used by individuals with active liver disease.

hands and feet. This risk is much higher where there is a vitamin B$_6$ (pyridoxine) deficiency (e.g., in diabetics, alcoholics, and during pregnancy). This nerve toxicity can be prevented or treated by taking oral vitamin B$_6$ supplements.

Isoniazid can slow the rate of breakdown of the blood thinner warfarin and such antiepileptic drugs as phenytoin, carbamazepine, and primidone.

Did You Know That ...?

The speed of isoniazid metabolism and inactivation by enzymes in the liver is genetically determined. Some 50 percent of whites and blacks and 80 to 90 percent of Asians and Eskimos are rapid metabolizers. The others are slow metabolizers. If they are given normal doses, drug levels build up, exposing them to an increased risk of nerve toxicity.

Rifampin

Rifampin is another valuable drug for TB, and when used with isoniazid can significantly reduce treatment time. Rifampin is also the most effective drug for treating leprosy.

Rifapentine and rifabutin are newer drugs used as substitutes for rifampin.

Common side effects include rash, fever, loss of appetite, nausea, and abdominal discomfort. Rifampin, in rare instances, causes liver toxicity, a risk increased in alcoholics.

Rifampin causes body fluids such as urine, saliva, sweat, and tears to turn red-orange in color, a harmless effect. Moreover, this drug causes permanent staining of soft contact lenses.

Rifampin speeds up the breakdown of many drugs that are metabolized by liver enzymes. Among these are the protease inhibitors used for HIV/AIDS. Rifampin also speeds the breakdown of oral contraceptives, increasing the risk of pregnancy. Patients should use another nonhormonal approach for contraception.

Pyrazinamide

The addition of pyrazinamide to isoniazid and rifampin shorten the needed treatment time.

Nausea, vomiting, diarrhea, and aching joints are common side effects. The most severe adverse effect is liver toxicity, and this risk increases when pyrazinamide is used with isoniazid and rifampin.

Ethambutol

Ethambutol's primary usefulness is when TB-causing bacteria are developing resistance to isoniazid, rifampin, and pyrazinamide.

Ethambutol can cause visual disturbances, which are usually reversible after the drug is discontinued. Drug therapy should be stopped if such effects occur.

The Least You Need to Know

♦ When taken as directed, drugs can cure active TB, prevent latent TB from spreading the disease to others, and provide protection against infection.

♦ Multiple oral drugs are used to treat TB, to prevent the development of microbial resistance, and to shorten the length of drug treatment.

♦ Isoniazid and rifampin are the primary first-line choice anti-TB drugs, with pyrazinamide and ethambutol commonly included as members of the multiple-drug treatment team.

Drugs Used for Tuberculosis

Generic Name	Trade Name	Generic Available
First-Line Choice Drugs		
Ethambutol	Myambutol	No
Isoniazid (INH)	Nydrazid	Yes
Pyrazinamide	—	Yes
Rifampin	Rifadin, Rimactane	Yes
Rifampin, Isoniazid, Pyrazinamide	Rifater	No
Rifapentine	Priftin	No
Second-Line Choice Drugs		
Capreomycin	Capastat	No
Cycloserine	Seromycin	No

continues

Drugs Used for Tuberculosis   (continued)

Generic Name	Trade Name	Generic Available
Ethionamide	Trecator-SC	No
Para-aminosalicylic acid (PAS)	Paser	No
Rifabutin	Mycobutin	No
Streptomycin	—	Yes

Typhoid Fever

Typhoid fever is a potentially life-threatening disease caused by Salmonella typhi, a bacterium that infects the gastrointestinal tract. This condition, also called enteric fever, is common in developing nations, affecting some 22 million people each year, with 200,000 deaths. There are about 400 cases each year in the United States, and most of these are picked up by travelers to Asia, Africa, and Latin America.

The typhoid bacterium comes from food or beverages that have been handled by individuals with the disease or from contaminated water used for drinking or for washing food. If you're looking for typhoid fever, your best bets are countries where hand washing is not common and where sewage contaminates water. Not all carriers show symptoms.

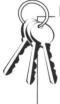

Did You Know That ...?

Mary Mallon, who'll go down in medical history as Typhoid Mary, was the first known "healthy carrier" in the United States. Working as a domestic cook in New York City early in the twentieth century, she was said to have infected 47 people with typhoid fever, 3 of whom died. To prevent her from infecting others, she was sent to live for a total of 26 years on North Brother Island in the East River near the Bronx.

The typhoid bacterium travels from the gastrointestinal tract to the blood. Common symptoms include a persistent high fever (102–106°F or 39–41°C), stomach pains, headache, fatigue, and loss of appetite. In severe cases, coma and shock may be present. In the absence of effective treatment, fever may continue for weeks or months. Complications of typhoid fever may lead to a 20 percent mortality rate.

Treatment and Prevention

Typhoid fever is very effectively treated with such antibacterial drugs as ampicillin, ciprofloxacin, and trimethoprim-sulfamethoxazole.

After treatment, patients show improvement within two to three days, although extended convalescent periods and relapses are not uncommon.

In addition to exercising caution when selecting food and drink, oral and injectable typhoid vaccines are available that are 50 to 80 percent effective in preventing the disease. They provide protection for two to five years. Vaccines must be completed at least one week prior to travel.

The Least You Need to Know

♦ When traveling to developing countries where the risk of typhoid fever exists, a typhoid vaccine may be considered and caution should be exercised when selecting food and drink.

♦ More than 99 percent of cases treated in a timely manner with antibacterial drugs are cured of this potentially fatal condition.

Drugs Used for Treatment of Typhoid Fever

Generic Name	Class	Trade Name	Generic Available
Ampicillin	Penicillin, Principen, Totacillin	Omnipen	Yes
Ciprofloxacin	Quinolones	Cipro	Yes
Trimethoprim + Sulfamethoxazole [co-trimoxazole; TMP-SMZ]	Sulfa-like	Bactrim, Cotrim, Septra	Yes

Appendix A

Glossary

absorption   Movement of a drug from its site of administration (usually the intestines) into the blood.

abstinence syndrome   *See* withdrawal syndrome.

ACE inhibitors   Angiotensin-converting enzyme inhibitors used for the treatment of a variety of heart and blood vessel conditions.

acetylcholine   Neurotransmitter in the autonomic nervous system and the brain.

acid reflux   Movement of acid backward (reflux) from the stomach into the esophagus, which may cause tissue damage and erosion and result in heartburn.

acute effect   Immediate response occurring after a single dose or a few doses. Opposite of chronic or long-term effects.

addiction   A state produced when a drug has been used repeatedly and in which the individual needs the drug to function normally. The absence of the drug results in a withdrawal syndrome.

adrenergic blockers   Drugs that block the effects of norepinephrine at its receptor site.

adverse effect   Unintended and undesirable drug effect that occurs at normal doses.

affective disorder   Disorders of mood or emotion (e.g., depression and mania).

agonist   A drug that binds to a tissue receptor and produces an effect.

AIDS Acquired immunodeficiency syndrome, in which the body's immune defense system breaks down and the individual is much more susceptible than normal to infection.

allergic reaction An adverse reaction, involving the immune system, that only occurs after more than one exposure to the drug. The severity of the reaction is not related to the dose of the drug. Also called a hypersensitivity reaction.

Alzheimer's disease Chronic condition in which there is a progressive loss of memory, ability to think, and ability to perform daily activities.

anabolic The buildup of body tissues.

analgesic A drug that relieves pain without causing the loss of consciousness.

androgenic Relating to the male sex hormone or a drug that increases male sex characteristics.

anemia A general term referring to a decrease in red blood cells.

angina pectoris Chest pain resulting from a partial and temporary interruption of the blood and oxygen supply to the heart muscle.

antagonist A drug that binds to a tissue receptor but produces no effect. In the presence of an antagonist, the effect of the agonist is reduced or prevented.

anti-arrhythmic A drug used to prevent or treat disorders of heart rhythm.

antibiotic A drug that kills or prevents the growth of microbes or cancer cells. It is often used more generally to refer to antimicrobial drugs.

anticholinergic drug A drug that blocks the effects of acetylcholine at its receptor site. *See* atropine-like effects.

anticoagulant A blood thinner that interferes with the clotting of blood.

antidepressants Drugs used for the treatment of depression.

antihistamines Drugs that block the effects of histamine at its H1 receptor site. Primarily used for the treatment of allergic conditions.

antihypertensives Drugs that reduce increased blood pressure.

anti-inflammatory drugs Drugs that reduces the heat, swelling, and redness seen during an inflammatory response to an infection or injury.

antipsychotics Drugs used for the treatment of schizophrenia and other psychoses. Also called neuroleptic drugs.

anxiety disorders A diverse group of mental disorders in which there is excessive worry, fears, and feelings of danger.

aphrodisiac   A drug that increases sexual desire or libido.

arrhythmia   An abnormal rhythm or rate at which the heart beats. Also called dysrhythmia.

arteriole   The smallest artery.

artery   Blood vessel that carries blood away from the heart.

arthritis   Inflammation (pain and swelling) of the joints. *See* osteoarthritis, rheumatoid arthritis.

asthma   Temporary collapse of the breathing tubes, reducing the flow of air into the lungs. Wheezing, coughing, and shortness of breath may result.

atherosclerosis   A type of hardening of the arteries in which the inner walls of arteries become lined with fatty deposits that restrict the flow of blood. (When this process involves small arteries, it is called arteriosclerosis.)

atria   The upper chambers of the heart.

atropine-like effects   Typically refers to the side effects caused by atropine and other anticholinergic drugs and some antihistamines. To a greater or lesser extent, these effects include dry mouth, blurred vision, difficulty in urinating, and an increased heart rate.

autoimmune disorders   Abnormality of the body's immune system in which it mistakes its own tissues for foreign tissues and attacks them.

autonomic nervous system   That branch of the nervous system that regulates the function of the heart, glands, and involuntary muscles, none of which are under conscious control.

benign prostatic hypertrophy (BPH)   Non-cancerous enlargement of the prostate gland.

benzodiazepines   Valium-like drugs that are used to relieve anxiety, induce sleep, relax muscles, and treat seizure disorders.

beta-blockers   Drugs that block the effects of norepinephrine at its beta-adrenergic receptor site. Very widely used group of drugs to treat high blood pressure, heart conditions, and other disorders.

bipolar disorder   Mood disorder in which the patient experiences periods of both depression and mania.

blood pressure   Measure of the pressure of blood exerted against the walls of blood vessels, expressed as two numbers. The upper number, systolic pressure, is the pressure in the arteries when the heart beats. The lower number, diastolic pressure, is the pressure in the arteries when the heart is relaxed and immediately before the next heartbeat.

body mass index   A measure of body weight based on height.

bone marrow   Inner hollow portion of bones where blood cells are manufactured.

bone mineral density   Measure of the thickness of bone, with thin bones increasing the susceptibility to fractures.

BPH   *See* benign prostatic hypertrophy.

bronchi   Breathing tubes that connect to the lungs.

bronchitis   Inflammation of the breathing tubes.

bronchodilators   Drugs used to widen the opening of the breathing tubes, as in the treatment of asthma.

calcium antagonists   Drugs used for the treatment of high blood pressure, angina pectoris, and abnormal heart rhythms. Also called calcium channel blockers (CCBs) and calcium blockers.

cancer   A general term referring to a group of diseases in which the body's normal cells become abnormal. The cancer cell (malignant neoplasm) grows and attacks other cells without restraint and travels to other parts of the body, where it grows into new malignant tumors.

cardiac output   Volume of blood pumped by the heart each minute.

central nervous system (CNS)   Brain and spinal cord.

cephalosporins   Widely used class of antibiotics.

chemical name   The precise name of a drug that describes its exact chemical structure.

chemotherapy   Use of drugs that are capable of destroying invading microbes and cancer cells, curing these conditions, without causing significant harm to the patient.

cholesterol   A fatty material both supplied by the diet and produced by the body. It is used for the manufacture of cell membranes, male and female sex hormones, and bile acids, which are needed for the breakdown and absorption of fats in the diet. When cholesterol lines arteries, it interferes with blood flow and increases the risk of heart attack and stroke.

chronic effect   Long-term response to multiple doses of a drug. Opposite of acute or short-term effects.

chronic obstructive pulmonary disease (COPD)   Conditions, such as asthma, emphysema, and chronic bronchitis, in which there is inadequate flow of air into the lungs.

clinical trial   Tests evaluating the effects of drugs or other procedures using human subjects.

CNS   *See* central nervous system.

compliance Taking your medicine, or following other directions given by your health-care provider.

contraception Preventing pregnancy by interfering with the fertilization of an egg by sperm.

contraindication A medical condition or drug that makes the use of another drug strongly inadvisable because of potentially serious consequences resulting from their interaction. This is the highest level of warning.

COPD *See* chronic obstructive pulmonary disease.

coronary artery disease Conditions resulting from atherosclerosis of the coronary arteries, insufficient blood flow, and inadequate supply of blood and oxygen to the heart muscle. Ultimately results in angina pectoris and heart attack.

corticosteroids *See* steroids.

COX-2 inhibitor A nonsteroidal anti-inflammatory drug (NSAID) that acts by selectively inhibiting the COX-2 enzyme.

cream Preparation applied to the skin in which the drug is contained in an oil and water base. Less greasy than ointments.

cumulative effects Drug effects that increase with repeated doses and that usually result from a drug buildup in the body.

cytotoxic drugs Anticancer drugs that act by killing cancer cells.

depressant General term referring to drugs that reduce the function of the central nervous system.

depression A mood disorder.

dermatitis Inflammation of the skin.

diabetes mellitus A common hormone disorder in which there is an excessively high level of blood sugar (also called hyperglycemia).

dietary supplement A general term referring to natural substances, such as plant products, vitamins, herbs, and minerals, that are intended to promote health and not claimed to cure specific medical conditions. Federal law classifies them as foods and not drugs.

dilation Widening of the diameter of a blood vessel or organ.

direct-to-consumer (DTC) ads Advertisements for prescription drugs appearing on TV and in the print media that are directed to the consumer (patient) of such drugs.

distribution Movement of a drug from the blood to the tissues and fluids of the body.

diuretic   A drug that increases the loss of salt and water in the urine. Also called water pill.

DMARDs   Disease-modifying antirheumatic drugs, used for the treatment of rheumatoid arthritis.

dopamine   A neurotransmitter in the brain. Plays a role in schizophrenia and Parkinson's disease.

double-blind trial   A clinical trial in which neither the investigator nor the test subject knows whether a drug or a placebo is being given.

drug   A chemical substance used to diagnose, prevent, or treat a medical condition or to alter the function of the body. Also called a medicine or pharmaceutical.

drug abuse   Use of a drug in such a manner or at such doses that it interferes with the user's physical or mental heath.

drug dependence   A state of psychological dependence, physical dependence, or both, resulting from drug use on a continuous basis.

drug-dosage form   Form in which an accurate dose of the active drug is administered to the patient (e.g., tablet, spray, suppository).

drug-drug interaction   The ability of one drug to modify the effectiveness or toxicity of another drug.

drug-food interaction   The ability of a food to modify the effectiveness of a drug.

effective dose   The dose of a drug that produces a specific effect. It is usually the therapeutic dose used for the treatment of disease.

elimination   Removal of a drug or its breakdown products from the body, most commonly, in the urine. Also called excretion.

-emia   Suffix meaning blood.

endocrine   Hormone. An endocrine gland makes hormones.

endogenous   Substance produced within the body.

endometrium   Inner lining of the uterus.

enzyme   A naturally occurring protein substance that speeds up the rate of chemical reactions in the body.

enzyme induction   Drugs or chemicals that increase the activity of drug metabolizing enzymes in the liver. This increases the rate at which drugs are chemically changed and usually inactivated and removed from the body.

erectile dysfunction   Impotence.

estrogen   A female sex hormone.

exogenous   A drug or chemical coming from outside the body.

FDA   United States Food and Drug Administration.

fibrinolytic drug   A drug that dissolves and breaks down blood clots. Also called a clot buster or clot dissolver.

GABA   Gamma-amino butyric acid, a central nervous system inhibitory neurotransmitter.

generic name   The official name used to designate a drug. This name can be used by anyone who markets the drug.

glaucoma   An eye condition in which there is excessive pressure in the fluid within the eye. If untreated, this can result in blindness.

glucose   Sugar.

glutamate   A central nervous system excitatory neurotransmitter.

Gram stain   A dye used to see and differentiate different types of bacteria.

H1 antagonist   Drug that blocks the effects of histamine at its H1 receptor site. Primarily used for the treatment of allergic conditions. Also called antihistamine.

H2 antagonist   Drug that blocks the effects of histamine at its H2 receptor site. Primarily used for the treatment of ulcer-related conditions in the gastrointestinal tract.

HDL   High-density lipoprotein (good cholesterol).

heart attack   Complete block in blood flow, disrupting the supply of oxygen and blood to the heart muscle.

heart failure   Condition in which the heart is no longer an effective pump sending blood around the body.

herpes   Virus responsible for causing cold sores and a sexually transmitted disease.

HIV   Human immunodeficiency virus, responsible for causing autoimmune deficiency syndrome (AIDS).

hormone   A chemical produced and released into the blood by an endocrine gland, and which acts at a distant location.

hormone replacement therapy   Used during menopause to replace estrogen which is absent or deficient.

hyper-   Prefix referring to overactivity or higher than normal levels.

hyperglycemia   Excessive levels of glucose (sugar) in the blood.

hypersensitivity reaction   *See* allergic reaction.

hypertension   High blood pressure.

hypo-   Prefix referring to under-activity or lower than normal levels.

hypodermic   Through the skin.

hypoglycemic drugs   Drugs used to lower elevated blood levels of glucose (sugar) in diabetes mellitus.

idiopathic condition   A medical condition arising from an unknown cause.

idiosyncratic reaction   A highly unusual drug response that may be extreme sensitivity to a low dose or insensitivity to a high dose. Often attributed to genetic influences.

inflammation   A defensive body reaction to infection or injury. Signs include redness, pain, heat, and swelling.

insomnia   Inability to sleep.

involuntary (smooth) muscle   Muscles not under conscious control, such as those lining blood vessels, breathing tubes, and the gastrointestinal tract.

ischemia   Interference of blood flow to an organ or blood vessel.

LDL   Low-density lipoprotein (bad cholesterol).

leukemia   General term referring to cancers of white blood cells.

leukocyte   White blood cell.

local effect   A drug effect limited to the location where the drug was administered.

lotion   Liquid suspensions of drugs that are not greasy.

mania   A mood disorder with excessive feelings of well-being (euphoria) and increased activity.

MAO   Monoamine oxidase, an enzyme. MAO inhibitors are used to treat depression.

Medicare Part D Prescription Drug Program   Voluntary government health insurance program, effective 2006, that is intended to reduce the cost of prescription drugs. Open to all individuals over 65 and the disabled.

medicine   Also called drug, medication, pharmaceutical.

melanoma   Skin cancer.

meningitis   Inflammation of the meninges, the tissue covering of the brain and spinal cord. Causes of inflammation include infections by bacteria and viruses.

menopause   Permanent ending of menstruation.

metabolism   Chemical change in a drug that often results in its inactivation. Metabolism also refers to chemical changes in food substances that produce energy.

metabolite   A breakdown product of a drug or body chemical.

metastasis   The spread of cancer cells from their original site to another location where they form a new tumor.

metered-dose inhaler   Handheld pressurized devise which, when activated, delivers a premeasured dose of a drug in a fine mist.

microbe (microorganism)   A microscopic organism such as bacterium, fungus, protozoan, and virus.

miotic   A drug that constricts the pupils.

modified-release preparations   Dosage forms (e.g., tablets, capsules, solutions, ointments) that release the active drug over an extended period of time rather than immediately. Such products make it possible to take the drug less frequently during the day.

mycoses   Fungal infections.

mydriatic   A drug that dilates (widens) the pupils.

narcotic   *See* opioids.

nerve   Elongated cells that receive impulses from other nerves and send impulses to other nerves and to the heart, muscles, and glands.

neuroleptic   Antipsychotic drug.

neurotransmitter   A chemical released from a nerve ending that carries a nerve impulse across a space (synapse) to another nerve or to a target tissue.

noncompliance   Failure to take medication or follow other treatments as have been directed by a health-care provider.

NSAIDs   Nonsteroidal anti-inflammatory drugs (e.g., aspirin).

ointment   The greasy base used to contain and apply drugs to the skin.

opioid   Naturally occurring or manufactured morphine-like drugs. Also called narcotics.

osteoarthritis   Chronic disease of the joints causing pain, stiffness, and loss of motion.

osteoporosis   Condition where bones become thin and brittle, making them more susceptible to fracture.

OTC   Over-the-counter (nonprescription) drugs.

otitis media   Middle ear infection.

parenteral   Given by injection.

Parkinson's disease   Disease of the nervous system in which the patient has tremors, moves slowly, and has a rigid posture.

peptic ulcers   Erosion of the inner layers of the stomach and small intestines by acid from the stomach.

pharmaceutical   Medicine or drug.

pharmacogenetics   Influence of genetic influences on the response to drugs.

pharmacokinetics   Study of the absorption, distribution, metabolism, and elimination of drugs after their administration. Fate of drugs in the body after they have been taken.

pharmacology   The scientific study of drugs and how they work.

physical dependence   Said to occur when the abrupt discontinuation of a drug produces a characteristic group of symptoms that are collectively termed a withdrawal syndrome.

placebo   An inactive substance that works because the subject believes or expects it to work.

platelet   Blood component essential for the formation of a clot.

pneumonia   General term referring to an infection of the lungs that may be caused by bacteria, viruses, or fungi.

progestin   A drug which produces effects like progesterone, a female sex hormone.

proprietary drug   A nonprescription or over-the-counter (OTC) medicine that is marketed directly to the public.

prostaglandins   Fatty acids that are released when cells are damaged. They produce a wide range of effects including pain, inflammation, and fever. Aspirin and related nonsteroidal anti-inflammatory drugs (NSAIDs) work by preventing the body's ability to manufacture prostaglandins.

prostate gland   Gland that surrounds the urethra, the tube that carries off urine from the bladder. Enlargement of the prostate interferes with the flow of urine.

protein   Naturally occurring substances composed of amino acid building blocks.

proton pump inhibitors (PPIs)   Drugs that prevent the secretion of acid in the stomach and are used to treat gastrointestinal tract ulcer disorders.

psychological dependence   A desire to continue to take a drug.

psychosis   A mental disorder in which there is a loss of touch with reality.

receptor   Specialized chemical groups on a cell with which a neurotransmitter or drug binds to produce an effect.

renal   Refers to kidney.

resistance   Response to an antimicrobial drug that makes microbes less sensitive or totally insensitive to that drug.

reuptake   Process by which a neurotransmitter is taken back into the nerve ending from which it was released. Reuptake removes the neurotransmitter away from its receptor site.

rheumatoid arthritis   The most common body-wide inflammatory condition in which joints become stiff, swollen, and painful.

serotonin   A neurotransmitter in the brain.

side effect   Unavoidable drug effect, in addition to the desired effect, that occurs at normal therapeutic doses.

single-blind   A clinical trial in which the investigator knows but the test subject doesn't know whether a drug or a placebo is being given.

skin patch   A patch that permits the drug to pass slowly through the skin and enter the blood in which it is distributed in the body.

SSRI   Selective serotonin-reuptake inhibitors, the most widely used class of drugs for the treatment of depression.

statins   The most widely used class of drugs for reducing elevated blood levels of cholesterol.

steroid   Chemicals found in the body and manufactured in the laboratory that have common characteristics in their chemistry. Many steroids are hormones and include the male and female sex hormones and cortisone-like chemicals produced by the adrenal gland. In this book, steroids refer to the latter chemicals (corticosteroids and glucocorticoids). These steroids are used to treat a very wide range of conditions, including inflammation.

stroke   Blockage of the blood supply to the brain.

subcutaneous   Under the skin.

sublingual   Under the tongue.

systemic   Body-wide effects.

teratogenic effects   A drug causing birth defects.

testosterone   Male sex hormone.

tetracyclines   A class of antibiotics that are effective against a wide range of infections caused by microbes.

therapeutic dose   Usual dose given to treat a medical condition.

thrombus   Blood clot abnormally present in the heart or a blood vessel.

tinea   Fungal (ringworm) infections of the skin, which include athlete's foot, jock itch, and ringworm of the scalp and body.

tolerance   Reduced effectiveness after repeated doses of a drug.

topical administration   Application of a drug to a body surface such as skin, lip, or eye.

toxicity   Undesirable effects that occur after an excessive drug dose has been taken.

trade name   A unique name used by a manufacturer to advertise and market their generic named drug. Also called brand name and proprietary name.

transdermal   A drug applied to the skin that passes through the skin layers and enters the blood.

triptans   A widely used class of drugs for migraine headaches.

tumor   A collection of new cells, which may be harmless (benign tumor) or cancerous (malignant tumor).

vasoconstriction   A narrowing of the inner diameter of a blood vessel.

vasodilation   A widening of the inner diameter of a blood vessel.

vein   Blood vessel that carries blood back to the heart.

ventricles   Lower chambers of the heart that pump blood into arteries, sending blood around your body or into the lungs.

vitamin   A chemical essential for health that must be provided by the diet.

withdrawal syndrome   Symptoms occurring after an individual has abruptly stopped taking a drug to which they have become dependent. The specific nature of the symptoms is dependent on the drug. Also called abstinence syndrome.

Resources

General

American Academy of Family
Physicians
www.familydoctor.org

Centers for Disease Control and
Prevention
1600 Clifton Rd,
Atlanta, GA 30333
1-800-311-3435
www.cdc.gov

National Institutes of Health
Bethesda, MD
www.nih.gov

National Library of Medicine
MedlinePlus
National Institutes of Health
8600 Rockville Pike
Bethesda, MD 20894
www.nlm.nih.gov/medlineplus/
print/organizations

U.S. Food and Drug
Administration
5600 Fishers Lane
Rockville MD 20857-0001
1-888-463-6332
www.fda.gov

Acne and Skin Conditions

National Institute of Arthritis and
Musculoskeletal and Skin Diseases
(NIAMS)
1 AMS Circle
Bethesda, MD 20892-3675
1-877-226-4267
www.niams.nih.gov

National Psoriasis Foundation
6600 SW 92nd Ave., Suite 300
Portland, OR 97223-7195
1-800-723-9166
www.psoriasis.org

AIDS

AIDS Action
1906 Sunderland Place NW
Washington, D.C. 20036
202-530-8030
www.aidsaction.org

AIDS Education Global Information
System
32234 Paseo Adelanto, Suite B
San Juan Capistrano, CA 92675
949-248-5843
www.aegis.com

AIDSinfo
PO Box 6303
Rockville, MD 20849-6303
1-800-448-0440
www.aidsinfo.nih.gov

Allergic, Asthma and Breathing Conditions

American Lung Association
New York, NY
1-800-586-4872
www.lungusa.org

Asthma and Allergy Foundation
of America
1233 20th Street, NW
Suite 402
Washington, D.C. 20036
202-466-7643
info@aafa.org

Alzheimer's Disease

Alzheimer's Association
225 N. Michigan Avenue, Suite 1700
Chicago, IL 60601
1-800-272-3900
www.alz.org

Alzheimer's Disease Education
and Referral (ADEAR) Center
PO Box 8250
Silver Spring, MD 20907-8250
1-800-438-4380
www.alzheimers.org

Arthritis

Arthritis Foundation
PO Box 7669
Atlanta, GA 30357-0669
1-800-568-4045
www.arthritis.org

Autism

Autism Society of America
7910 Woodmont Avenue, Suite 300
Bethesda, MD 20814-3067
1-800-328-8476
www.autism-society.org

Bladder and Prostate Conditions

National Kidney and Urologic Diseases
Information Clearinghouse
3 Information Way
Bethesda, MD 20892–3580
1-800–891–5390
kidney.niddk.nih.gov

Cancer

American Cancer Society
1-800-227-2345
www.cancer.org

National Cancer Institute
Bethesda, MD
1-800-422-6237
www.cancer.gov

National Coalition for Cancer
Survivorship
1010 Wayne Avenue, Suite 770
Silver Spring, MD 20910
301-650-9127
www.canceradvocacy.org

Diabetes Mellitus

American Diabetes Association
ATTN: National Call Center
1701 North Beauregard Street
Alexandria, VA 2231
1-800-342-2383
www.diabetes.org

National Diabetes Education Program
Bethesda, MD
www.ndep.nih.gov

National Diabetes Information
Clearinghouse
1 Information Way
Bethesda, MD 20892–3560
1-800–860–8747
diabetes.niddk.nih.gov

Digestive Conditions and Peptic Ulcers

Crohn's & Colitis Foundation
of America Inc
386 Park Avenue South, 17th Floor
New York, NY 10016-8804
1-800-932-2423
www.ccfa.org

International Foundation for Functional
Gastrointestinal Disorders
PO Box 170864
Milwaukee, WI 53217-8076
1-888-964-2001
www.iffgd.org

National Digestive Diseases Information
Clearinghouse
2 Information Way
Bethesda, MD 20892-3570
1-800-891-5389
www.digestive.niddk.nih.gov/
ddiseases/pubs/facts

National Institute of Diabetes and
Digestive and Kidney Diseases
Office of Communications and Public
Liaison, NIDDK, NIH,
Building 31, Room 9A04
31 Center Drive, MSC 2560
Bethesda, MD 20892-2560
www.niddk.gov

Family Planning

Planned Parenthood of America
New York, NY
www.plannedparenthood.org

Glaucoma and Eye Disorders

National Eye Institute
2020 Vision Place
Bethesda, MD 20892-3655
301-496-5248
www.nei.nih.gov

Heart and Blood Vessel Conditions

American Heart Association
7272 Greenville Avenue
Dallas, TX 75231
1-800-242-8721
www.americanheart.org

National Heart, Lung, and Blood
Institute (NHLBI)
Health Information Center
Attention: Web Site
PO Box 30105
Bethesda, MD 20824-0105
301-592-8573
www.nhlbi.gov

Vascular Disease Foundation
1075 S. Yukon, Suite 320
Lakewood, Colorado 80226
1-866-723-4636
www.vdf.org

Infectious (Bacterial, Fungal, Viral) Diseases

Centers for Disease Control and
Prevention
1600 Clifton R.
Atlanta, GA 30333
1-800-311-3435
www.cdc.gov

National Institute of Allergy and
Infectious Diseases
Bethesda, MD
301-496-5717
www.niaid.nih.gov

Mental Health/Behavioral Disorders

National Institute of Mental Health
(NIMH)
Public Information and Communications
Branch
6001 Executive Boulevard,
Room 8184, MSC 9663
Bethesda, MD 20892-9663
1-866-615-6464
www.nimh.nih.gov

National Mental Health Association
2001 N. Beauregard Street, 12th Floor
Alexandria, VA 22311
703-684-7722
www.nmha.org

Pain and Headaches

American Council for Headache
Education
19 Mantua Road
Mt. Royal, NJ 08061
856-423-025
www.achenet.org

American Chronic Pain Association
(ACPA)
PO Box 850
Rocklin, CA 95677-0850
1-800-533-3231
www.theacpa.org

National Institute of Neurological
Disorders and Stroke
National Institutes of Health
Bethesda, MD 20892
www.ninds.nih.gov/disorders/chronic_pain

Parkinson's Disease

National Parkinson Foundation, Inc.
1501 N.W. 9th Avenue
Bob Hope Road
Miami, Florida 33136-1494
1-800-327-4545
www.parkinson.org

Parkinson's Disease Foundation
1359 Broadway, Suite 1509
New York, NY 10018
1-800-457-6676
www.pdf.org

Sexually Transmitted Diseases

American Social Health Association
PO Box 13827
Research Triangle Park, NC 27709
919-361-8400
www.ashastd.org

Centers for Disease Control
and Prevention
1600 Clifton Rd.
Atlanta, GA 30333
1-800-311-3435
www.cdc.gov/nchstp/disease

Stroke

American Stroke Association
7272 Greenville Avenue
Dallas, TX 75231
1-888-478-7653
www.strokeassociation.org

National Stroke Association
9707 E. Easter Lane
Englewood, CO 80112
1-800-787-6537
www.stroke.org

NIH Neurological Institute
PO Box 5801
Bethesda, MD 20824
1-800-352-9424
www.ninds.nih.gov/disorders/stroke

Index

A

U-V

W-X-Y-Z

Drug Index

A

Abacavir (ABC)
for AIDS/HIV, 92
Abbokinase. *See* Urokinase, 160
Abitrexate. *See* Methotrexate, 306
Acarbose
for diabetes, 214
Accolate. *See* Zafirlukast, 115
Accupril. *See* Quinapril, 267, 291
Accutane. *See* Isotretinoin, 84, 86
Acebutolol
for heart conditions, 268
for heart disease, 269
for high blood pressure, 291
Aceon. *See* Perindopril, 291, 405
Acetaminophen
for pain, 354
Acetazolamide
for glaucoma, 243
Acetohexamide
for diabetes, 214
Achromycin V, *See* Tetracycline, 86
Aciphex. *See* Rabeprazole, 279
Acitretin
for acne, 86
for psoriasis, 379

Aclometasone
for eczema, 221
for inflammation, 300
for psoriasis, 378
Aclovate. *See* Alclometasone, 221, 300, 378
Activase. *See* Alteplase, 160, 269, 405
Activella. *See* Estrogen + progestin, 326
Actonel. *See* Risedronate, 345
Actos. *See* Pioglitazone, 214
Acyclovir
for herpes, 281
for STDs (sexually transmitted diseases), 395
Adalat. *See* Nifedipine, 269, 291, 365
Adalimimab
for rheumatoid arthritis, 385
Adapalene
for acne, 86
Adderall. *See* Amphetamine salts, 119, 122
Adenocard. *See* Adenosine, 270
Adenosine
for heart conditions, 270
Adipex-P. *See* Phentermine, 337
Adriamycin. *See* Doxorubicin, 183
Adrucil. *See* Fluorouracil (5-FU), 182

Advair Diskus. *See* Fluticasone/Salmeterol, 115
Advil. *See* Ibuprofen, 247, 300, 342, 354, 385
Afrin. *See* Oxymetazoline, 96
Agenerase. *See* Amprenavir, 92
Aggrenox. *See* Aspirin + dipyridamole, 365, 405
Akarpine. *See* Pilocarpine, 243
AKBeta. *See* Levobunolol, 242
AKPro. *See* Dipivefrin, 243
Albuterol
for asthma, 115
Aldactone. *See* Spironolactone, 270, 291, 368
Aldara. *See* Imiquimod, 184
Aldesleukin (IL-2, Interleukin-2)
for cancer, 184
Aldomet. *See* Methyldopa, 292
Alemtuzumab
for cancer, 184
Alendronate
for osteoporosis, 345
Alesse. *See* Estrogen + progestin, 197, 225
Aleve. *See* Naproxen, 222, 247, 300, 342, 355, 385
Alfuzosin
for prostate enlargement, 374
Alimta. *See* Permetrexed, 182

I-J-K